SURGICAL TECHNIQUES IN OTOLARYNGOLOGY HEAD AND NECK SURGERY

Series Editor: **Robert T Sataloff** MD DMA FACS

HEAD AND NECK SURGERY

SURGICAL TECHNIQUES IN OTOLARYNGOLOGY HEAD AND NECK SURGERY

Series Editor: **Robert T Sataloff** MD DMA FACS

HEAD AND NECK SURGERY

Author

David Goldenberg MD FACS

Chief, Division of Otolaryngology—Head and Neck Surgery
Steven Baron Professor of Surgery and Medicine
Division of Otolaryngology—Head and Neck Surgery
The Penn State University
Milton S Hershey Medical Center
Hershey, Pennsylvania, USA

JAYPEE *The Health Sciences Publisher*

Philadelphia | New Delhi | London | Panama

Jaypee Brothers Medical Publishers (P) Ltd

Headquarters

Jaypee Brothers Medical Publishers (P) Ltd
4838/24, Ansari Road, Daryaganj
New Delhi 110 002, India
Phone: +91-11-43574357
Fax: +91-11-43574314
Email: jaypee@jaypeebrothers.com

Overseas Offices

J.P. Medical Ltd
83, Victoria Street, London
SW1H 0HW (UK)
Phone: +44-2031708910
Fax: +02-03-0086180
Email: info@jpmedpub.com

Jaypee-Highlights.
Medical Publishers Inc
City of Knowledge, Bld. 237
Clayton, Panama City, Panama
Phone: +1 507-301-0496
Fax: +1 507-301-0499
Email: cservice@jphmedical.com

Jaypee Medical Inc.
325 Chestnut Street
Suite 412
Philadelphia, PA 19106, USA
Phone: +1 267-519-9789
E-mail: support@jpmedus.com

Jaypee Brothers
Medical Publishers (P) Ltd
17/1-B Babar Road, Block-B
Shaymali, Mohammadpur
Dhaka-1207, Bangladesh
Mobile: +08801912003485
Email: jaypeedhaka@gmail.com

Jaypee Brothers
Medical Publishers (P) Ltd
Shorakhute, Kathmandu
Nepal
Phone: +00977-9841528578
Email: jaypee.nepal@gmail.com

Website: www.jaypeebrothers.com
Website: www.jaypeedigital.com

Inquiries for bulk sales may be solicited at: jaypee@jaypeebrothers.com

Surgical Techniques in Otolaryngology–Head and Neck Surgery: Head and Neck Surgery

First Edition: 2016
ISBN 978-93-5152-807-4
Printed at: Ajanta Offset & Packagings Ltd., New Delhi

Dedication

This book is dedicated to my parents, Sarah and Dr Herb Goldenberg, whose love, dedication and drive have helped shape me; to my wife, Dr Renee Flax-Goldenberg, who is an invaluable partner and inspiration in my life; and to my beloved children, Michael, Ellie and Dana, who are a constant source of pride, joy and laughter.

David Goldenberg

Contributors

Ralph Abi-Hachem MD
Department of Otolaryngology—
Head and Neck Surgery
University of Miami/
Jackson Memorial Hospital
Miami, Florida, USA

Sun M Ahn MD
Department of Otolaryngology—
Head and Neck Surgery
Johns Hopkins Medical Institutes
Baltimore, Maryland, USA

Genevieve A Andrews MD
Assistant Professor of Surgery
Division of Otolaryngology—
Head and Neck Surgery
Penn State College of Medicine and
Milton S Hershey Medical Center
Hershey, Pennsylvania, USA

Kim Atiyeh MD
Department of Otolaryngology—
Head and Neck Surgery
New York University Medical Center
New York, New York, USA

Darrin V Bann MD PhD
Division of Otolaryngology—
Head and Neck Surgery
Penn State College of Medicine and
Milton S Hershey Medical Center
Hershey, Pennsylvania, USA

J Kenneth Byrd MD
Assistant Professor of Otolaryngology
Department of Otolaryngology—
Head and Neck Surgery
Georgia Regents University
Augusta, Georgia, USA

Irina M Chaikhoutdinov MD
Division of Otolaryngology—
Head and Neck Surgery
Penn State College of Medicine and
Milton S Hershey Medical Center
Hershey, Pennsylvania, USA

Jason YK Chan MBBS
Assistant Professor
Department of Otorhinolaryngology—
Head and Neck Surgery
Chinese University of Hong Kong
Shatin, Hong Kong, SAR

Steven S Chang MD
Senior Staff Surgeon
Department of Otolaryngology—
Head and Neck Surgery
Henry Ford Health System
Detroit, Michigan, USA

Garret W Choby MD
Department of Otolaryngology—
Head and Neck Surgery
University of Pittsburgh Medical Center
Pittsburgh, Pennsylvania, USA

David Cognetti MD
Associate Professor
Department of Otolaryngology—
Head and Neck Surgery
Thomas Jefferson University
Philadelphia, Pennsylvania, USA

Joseph Curry MD
Assistant Professor
Department of Otolaryngology—
Head and Neck Surgery
Jefferson University
Philadelphia, Pennsylvania, USA

Robert Deeb MD
Senior Staff Surgeon
Department of Otolaryngology—
Head and Neck Surgery
Henry Ford Health System
Detroit, Michigan, USA

Robert L Ferris MD PhD FACS
Professor
Department of Otolaryngology—
Head and Neck Surgery
University of Pittsburgh
Pittsburgh, Pennsylvania, USA

Frank G Garritano MD
Division of Otolaryngology—
Head and Neck Surgery
Penn State College of Medicine and
Milton S Hershey Medical Center
Hershey, Pennsylvania, USA

Jonathan Giurintano MD
Department of Otolaryngology—
Head and Neck Surgery
University of Tennessee Health
Science Center
Memphis, Tennessee, USA

David Goldenberg MD FACS
Chief, Division of Otolaryngology—
Head and Neck Surgery
Steven Baron Professor of
Surgery and Medicine
Division of Otolaryngology—
Head and Neck Surgery
Penn State College of Medicine and
Milton S Hershey Medical Center
Hershey, Pennsylvania, USA

Richard Goldman MD
Assistant Professor
Department of Otolaryngology—
Head and Neck Surgery
University of Kentucky
Lexington, Kentucky, USA

Head and Neck Surgery

Bradley J Goldstein MD PhD FACS
Associate Professor of Otolaryngology
University of Miami
Miller School of Medicine
Miami, Florida, USA

Neerav Goyal MD MPH
Assistant Professor of Surgery
Division of Otolaryngology—
Head and Neck Surgery
Penn State College of Medicine and
Milton S Hershey Medical Center
Hershey, Pennsylvania, USA

Theresa Guo MD
Department of Otolaryngology—
Head and Neck Surgery
Johns Hopkins Medical Institutes
Baltimore, Maryland, USA

Francis Hall MBChB FRACS
Department of Otolaryngology—
Head and Neck Surgery
Henry Ford Hospital
Detroit, Michigan, USA

Gina D Jefferson MD
Department of Otolaryngology
University of Illinois
College of Medicine at Chicago
Chicago, Illinois, USA

Ali Khaku MD MBA
Division of Otolaryngology—
Head and Neck Surgery
Penn State College of Medicine and
Milton S Hershey Medical Center
Hershey, Pennsylvania, USA

Ian Lee MD
Department of Neurosurgery
Henry Ford Hospital
Detroit, Michigan, USA

Adam Luginbuhl MD
Assistant Professor
Jefferson University
Philadelphia, Pennsylvania, USA

Marcus J Magister MD
Department of Otolaryngology—
Head and Neck Surgery
Penn State College of Medicine and
Milton S Hershey Medical Center
Hershey, Pennsylvania, USA

David Myssiorek MD FACS
Professor
Department of Otolaryngology—
Head and Neck Surgery
New York University Medical Center
New York, New York, USA

Jason G Newman MD FACS
Associate Professor
Hospital of the University of
Pennsylvania
Pennsylvania Hospital
Philadelphia, Pennsylvania, USA

Benjamin Oberman MD
Division of Otolaryngology—
Head and Neck Surgery
Penn State College of Medicine and
Milton S Hershey Medical Center
Hershey, Pennsylvania, USA

Rosemary B Ojo MD
University of Miami
Miller School of Medicine
Miami, Florida, USA

Ryan Orosco MD
Division of Otolaryngology
University of California San Diego
San Diego, California, USA

Mihir R Patel MD
Assistant Professor
Department of Otolaryngology
Emory University School of Medicine
Atlanta, Georgia, USA

Vijay A Patel MD
Division of Otolaryngology—
Head and Neck Surgery
Penn State College of Medicine and
Milton S Hershey Medical Center
Hershey, Pennsylvania, USA

Chris R Roxbury MD
Department of Otolaryngology—
Head and Neck Surgery
Johns Hopkins Medical Institutes
Baltimore, Maryland, USA

Liat Shama MD
Assistant Professor
Department of Surgery
University of New Mexico
Albuquerque, New Mexico, USA

Courtney B Shires MD
Assistant Professor
Department of Otolaryngology—
Head and Neck Surgery
University of Tennessee
Memphis, Tennessee, USA

Steven M Sperry MD
Assistant Professor
Department of Otolaryngology
University of Iowa
Iowa City, Iowa, USA

Alexander C Vlantis FCSHK
Associate Professor
Department of Otorhinolaryngology—
Head and Neck Surgery
The Chinese University of Hong Kong
Shatin, Hong Kong, SAR

Barry L Wenig MD MPH FACS
Francis L Lederer Professor
Department of Otolaryngology
University of Illinois
Chicago, Illinois, USA

Eddy WY Wong FRCSEd (ORL)
Associate Consultant
Department of Otolaryngology—
Head and Neck Surgery
Prince of Wales Hospital
Shatin, Hong Kong, SAR

Jacqueline Wulu MD
Department of Otolaryngology—
Head and Neck Surgery
Boston University Medical Center
Boston, Massachusetts, USA

Foreword

Surgical Techniques in Otolaryngology—Head and Neck Surgery is a six-volume compendium. In addition to being an integral component of the compendium, each volume was written to stand alone, as well. The volumes in this work include Atlases of Otologic and Neurotological Surgery, Rhinologic and Sinus Surgery, Laryngeal Surgery, Facial Plastic and Reconstructive Surgery, Pediatric Otolaryngologic Surgery, and Head and Neck Surgery. The authors of each volume have included not only background information and step-by-step details of surgical technique, but also "pearls" gleaned through vast experience. Each volume contains extensive illustrations and intraoperative photographs that illustrate and simplify the techniques described.

Surgical Techniques in Otolaryngology—Head and Neck Surgery is intended to provide clinicians with thorough, accessible and clinically useful details of surgery for nearly all disorders cared for by otolaryngologists. The work also serves as a companion to Sataloff's six-volume *Comprehensive Textbook of Otolaryngology—Head and Neck Surgery,* which was written simultaneously with the compendium on surgical techniques. Hopefully, *Surgical Techniques* will prove useful for otolaryngologists by making it easier to provide (and teach) state-of-the-art otolaryngologic surgery.

Robert T Sataloff MD DMA FACS
Series Editor
Professor and Chairman
Department of Otolaryngology—Head and Neck Surgery
Senior Associate Dean for Clinical Academic Specialties
Drexel University College of Medicine
Philadelphia, Pennsylvania, USA

Preface

Our aim in writing this book is to provide a highly illustrated reference for surgeons of all stages trying to get organized before they observe, assist, or perform a head and neck oncologic surgery procedure. Many textbooks and articles are exhaustive about the indications for a procedure and the expected outcomes, but lack operational details such as patient positioning or instrument choice. The authors and coauthors endeavored to describe how they approach some of the commonly performed ablative head and neck procedures, whether open or endoscopic. Whenever pictures or drawings are illustrative, we included them.

The chapters in this Atlas are intended to capture the small anatomic and procedural details that are often left out of the main textbook references. Much of this information gets passed down from attending to fellow, to senior resident, to junior resident, etc.

As technology and medicine advance, we anticipate that revisions and updates will be necessary. We hope this work will be helpful to neophytes and older surgeons alike. We welcome your feedback so that future editions may fill a specific gap on your library shelf.

David Goldenberg MD FACS

Acknowledgments

The writing of a medical textbook takes the effort of many individuals. I would like to thank all of the section editors, authors and coauthors who have contributed time and effort to finish this Atlas. I would also like to thank the entire staff at Jaypee Brothers who helped us along the way, especially Joe Rusko, Marco Ulloa and Thomas Gibbons.

I am very grateful to Dr Robert T Sataloff for affording me the opportunity to contribute to his Atlas series and for his guidance and mentorship.

Contents

Section 1: Sinonasal Cancer

Section Editor: *Francis Hall*

Section 2: Oral Cavity and Oropharynx
Section Editor: *Steven S Chang*

Section 4: Neck Dissections
Section Editor: *Neerav Goyal*

Section 5: Thyroid
Section Editor: *Neerav Goyal*

Section 6: Salivary and Parapharyngeal Space Tumors
Section Editor: *Jason G Newman*

Section 7: Surgery for Skin Cancer

Section Editor: *Genevieve A Andrews*

Section 1

Sinonasal Cancer

Section Editor: ***Francis Hall***

Chapters

CHAPTER 1

Medial Maxillectomy

Robert Deeb

OVERVIEW

Medial maxillectomy involves the removal of the lateral nasal wall, including the inferior turbinate, the medial 1/3-1/2 of the inferior orbital floor, and usually includes the removal of the middle turbinate and ethmoid cavity. The extent of the resection is somewhat dependent on the extent and natural history of the disease process being treated (Figs. 1.1A and B).

A medial maxillectomy can be accomplished through a variety approaches. The classic approach is via lateral rhinotomy. It is important to note that a lateral rhinotomy is not in itself a procedure, but instead is an incision used to perform a medial maxillectomy. It is also a portion of an incision used in larger maxillectomy procedures, such as the Weber-Ferguson incision for a complete maxillectomy. The lateral rhinotomy approach allows for a largely en bloc resection of the tumor.

Medial maxillectomy can also be performed via a midfacial degloving approach that was first described in 1974.[1] The midfacial degloving approach can be performed alone or as a part of larger craniofacial approaches. Of note there are several variations of the medial maxillectomy procedure that have been described.[2–4] The exposure afforded by the midfacial degloving approach alone is somewhat limited.

The advent of endoscopes has allowed for the development of the endoscopic medial maxillectomy procedure. This procedure is performed in its entirety transnasally and requires a variety of endoscopes as well as specialized instrumentation used to perform functional endoscopic sinus surgery. This procedure is discussed in Chapter 2.

INDICATIONS

The most common indication for medial maxillectomy is for the removal of benign and malignant lesions arising from the lateral nasal sidewall, nasal septum, maxillary antrum, ethmoid cavity, and lacrimal sac. The most

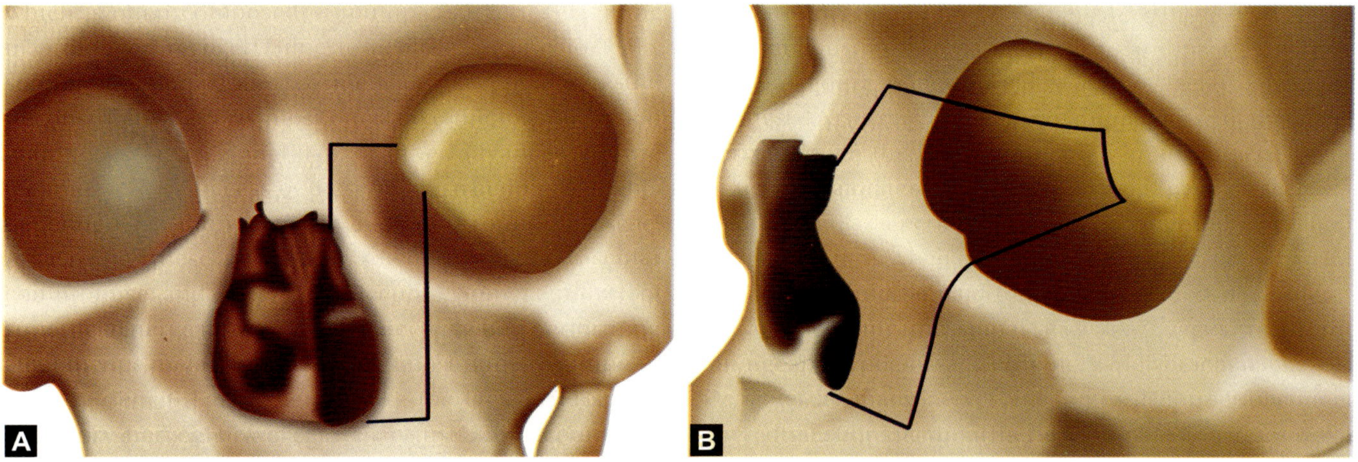

Figs. 1.1A and B: The extent of the resection is of medial maxillectomy.

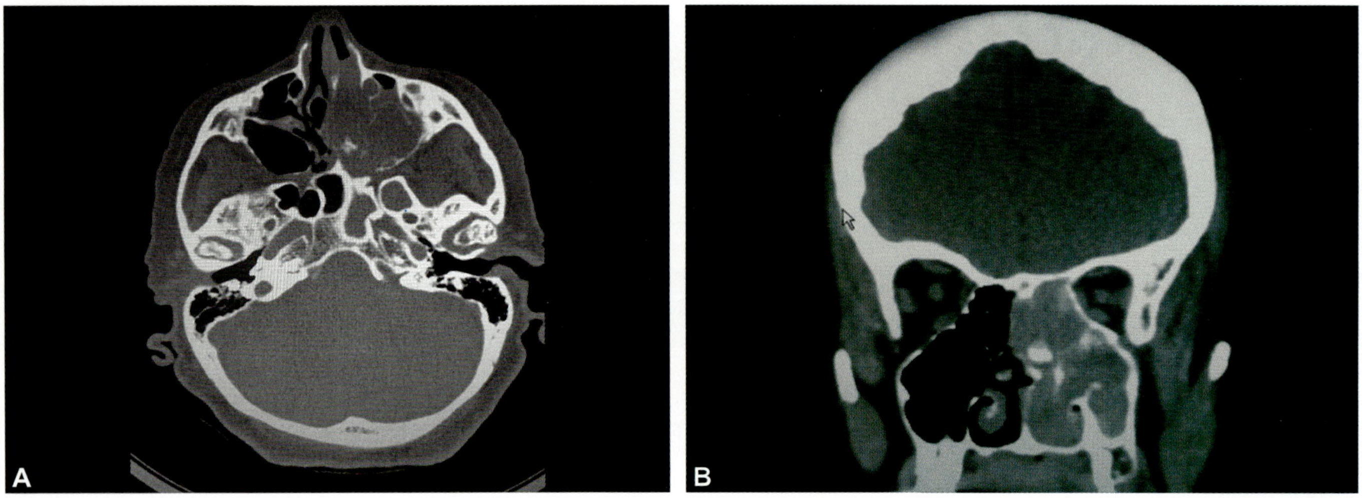

Figs. 1.2A and B: Axial and coronal CT scans showing an inverted papilloma arising from the lateral nasal wall.

common lesion encountered in these areas is inverted papilloma (Figs. 1.2A and B).

Inverted papilloma is a benign but aggressive sinonasal tumor that generally arises from the lateral nasal wall.

Its overall incidence is 0.5–4% of all primary nasal tumors.[11] The primary concern in treating this condition is related to its propensity for local destruction as well as a known rate of malignant degeneration. A study by Phillips et al. found a malignancy rate of 7%, all of which was squamous cell carcinoma.[5]

The recurrence rate of these lesions is highly variable. A study by Bielamowicz et al. showed that regardless of the operative approach the recurrence rate ranges from 20% to 47%.[12] Lawson et al. reported a recurrence rate of 13.8% in their cohort of patients treated with the lateral rhinotomy approach. The average interval to recurrence was 56 months, which highlights the importance of long-term surveillance in these patients.[6] Waitz and Wigand showed a recurrence rate of approximately 18% in patients treated via the endoscopic approach, while Sadeghi et al. reported no recurrences after their description of the transnasal endoscopic medial maxillectomy.[10,13] It should be noted that the latter report had a mean follow-up period of only 16.8 months.

The extent of the disease process dictates the extent of the surgical resection. The classical approach advocated for many years was the medial maxillectomy performed via a lateral rhinotomy incision.[6] Conservative surgery has been proposed by Lawson et al. as an effective therapy in highly selected cases.[7] Additionally, endoscopic excision has been advocated as being equally efficacious to the traditional open approaches.[8,9] Certainly the past few years has seen a surge in the use of endoscopic techniques in the treatment of this disease process that has become known as transnasal endoscopic medial maxillectomy.[10]

A variety of other conditions can be treated with a medial maxillectomy. These include lacrimal sac tumors, nasal septal tumors, minor salivary gland tumors, and early malignancies of the sinonasal cavity such as squamous cell carcinoma and adenocarcinoma. Medial maxillectomy is sometimes performed as part of a larger procedure such as a craniofacial resection for esthesioneuroblastoma or other skull-based tumors.

SURGICAL TECHNIQUES

Lateral Rhinotomy

The patient is placed in the supine position and administered general anesthesia via orotracheal intubation. The entire face is left exposed. Lacrilube and temporary tarsorrhaphy sutures are placed to protect the globe. Proposed incision is marked superior to the medial canthus, at a point horizontally halfway between the medial canthus and the midline nasal dorsum, down the lateral nasal sidewall and around the nasal ala. The incision can be curved into the nasal cavity or may be extended vertically down the philtrum of the lip for added exposure (Fig. 1.3).

It is important that the incision lie at the junction of the lateral nasal wall and the medial check subunits, as

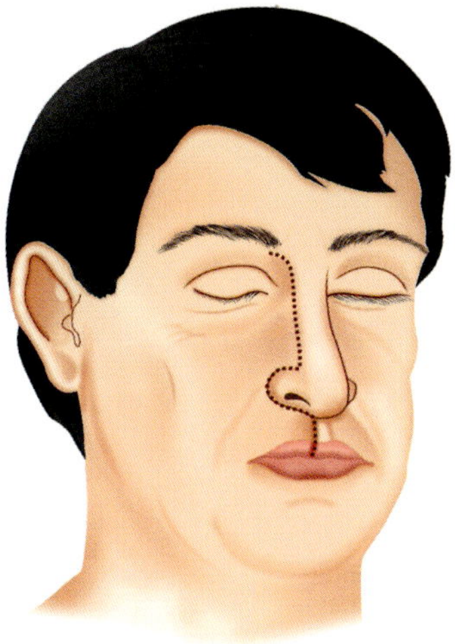

Fig. 1.3: The incision can be curved into the nasal cavity or may be extended vertically down the philtrum of the lip for added exposure.

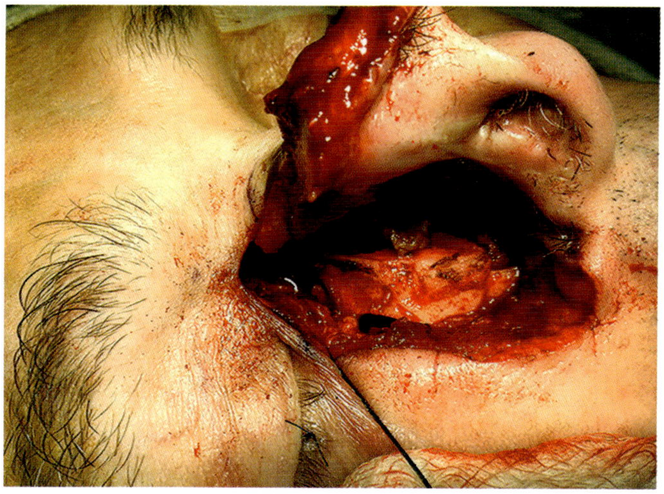

Fig. 1.4: The anterior ethmoid artery can be cauterized with bipolar cautery to avoid bleeding.

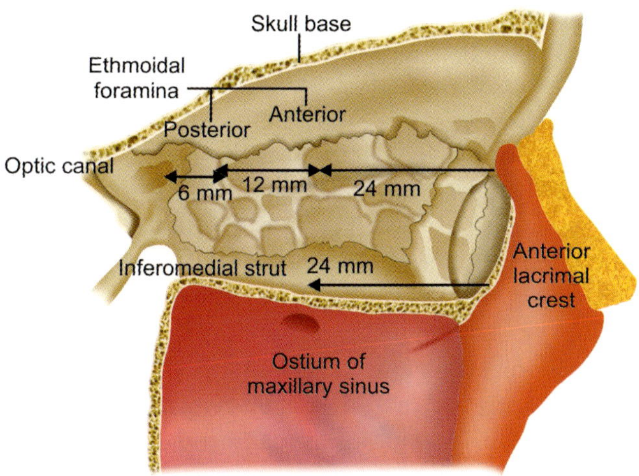

Fig. 1.5: Of note the posterior ethmoid artery is ~1 cm posterior and in the same plane as the anterior ethmoid artery.

this will aid in camouflaging the scar. If the lip is to be split the vermillion border should be carefully marked to assist in closure.

The proposed incision is infiltrated with 1% lidocaine containing 1:100,000 epinephrine for hemostasis.

Incision is made and carried down through the skin, subcutaneous tissue, and periosteum. The periorbita is incised and dissection is continued intraorbitally until the anterior ethmoid artery is encountered. This entails dissected free the attachments of the medial canthal tendon as well as teasing the lacrimal sac out of the lacrimal fossa. The medial canthal tendon can be tagged with a 4-0 silk suture to aid in closure. The anterior ethmoid artery can be cauterized with bipolar cautery to avoid bleeding (Fig. 1.4). The dissection generally does not have to extend far beyond the anterior ethmoid artery. Of note, the posterior ethmoid artery is ~1 cm posterior and in the same plane as the anterior ethmoid artery (Fig. 1.5).

Of note, a line connecting these two arteries approximates the frontoethmoidal suture line. Dissection should remain below this suture line at all times. Dissection above this plane may lead to inadvertent entry into the intracranial cavity.

Once the lacrimal sac has been extracted from the fossa the lacrimal duct should be incised flush with the bony canal as it enters. The sac can be marsupialized by incising it and suturing the incised ends posteriorly (Figs. 1.6A and B).

The medially third of the floor of the orbit should be exposed in a subperiorbital plane from the infraorbital neurovascular bundle medially.

The entire ascending process of the maxilla should be exposed in subperiosteal plane. Care should be taken to avoid injury to the infraorbital nerve.

Once the ascending process of the maxilla and the medial aspect of the inferior orbital floor and rim are exposed, the nasal cavity can be entered at the pyriform aperture. This allows access for the subsequent osteotomies. The exact location of the tumor will dictate whether both the inferior and middles turbinates will be removed.

The anterior aspect of the maxillary sinus is entered with an osteotome at the level of the canine fossa. A bony cut is made along the floor of the nose through the bone separating the nasal cavity from the maxillary sinus at a

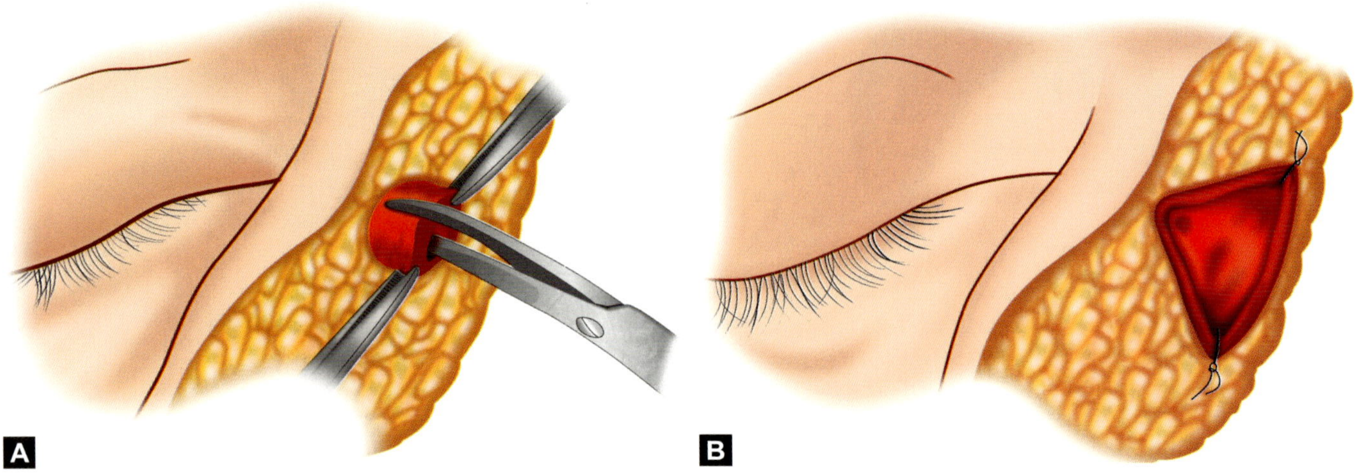

Figs. 1.6A and B: The sac can be marsupialized by incising it and suturing the incised ends posteriorly.

point inferior to the inferior turbinate. This can be done with an osteotome or a heavy scissor with one tine in the nose and one in the sinus.

Additional osteotomies are as follows: (1) along the frontoethmoidal suture line being sure to stay inferior to the anterior ethmoid artery and (2) along the medial floor of the orbit, this osteotomy should connect with the previous two osteotomies (Figs. 1.7A to C).

Soft tissue attachments are freed with heavy scissors and hemostasis is obtained. This should lead to an en bloc removal of the lateral nasal wall. Brisk bleeding is sometimes encountered at this point due to branches of the internal maxillary artery.

After removal of the en block specimen, the mucosa of the antrum should be stripped. A frontosphenoethmoidectomy may be performed at this point. Frontal sinus can be entered using a Kerrison rongeur and biting the bone directly superior to the lacrimal fossa. This allows safe entry into the sinus without violating the skull base. Additional disease involving the frontal sinus is then removed. This also widens the region of the frontal recess so as to prevent subsequent mucocele formation.

Ethmoid bony septations and mucosa can be removed with combination of upcutting and biting instruments.

The cavity is packed with 0.5-in. vaselineated gauze. The wound is closed in a layered fashion. Meticulous reapproximation of the periorbita, which is guided by the previously tagged medial canthal tendon, will allow for accurate positioning of the medial canthus. Subcutaneous tissue and skin are closed meticulously as well. If the lip has been split, a layered closure of the inner mucosa, muscle, subcutaneous tissue, and skin must be performed.

Bacitracin ointment is applied to the suture line and tarsorrhaphy sutures are removed. The pharynx is suctioned to clear any blood and the patient is extubated.

Midfacial Degloving

The patient is placed in the supine position and administered general anesthesia via orotracheal intubation. The entire face is left exposed. Lacrilube and temporary tarsorrhaphy sutures are placed to protect the globe.

One percent lidocaine containing 1:100,000 epinephrine is injected along the caudal septum, intercartilaginous space, and in the upper gingivolabial sulcus.

Full transfixion incision is made and is connected to bilateral intercartilaginous incisions. Incision is also made along the upper gingivolabial sulcus from approximately canine to canine. This incision is connected to the full transfixion incision (Fig. 1.8). The connection requires additional incisions along the nasal floor bilaterally. Care should be taken to place these incisions posterior to the vestibular lining to minimize the risk of postoperative vestibular stenosis. The soft tissues of the bilateral midface and nasal tip are then elevated in a subperiosteal plane. Care is taken not to injure the inferior orbital nerves.

Once the midface has been exposed, the osteotomies can take place as described above. Again the extent of the tumor will dictate the exact placement of the cuts.

Upon en bloc removal of the specimen, hemostasis is obtained. Sublabial incision is closed with 3-0 chromic gut sutures being sure to close the muscle layer. Transfixion incision is closed with 4-0 chromic gut sutures. The

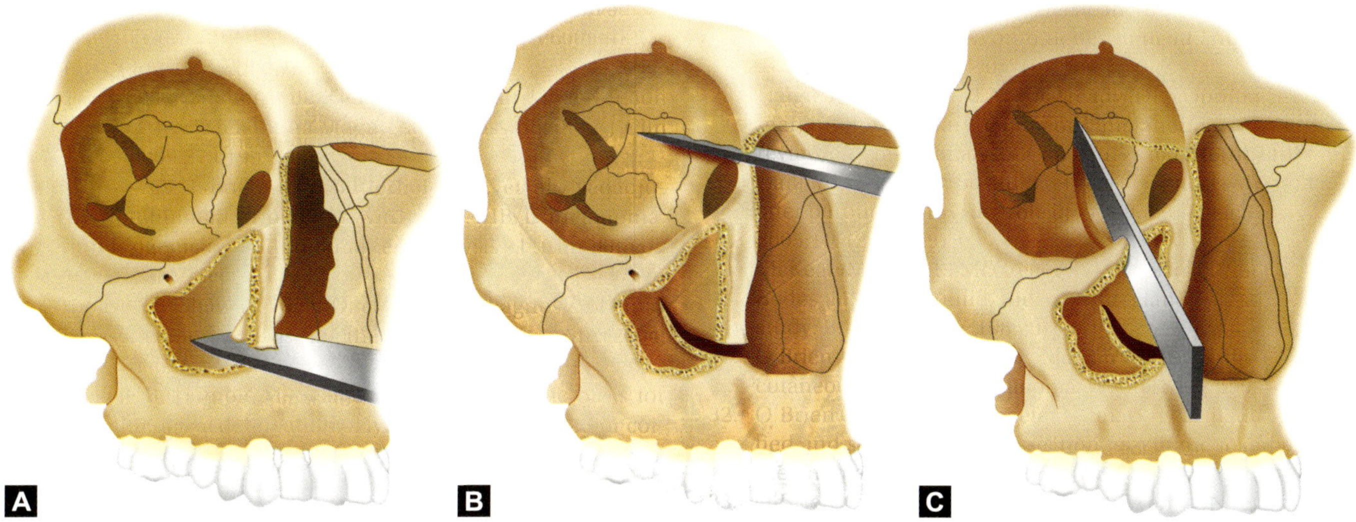

Figs. 1.7A to C: Along the medial floor of the orbit; this osteotomy should connect with the previous two osteotomies.

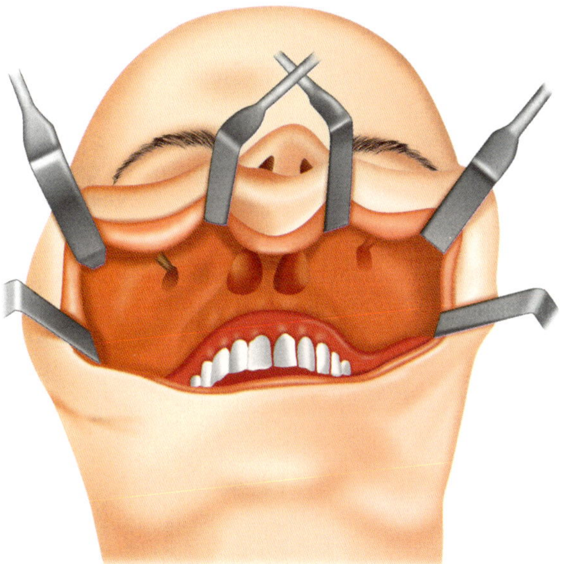

Fig. 1.8: Midface degloving approach.

incisions of the nasal floor are closed meticulously as well. The intercartilaginous incision does not require closure.

The stomach contents are suctioned and the cavity is packed with vaselineated gauze for a period of 2–3 days. The patient is extubated.

POSTOPERATIVE CARE

The patient is generally admitted to the hospital for approximately 2–4 days. The packing is removed from the nasal cavity on postoperative day 3. Facial incision lines are kept moist with bacitracin ointment. If an intraoral incision was made, chlorhexidine (Peridex) mouth rinse is used. Vision and neurologic checks are generally performed for the first 24 hours postoperatively.

A regular diet is acceptable and the patient should be encouraged to ambulate. After removal of the nasal packing, saline nasal irrigation should be performed twice daily. After discharge from the hospital, the patient is seen in 1–2 weeks in the outpatient setting. The incision is checked for proper healing. Nasal endoscopy is performed with gentle debridement of any crusts or clots. Saline nasal irrigation should be continued for several weeks.

COMPLICATIONS

The most feared complications involve injury to the globe or violation of the skull base. The osteotomies in and around the orbit must be done with care. It is important to stay medial to the infraorbital nerve so as to leave enough orbital floor to prevent enophthalmos. Direct injury to the globe or optic nerve with the osteotome is a possibility as well. A full ophthalmologic examination should be performed in the immediate postoperative period. If there is any concern for an ocular complication, an ophthalmologist should be consulted. Orbital complications include blindness (rare), enophthalmos, ectropion, entropion, asymmetry, and epiphora.

Epiphora is likely a result of improper marsupialization of the lacrimal sac. If it occurs a dilational procedure, with or without stents may be necessary.

Asymmetry may result from malalignment of the medial canthal tendon during closure. Meticulous reapproximation of the orbital septum generally results in proper positioning.

Violation of the skull base may result in cerebrospinal fluid leak. If this complication is recognized intraoperatively it should be repaired immediately. If it is a delayed leak, the patient may require a return to the operating room for repair.

Postoperative bleeding is a possibility as well. If it is minor a small amount of hemostatic packing material can be placed. A massive bleed warrants return to the operating room for exploration. This can generally be performed endoscopically. Significant bleeding may be from the sphenopalatine artery or one of its branches and formal ligation may be necessary. Note that this complication may be delayed by several weeks.

REFERENCES

1. Casson PR, Bonanno PC, Converse KM. The mid-facial degloving procedure. Plast Reconstr Surg. 1974;53:102-3.
2. Buchwald C, Bonding P, Kirkby B, et al. Modified midfacial degloving: a practical approach to extensive bilateral benign tumors of the nasal cavity and paranasal sinuses. Rhinology. 1995;33:39-42.
3. Krause GE, Jafek BW. A modification of the midface degloving technique. Laryngoscope. 1999;109:1781-4.
4. Jeon SY, Jeong JH, Kim HS, et al. Hemifacial degloving approach for medial maxillectomy: a modification of midfacial degloving approach. Laryngoscope. 2003;113:754-6.
5. Phillips PP, Gustafson RO, Facer GW. The clinical behavior of inverting papilloma of the nose and paranasal sinuses: report of 112 cases and review of the literature. Laryngoscope.1990;100(5):463-9.
6. Lawson W, Ho BT, Shaari CM, et al. Inverted papilloma: a report of 112 cases. Laryngoscope. 1995;105:282-8.
7. Lawson W, Biller HF, Jacobsen A, et al. The role of conservative surgery in the management of inverted papilloma. Laryngoscope. 1983;93:148-55.
8. Kraft M, Simmen D, Kaufmann T, et al. Long term results of endonasal sinus surgery in sinonasal papillomas. Laryngoscope. 2003;113:1541-7.
9. Chee LWJ, Sethi DS. The endoscopic management of sinonasal inverted papillomas. Clin Otolaryngol. 1999;24:61-6.
10. Sadeghi N, al-Dhahri S, Manoukian JJ. Transnasal endoscopic medial maxillectomy for inverting papilloma. Laryngoscope. 2003;113:749-53.
11. Skolnik EM, Loewy A, Friedman JE. Inverted Papilloma of the nasal cavity. Arch Otolaryngol. 1966;84:61-7.
12. Bielamowicz S, Calcaterra TC, Watson D. Inverting papilloma of the head and neck: the UCLA update. Otolaryngol Head Neck Surg. 1993;109:71-6.
13. Waitz G, Wigand ME. Result of endoscopic sinus surgery for the treatment of inverted papilloma. Laryngoscope. 1992; 102:917-22.

CHAPTER

2

Endoscopic Medial Maxillectomy

Liat Shama, Francis Hall

EVOLUTION

Endoscopic medial maxillectomy (EMM) has evolved as a treatment for recalcitrant chronic sinusitis as well as benign and malignant sinonasal tumors in parallel with endoscopic skull base surgery. It has been used to treat benign pathology such as inverted papilloma (IP) and juvenile nasopharyngeal angiofibroma (JNA) as well as malignant pathology in a limited fashion. Endoscopic medial maxillectomy is the current standard of care for resection of tumors fully accessible and resectable with endoscopic techniques, following a trend toward minimally invasive techniques.[1-14] Many lesions require open resection; those are beyond the scope of this chapter. For some lesions resected with open approach, endoscopic assistance may be of value.

With respect to tumors involving the maxillary sinus, especially IP, resection has evolved from open techniques such as lateral rhinotomy or midface degloving or open maxillectomy to endoscopic techniques.[15-20] Historically, the technique of EMM included resection of the entire lateral nasal wall including the nasolacrimal duct, inferior turbinate; it has evolved to preserve these structures when possible.[3,11,15,21-23] Modification of the EMM is possible, especially with benign tumors or chronic disease, allowing for preservation of the nasolacrimal duct and/or partial preservation of the inferior turbinate, and is known as a modified endoscopic medial maxillectomy (MEMM).[13]

INDICATIONS

Endoscopic medial maxillectomy is ideal for tumors involving the lateral wall of the nasal cavity and/or medial maxillary sinus (Figs. 2.1 and 2.2). Historically, this procedure was used as a treatment for recalcitrant maxillary sinusitis and for removal of IP.[24] Endoscopic medial maxillectomy allows for irrigation and topical application of medications that may improve disease in patients with recalcitrant maxillary sinusitis. This is especially important in cases in which the patient has altered mucociliary transport and requires irrigation. Prolapsed fat after endoscopic orbital decompression may necessitate endoscopic maxillary antrostomy for a wider cavity.[25] Endoscopic medial maxillectomy can also be used for selected malignant tumors involving the lateral wall of the maxillary sinus or the medial wall of the maxillary sinus. It is widely used for benign lesions of the maxillary sinus such as IP; resection of this pathology is the basis for the majority of the literature on this procedure.

Outcomes have been compared between open and endoscopic approaches for IP. Endoscopic procedures are associated with decreased rates of complications and similar if not lower recurrence rates than open procedures.[15,26] Endoscopic medial maxillectomy is generally the recommended approach for resection of most cases of IP, and allows for sufficient visualization for endoscopic surveillance.[25-30] The EMM has been shown to be safe and effective for treatment of pathology such as IP and JNA, with recurrence rates similar to open procedures and lower complication rates than open approaches.[1,6,7,9,10,14,22,29] The endoscopic approach allows for better visualization and can utilize image guidance. Its utility is lower for tumors in the anterolateral maxillary sinus and may not allow for visualization of some lesions of the frontal sinus.[6]

Another pathology for which this modality of tumor removal has been widely utilized is JNA. Although JNA is not always completely resectable with the endoscopic approach, selected cases may be ideal. Often preoperative

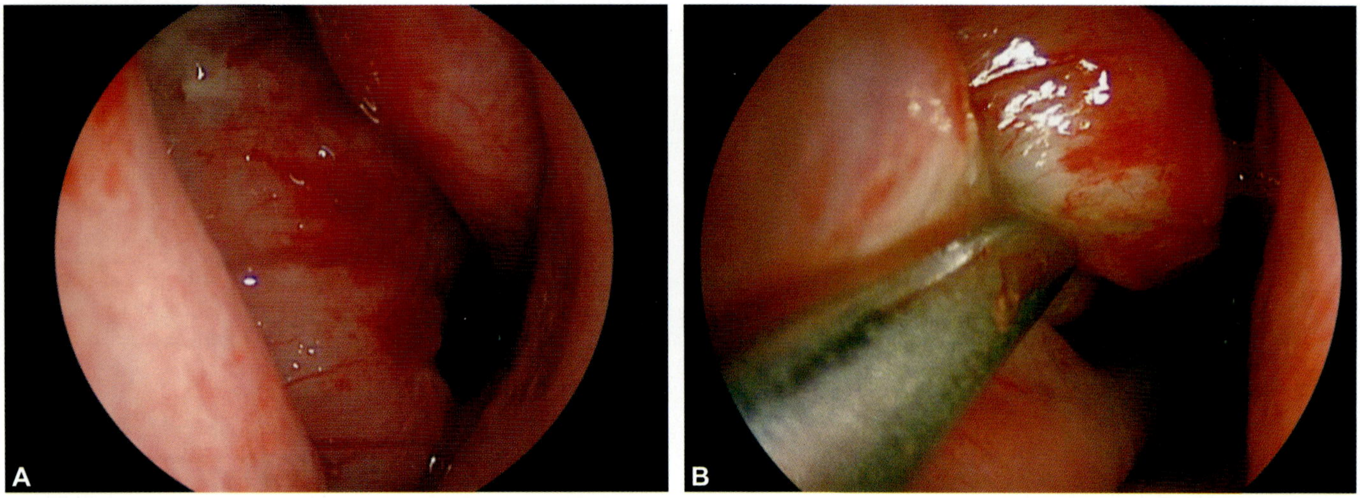

Figs. 2.1A and B: Tumor shown involves the medial wall of the maxillary sinus, extending into the nasal cavity.

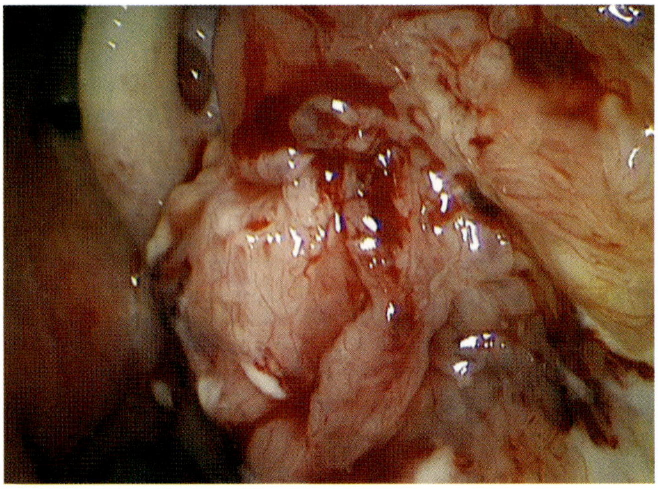

Fig. 2.2: Recurrent papilloma involving the lateral wall of the nasal cavity.

embolization is used to improve hemostasis during surgery.[31-33] Ligation of various arteries, including the sphenopalatine and/or internal maxillary artery, may be necessary. Careful review of imaging is imperative to determine if this will be the best approach. Both open and endoscopic approaches may be beneficial.[31]

The decision of which approach to use is preceded by careful review of imaging to determine whether both approaches allow for adequate resection of the tumor. Malignant tumors can be resected in this fashion as well, although endoscopic approach is not necessarily the standard of care. Endoscopic approach should be used only in cases in which it does not compromise the principles of oncologic resection.

IMAGING

Both CT and MRI imaging have a role in the preparation for surgery. CT delineates the bony anatomy; MRI will highlight the soft tissue components and involvement. Use of both modalities will allow for determination of the best possible approach to the removal of the tumor. These should be reviewed in depth prior to deciding the approach and prior to the surgery for planning purposes.[34] Defining the extent of tumor allows for determination of the best approach and for careful planning of resection. Endoscopic removal of the medial wall of the maxilla allows for access to the anterior, posterior, and lateral walls of maxillary sinus.[14,35-37] Determination of whether or not the tumor is resectable endoscopically depends on imaging and preoperative endoscopy.[38] Review of imaging may allow for preoperative determination of point of attachment if not already determined on preoperative endoscopy, as it is an important step in the resection.[30] This is especially relevant in cases of IP. However, imaging may not be able to decisively determine the point of origin as bone destruction may occur from growth of the tumor.[14]

CONTRAINDICATIONS

Involvement of medial maxillary wall was previously thought to be a contraindication to an endoscopic resection; this has recently been shown not to be the case.[5,6,11,35,38-42] Endoscopic medial maxillectomy as the sole procedure is absolutely contraindicated in cases in which the tumor cannot be removed completely and safely endoscopically. In these cases, an open approach is recommended, possibly with endoscopic assistance.

EQUIPMENT AND SETUP

Equipment and room setup for EMM uses the standard setup for endoscopic sinus surgery. As with most surgical cases, routinizing the setup and flow of events leads to a controlled environment that provides for a smooth flow of events, setting the stage for minimizing errors. Surgical technicians and scrub nurses should be familiar with the equipment and room setup. Instruments normally used for endoscopic sinus surgery are used for this procedure, including angled endoscopes, bipolar suction forceps, and a drill as needed. Endoscopic clip appliers may be advantageous as well in cases of vascular tumors.

Endoscopic medial maxillectomy for tumor resection should utilize image guidance. Image guidance, or computer-assisted navigation, has evolved over many years to the current devices that are versatile and accurate to within 2 mm.[30] Although these devices are not a substitute for thorough knowledge of sinonasal anatomy, there is a possibility for more complete surgery with the use of these devices as additional information is available to the surgeon. Although intraoperative imaging is available, it has yet to be widely incorporated into the realm of endoscopic sinus surgery. The main limitation of image guidance is that the images are obtained preoperatively and are therefore not an accurate reflection of any changes applied during surgery. While not routinely used for maxillary antrostomy, image guidance is both useful and strongly recommended for EMM, especially in cases of tumor resection.

OPERATIVE STEPS

The nasal cavities are topically anesthetized and decongested with various agents on cottonoid pledgets. Diluted 4% cocaine, high concentration epinephrine (1:1,000), and Afrin have all been used to improve hemostasis. Thereafter, intranasal injections are undertaken with a mixture of usually 1–2% lidocaine with 1:80,000–100,000 of epinephrine. Often, especially with extended maxillary sinus procedures, pterygopalatine fossa block is performed transorally through the greater palatine canal usually with 1% lidocaine with 1:100,000 of epinephrine.

MAXILLARY ANTROSTOMY

Endoscopic medial maxillectomy begins with a large middle meatal maxillary antrostomy (Fig. 2.3). This is generally done widely for access to the entirety of the maxillary sinus as well as to the medial wall of the maxilla. More importantly, it allows for identification and visualization of the medial and inferior orbital walls that decrease the chance of injury to the orbit. The middle turbinate is medialized or resected, with care taken superiorly so as not to fracture the lateral lamella or cribriform plate. If a concha bullosa is present, it is either partially resected and medialized or fully resected. If the middle turbinate or concha bullosa is resected, the sphenopalatine artery should be cauterized along the basal lamella to prevent bleeding.

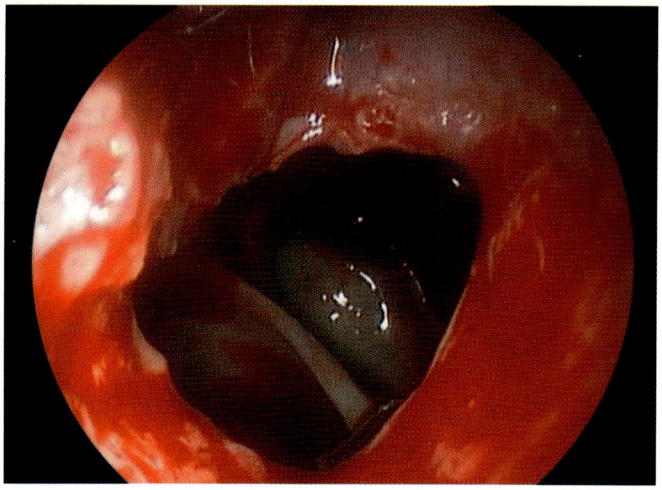

Fig. 2.3: Endoscopic medial maxillectomy begins with a large middle meatal maxillary antrostomy.

The most important step in performing a maxillary antrostomy is identification and opening of the natural ostium of the maxillary sinus that requires removal of the uncinate process (Fig. 2.4). The uncinate process should be removed entirely and to its most superior attachment. The anterior attachment is the posterior aspect of the lacrimal bone. Posteriorly and inferiorly, the uncinate attaches to the ethmoidal process of the inferior turbinate bone. Removal of the uncinate process is generally done in a retrograde fashion. It is removed completely and superiorly to the skull base or its most superior attachment; various superior attachment points have been described and will likely be apparent on preoperative review of imaging. Mucosa is preserved inferiorly if possible during removal of the bony portion of the uncinate process. The ostium is extended posteriorly to the perpendicular plate of the palatine bone if necessary. If the posterior fontanelle is encountered, it is incorporated into the surgical ostium.

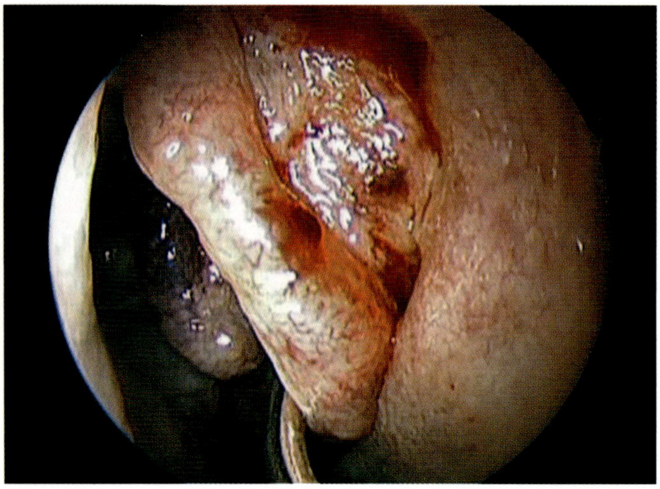

Fig. 2.4: The most important step in performing a maxillary antrostomy is identification and opening of the natural ostium of the maxillary sinus which requires removal of the uncinate process.

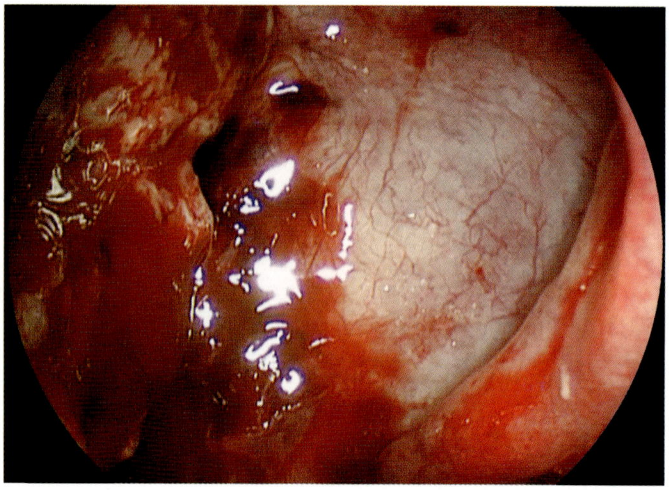

Fig. 2.5: The extent of the procedure depends on the extent of the lesion that is being resected; wide maxillary antrostomy is shown.

ENDOSCOPIC MEDIAL MAXILLECTOMY

After completion of the maxillary antrostomy, there are several variations to performing the EMM. The extent of the procedure depends on the extent of the lesion that is being resected (Fig. 2.5). If the procedure is done for recalcitrant maxillary sinusitis, it may be possible to spare the nasolacrimal duct and inferior turbinate, whereas for some tumors, it may not be possible nor advisable especially if the tumor is malignant and/or involves these structures or is located such that modification will preclude endoscopic surveillance.

A more invasive procedure is indicated in cases of neoplasm such as IP, the most commonly described indication for EMM.[5,6,10,22,35,43] This includes complete removal of the inferior turbinate, the nasolacrimal duct, and the entire medial maxillary wall. The margins of the EMM include floor of nose inferiorly, posterior wall of maxillary sinus posteriorly, floor of orbit superiorly, and anterior maxillary wall anteriorly. Nasolacrimal duct removal is necessary to visualize the anterior maxillary wall. Complete ethmoidectomy is then performed as well as sphenoidotomy if indicated, followed by a dacryocystorhinostomy to decrease the chance of nasolacrimal duct stenosis.[44]

As many tumors of the maxillary sinus and pterygopalatine fossa may involve the ethmoid and sphenoid sinuses; these sinuses should be addressed as well. Traditionally, complete ethmoidectomy, exposing the lamina papyracea, fovea ethmoidalis, sphenoid rostrum, is performed as part of the EMM. This allows for identification of the skull base and allows for examination of the sinonasal cavity to determine if gross tumor is present. This will allow for more complete removal of tumor. The extent of these adjunct procedures can be adjusted as necessary.

The inferior turbinate is medialized and removed by crushing the anterior head of the turbinate just distal to its junction with the lateral nasal wall. Turbinate scissors are then used to cut the inferior turbinate to its insertion point along the lateral nasal wall (Fig. 2.6A). Next, the mucosa is incised from just below the orbit to through the cut portion of the inferior turbinate to the floor of the nose (Fig. 2.6B). The cut is then extended from the inferior meatus and nasal floor junction to the posterior wall of the maxillary sinus.[14,45] After mucosal elevation, osteotomy cuts are made on the lateral nasal wall from the inferior meatus to the floor of the nose.[42] If necessary, a drill may be used to further remove bone. At this point, the nasal wall, including the tumor, is mobilized medially. Anteriorly, the nasolacrimal duct will be attached to the specimen. At this point, consideration of incising and opening the nasolacrimal duct with possible catheterization should be undertaken, as it may prevent epiphora.[14,37,46-48] It has been advocated that incision and opening of the nasolacrimal duct is not necessary in all cases and should be reserved for select cases such as tumors involving the medial buttress.[42] As the contents are separated posteriorly from the maxillary sinus, the

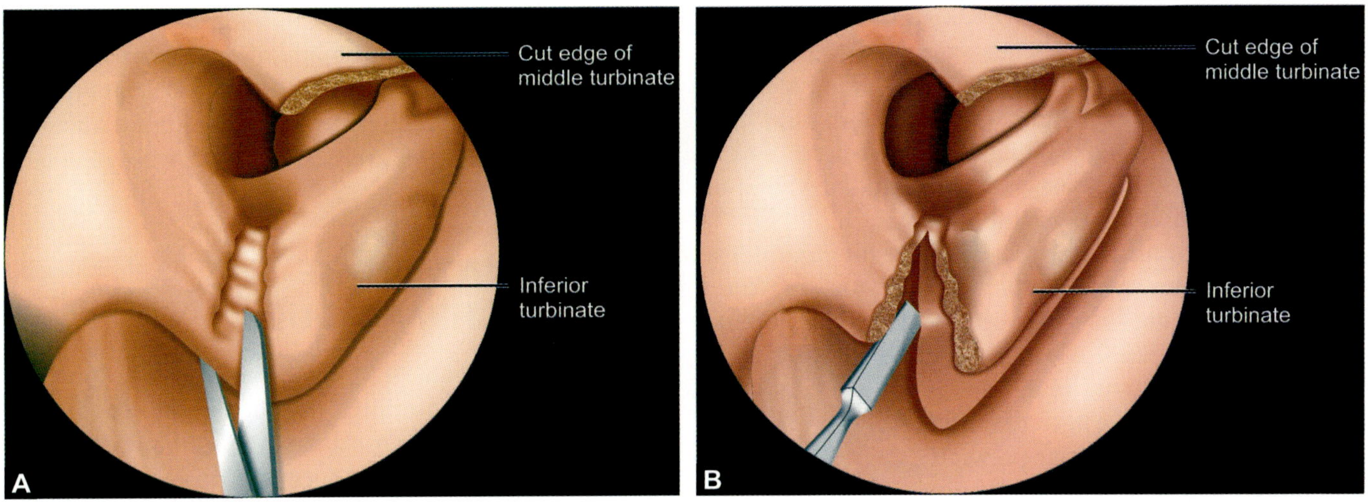

Figs. 2.6A and B: (A) Turbinate scissors are then used to cut the inferior turbinate to its insertion point along the lateral nasal wall. (B) Next, the mucosa is incised from just below the orbit to through the cut portion of the inferior turbinate to the floor of the nose.

sphenopalatine artery is cauterized if it was not previously addressed. Further dissection is taken inside the now fully accessible maxillary sinus if necessary. The floor of the nose should be level with the inferior extent of the maxillectomy.[24] Angled endoscopes should allow for full visualization of the maxillary sinus. If further tumor is encountered and inaccessible or if the entire maxillary sinus cannot be visualized, canine fossa puncture can be performed. This will allow for improved visualization and/or instrumentation of tumors or pathology within the maxillary sinus.[25,36,49]

In situations requiring further exposure to visualize the anterior face of the maxillary sinus, resection of pyriform aperture will further maximize access to the maxillary sinus.[42,45,50,51] An anterior cut of the attachment of the head of the inferior turbinate on the mucosa covering the frontal process of the maxilla is made. Mucosa is removed and the free margin of pyriform aperture is exposed. Mucosa and periosteum is elevated until the infraorbital nerve is appreciated. The anterior wall of maxillary sinus is then drilled or removed with an osteotome. This includes the frontal process of the maxilla. This maximizes exposure to the maxillary sinus including the anterior and medial walls.[42,50] A trans-septal approach may be employed as well to increase access to the maxillary sinus. This is performed using a contralateral hemitransfixion incision and ipsilateral horizontal septal mucosal flap in nonapposing portions of the septum. Cartilaginous cuts then allow the passage of instruments that further increases access to the maxillary sinus.[45]

With traditional EMM, the nasolacrimal duct is violated; dacryocystorhinostomy should be considered as it may prevent epiphora. The nasolacrimal duct may be opened with oblique transection to prevent stenosis and epiphora. This is appropriate for tumors involving the medial buttress of the maxillary sinus. However, in cases in which this is not necessary, modified EMM avoids the need for stenting and/or dacryocystorhinostomy and has been shown to be both safe and effective.[13,24,25,52] The EMM with and without dacryocystorhinostomy has been studied; epiphora rates have been shown to be similar. Therefore, dacryocystorhinostomy not necessitated if the nasolacrimal sac can be preserved.[11,42] However, the study was small so the conclusion is not necessarily proven. However, this reflects a trend toward preservation of the nasolacrimal duct.

MODIFIED EMM

Historically, EMM was defined as an en bloc resection including the lateral nasal wall, inferior turbinate, nasolacrimal duct, middle turbinate with complete ethmoidectomy, generally for recalcitrant maxillary mucosal disease and/or mucociliary flow dysfunction.[42,44,46,53] Several variations from the original procedure have been proposed. More recent modifications of this procedure include preserving the inferior turbinate as well as the nasolacrimal duct.

In cases of recalcitrant maxillary sinusitis or smaller tumors that allow for conservative resection, modifications of the EMM have been proposed as the compromise of nasolacrimal duct and inferior turbinate functions may lead to complications and decreased quality of life. Injury to the nasolacrimal duct may cause stenosis and epiphora.[25] Removal of the inferior turbinate may decrease temperature and humidification of nasal airflow and perhaps modify the nasal airflow. This may lead to empty nose sensation as well as atrophic rhinitis.[25,54-56] Modifications of an EMM may decrease the need for a dacryocystorhinostomy and the alteration of nasal function such as humidification and turbulence.[25,57,58] Several approaches to MEMM with complete or partial preservation of the inferior turbinate and/or preservation of the nasolacrimal duct have been described.

With respect to oncologic principles, the volume of the maxillary sinus made inaccessible by various structures including the nasolacrimal duct and inferior turbinate was analyzed. Up to 64% of volume is inferior to the inferior turbinate that necessitates removal or shift of the inferior turbinate to access the maxillary sinus. Five percent of the nasal volume is anterior to the nasolacrimal duct. This requires modification of preoperative plan depending on location of tumor to allow for optimal visualization and resection of tumor.[15] However, a study showed that preservation of the nasolacrimal duct and inferior turbinate reduces exposure to maxillary sinus; visualization of 70% of the maxillary sinus mucosa is blocked by inferior turbinate and nasolacrimal duct, the majority of which is obstructed by the inferior turbinate.[15] Therefore, MEMM should be used with caution in cases of tumors, especially malignancy.

PRESERVATION OF THE INFERIOR TURBINATE

Several methods have been described to preserve the inferior turbinate as part of a MEMM. In an MEMM with preservation of the inferior turbinate, the anterior two thirds of the inferior turbinate is medially displaced and cut and secured medially out of the operative field. The posterior third of the inferior turbinate and its blood supply are preserved. After completion of the remainder of the procedure and removal of the tumor, the interior turbinate is sutured into its original position.[59-61] This preserves the functionality of the inferior turbinate and decreases the risk of bleeding.[62] The inferior turbinate can also be shifted medially with removal of tumor posterior to the nasolacrimal duct. A flap is elevated over frontal process of maxilla, revealing underlying bone and nasolacrimal duct, which may be preserved. Inverted papilloma, or other tumors, can then be removed in subperiosteal plane.[59,60] The inferior turbinate, nasolacrimal duct, and nasal mucosa can be shifted medially as well. This requires removal of tumor posterior to the nasolacrimal duct that may require piecemeal excision and/or the use of angled endoscopes.[60]

PRESERVATION OF THE NASOLACRIMAL DUCT

The technique for an MEMM generally involves elevation of a mucosal flap anteriorly including the mucosa of the inferior turbinate, which exposes and allows for preservation of the nasolacrimal duct. The posterior aspect of the inferior turbinate is preserved.[28] The nasolacrimal duct and lacrimal bone can be shifted superiorly as well to allow for removal of medial maxillary wall, and then is shifted inferiorly into its original place.[63]

PTERYGOPALATINE AND INFRATEMPORAL FOSSA

Extended EMM allows for transantral access to the pterygomaxillary and pterygopalatine fossa that provides access for resection of tumors in this region, usually a JNA. This would be performed after ethmoidectomy, EMM (and in some cases, wide middle meatal antrostomy) to provide access to posterior wall of maxillary sinus. The posterior wall of the maxillary sinus is then removed as necessary to access the tumor.[42,64]

Access to the pterygopalatine fossa can be achieved through a wide middle meatal antrostomy and at least a partial inferior turbinate resection. Removal of the bone of the posterior wall of the maxillary sinus will provide transantral access to the pterygopalatine fossa.[36,42,64] For access to the infratemporal fossa, EMM is necessary. Removal of this lesion has evolved from an open to an endoscopic route; improved with the advent of preoperative embolization.[36] This route has been shown to be both safe and effective for removal of JNA.[31,35]

POSTOPERATIVE CARE

Postoperative care is generally minimal. Meticulous surgical technique and maintenance of hemostasis set the stage for healing with minimal scarring and postoperative complications. Frequent nasal saline irrigations postoperatively improve circumstances for debridement.

Prevention of lateralization of middle turbinate (if not removed) may be done in a variety of ways. Merocel sponge placement, steroid-eluting implant placement, and finger cot (Merocel sponge sutured inside glove) placement prevent lateralization of middle turbinate and require removal.

Complications include bleeding, scarring, and residual tumor. Bleeding can be prevented with cauterization posteriorly along the basal lamella. Synechiae can be prevented with limitation of mucosal trauma. Persistent disease, ostial stenosis, lacrimal injury, orbital injury, bleeding, and recirculation can be prevented with meticulous operative technique and careful surgical planning including review of images preoperatively and use of image-guidance technology.

SUMMARY

Endoscopic medial maxillectomy is ideal for selected tumors of the maxillary sinus and lateral nasal wall. It may be modified to preserve structures that may improve quality of life. Evidence has shown that this procedure is safe and effective for tumors in selected patients. When selected, it should be modified as necessary, provided the ultimate goals of the surgical procedure, including oncologic resection, can be obtained. The EMM can be extended for tumors in the infratemporal fossa as well.

REFERENCES

1. Busquets JM, Hwang PH. Endoscopic resection of sinonasal inverted papilloma: a meta-analysis. Otolaryngol Head Neck Surg. 2006;134(3):476-82.
2. Han JK, Smith TL, Loehrl T, et al. An evolution in the management of sinonasal inverting papilloma. Laryngoscope. 2001;111(8):1395-400.
3. Kamel RH. Conservative endoscopic surgery in inverted papilloma. Preliminary report. Arch Otolaryngol Head Neck Surg. 1992;118(6):649-53.
4. Lawson W, Kaufman MR, Biller HF. Treatment outcomes in the management of inverted papilloma: an analysis of 160 cases. Laryngoscope. 2003;113(9):1548-56.
5. Lund VJ. Optimum management of inverted papilloma. J Laryngol Otol. 2000;114(3):194-7.
6. Sautter NB, Cannady SB, Citardi MJ, et al. Comparison of open versus endoscopic resection of inverted papilloma. Am J Rhinol. 2007;21(3):320-3.
7. Schlosser RJ, Mason JC, Gross CW. Aggressive endoscopic resection of inverted papilloma: an update. Otolaryngol Head Neck Surg. 2001;125(1):49-53.
8. Stammberger H, Anderhuber W, Walch C, et al. Possibilities and limitations of endoscopic management of nasal and paranasal sinus malignancies. Acta Otorhinolaryngol Belg. 1999;53(3):199-205.
9. Thaler ER, Lanza DC, Tufano RP. Inverted papilloma: an endoscopic approach. Oper Tech Otolaryngol Head Neck Surg. 1999;10(2):8.
10. Tufano RP, Thaler ER, Lanza DC, et al. Endoscopic management of sinonasal inverted papilloma. Am J Rhinol. 1999; 13(6):423-6.
11. Waitz G, Wigand ME. Results of endoscopic sinus surgery for the treatment of inverted papillomas. Laryngoscope. 1992;102(8):917-22.
12. Winter M, Rauer RA, Gode U, et al. [Inverted papilloma of the nose and paranasal sinuses. Long-term outcome of endoscopic endonasal resection]. Hno. 2000 Aug;48(8): 568-72.
13. Woodworth BA, Parker RO, Schlosser RJ. Modified endoscopic medial maxillectomy for chronic maxillary sinusitis. Am J Rhinol. 2006;20(3):317-9.
14. Wormald PJ, Ooi E, van Hasselt CA, et al. Endoscopic removal of sinonasal inverted papilloma including endoscopic medial maxillectomy. Laryngoscope. 2003;113(5):867-73.
15. Tanna N, Edwards JD, Aghdam H, et al. Transnasal endoscopic medial maxillectomy as the initial oncologic approach to sinonasal neoplasms: the anatomic basis. Arch Otolaryngol Head Neck Surg. 2007;133(11):1139-42.
16. Lane AP, Bolger WE. Endoscopic management of inverted papilloma. Curr Opin Otolaryngol Head Neck Surg. 2006;14(1):14-8.
17. Sachs ME, Conley J, Rabuzzi DD, et al. Degloving approach for total excision of inverted papilloma. Laryngoscope. 1984;94(12 Pt 1):1595-8.
18. Bielamowicz S, Calcaterra TC, Watson D. Inverting papilloma of the head and neck: the UCLA update. Otolaryngol Head Neck Surg. 1993;109(1):71-6.
19. Myers EN, Fernau JL, Johnson JT, et al. Management of inverted papilloma. Laryngoscope. 1990;100(5):481-90.
20. Price JC, Holliday MJ, Johns ME, et al. The versatile midface degloving approach. Laryngoscope. 1988;98(3):291-5.
21. Sham CL, Woo JK, van Hasselt CA. Endoscopic resection of inverted papilloma of the nose and paranasal sinuses. J Laryngol Otol. 1998;112(8):758-64.
22. Stankiewicz JA, Girgis SJ. Endoscopic surgical treatment of nasal and paranasal sinus inverted papilloma. Otolaryngol Head Neck Surg. 1993;109(6):988-95.
23. Tomenzoli D, Castelnuovo P, Pagella F, et al. Different endoscopic surgical strategies in the management of inverted papilloma of the sinonasal tract: experience with 47 patients. Laryngoscope. 2004;114(2):193-200.
24. Wang EW, Gullung JL, Schlosser RJ. Modified endoscopic medial maxillectomy for recalcitrant chronic maxillary sinusitis. Int Forum Allergy Rhinol. 2011;1(6):493-7.
25. Konstantinidis I, Constantinidis J. Medial maxillectomy in recalcitrant sinusitis: when, why and how? Curr Opin Otolaryngol Head Neck Surg. 2014;22(1):68-74.

26. Jurado-Ramos A, Jodas JG, Romero FR, et al. Endoscopic medial maxillectomy as a procedure of choice to treat inverted papillomas. Acta Otolaryngol. 2009;129(9):1018-25.
27. Krouse JH. Endoscopic treatment of inverted papilloma: safety and efficacy. Am J Otolaryngol. 2001;22(2):87-99.
28. Nakayama T, Asaka D, Okushi T, et al. Endoscopic medial maxillectomy with preservation of inferior turbinate and nasolacrimal duct. Am J Rhinol Allergy. 2012;26(5):405-8.
29. Philpott CM, Dharamsi A, Witheford M, et al. Endoscopic management of inverted papillomas: long-term results—the St. Paul's Sinus Centre experience. Rhinology. 2010; 48(3):358-63.
30. Rutherford KD, Brown SM. Endoscopic resection of maxillary sinus inverted papillomas with inferior turbinate preservation. Otolaryngol—Head Neck Surg. 2010;142(5): 760-2.
31. Douglas R, Wormald PJ. Endoscopic surgery for juvenile nasopharyngeal angiofibroma: where are the limits? Curr Opin Otolaryngol Head Neck Surg. 2006;14(1):1-5.
32. Fagan JJ, Snyderman CH, Carrau RL, et al. Nasopharyngeal angiofibromas: selecting a surgical approach. Head Neck. 1997;19(5):391-9.
33. Ungkanont K, Byers RM, Weber RS, et al. Juvenile nasopharyngeal angiofibroma: an update of therapeutic management. Head Neck. 1996;18(1):60-6.
34. Kennedy DW, Ramakrishnan V. Functional endoscopic sinus surgery: concepts, surgical indications, and techniques. In: Kennedy DW, Hwang PH (Eds). Rhinology: Diseases of the Nose, Sinuses, Skull Base. New York: Thieme Medical Publishers, Inc; 2012. pp. 306-35.
35. Sukenik MA, Casiano R. Endoscopic medial maxillectomy for inverted papillomas of the paranasal sinuses: value of the intraoperative endoscopic examination. Laryngoscope. 2000;110(1):39-42.
36. Wormald PJ. Endoscopic Sinus Surgery: Anatomy, Three-Dimensional Reconstruction, and Surgical Technique, 2nd edition. New York: Thieme Medical Pulishers, Inc; 2008.
37. Wormald PJ, Van Hasselt A. Endoscopic removal of juvenile angiofibromas. Otolaryngol Head Neck Surg. 2003; 129(6):684-91.
38. Keles N, Deger K. Endonasal endoscopic surgical treatment of paranasal sinus inverted papilloma—first experiences. Rhinology. 2001;39(3):156-9.
39. Karkos PD, Fyrmpas G, Carrie SC, et al. Endoscopic versus open surgical interventions for inverted nasal papilloma: a systematic review. Clin Otolaryngol. 2006;31(6):499-503.
40. McCary WS, Gross CW, Reibel JF, et al. Preliminary report: endoscopic versus external surgery in the management of inverting papilloma. Laryngoscope. 1994;104(4):415-9.
41. Myers EN, Petruzzelli GJ. Endoscopic sinus surgery for inverting papillomas. Laryngoscope. 1993;103(6):711.
42. Stamm A, Toledo R, Nogueira J, et al. Endoscopic maxillary sinus surgery: from minimal to maximal. In: Duncavage J, Becker S (Eds). The Maxillary Sinus: Medical and Surgical Management. New York: Thieme Medical Pulishers, Inc; 2011. pp. 172-8.
43. Chee LW, Sethi DS. The endoscopic management of sinonasal inverted papillomas. Clinical otolaryngology and allied sciences. 1999;24(1):61-6.
44. Casiano R, Herzallah I, Anstead A, et al. Advanced endoscopic sinonasal dissection. In: Casiano R (Ed.) Endoscopic Sinonasal Dissection Guide. New York: Thieme Medical Publishers, Inc; 2012. pp. 59-99.
45. Seiberling K, Wormald PJ. Benign sinonasal tumors. In: Kennedy DW (Ed). Rhinology: Diseases of the Nose, Sinuses, and Skull Base. New York: Thieme Medical Publishers, Inc; 2012. p. 394-408.
46. Sadeghi N, Al-Dhahri S, Manoukian JJ. Transnasal endoscopic medial maxillectomy for inverting papilloma. Laryngoscope. 2003;113(4):749-53.
47. Sadeghi N, Joshi A. Management of the nasolacrimal system during transnasal endoscopic medial maxillectomy. Am J Rhinol Allergy. 2012;26(2):e85-8.
48. Vrabec DP. The inverted Schneiderian papilloma: a 25-year study. Laryngoscope. 1994;104(5 Pt 1):582-605.
49. Sathananthar S, Nagaonkar S, Paleri V, et al. Canine fossa puncture and clearance of the maxillary sinus for the severely diseased maxillary sinus. Laryngoscope. 2005;115(6): 1026-9.
50. Lim SC, Lee JK, Yoon TM. Extended endoscopic medial maxillectomy for sinonasal neoplasms. Otolaryngol Head Neck Surg. 2008;139(2):310-2.
51. Smith W, Lowe D, Leong P. Resection of pyriform aperture: a useful adjunct in nasal surgery. J Laryngol Otol. 2009; 123(1):123-5.
52. Virgin FW, Rowe SM, Wade MB, et al. Extensive surgical and comprehensive postoperative medical management for cystic fibrosis chronic rhinosinusitis. Am J Rhinol Allergy. 2012;26(1):70-5.
53. Rodriguez MJ, Sargi Z, Casiano RR. Extended maxillary sinusotomy in isolated refractory maxillary sinus disease. Otolaryngol Head Neck Surg. 2007;137(3):508-10.
54. Chen XB, Lee HP, Chong VF, et al. Numerical simulation of the effects of inferior turbinate surgery on nasal airway heating capacity. Am J Rhinol Allergy. 2010;24(5):e118-22.
55. Chen XB, Leong SC, Lee HP, et al. Aerodynamic effects of inferior turbinate surgery on nasal airflow—a computational fluid dynamics model. Rhinology. 2010;48(4):394-400.
56. Modrzynski M. Hyaluronic acid gel in the treatment of empty nose syndrome. Am J Rhinol Allergy. 2011;25(2):103-6.
57. Kastl KG, Rettinger G, Keck T. The impact of nasal surgery on air-conditioning of the nasal airways. Rhinology. 2009;47(3):237-41.
58. Lee HP, Garlapati RR, Chong VF, et al. Comparison between effects of various partial inferior turbinectomy options on nasal airflow: a computer simulation study. Computer methods in biomechanics and biomedical engineering. 2013;16(1):112-8.
59. Gras-Cabrerizo JR, Massegur-Solench H, Pujol-Olmo A, et al. Endoscopic medial maxillectomy with preservation of inferior turbinate: how do we do it? Eur Arch Otorhinolaryngol. 2011;268(3):389-92.

60. Suzuki M, Nakamura Y, Nakayama M, et al. Modified transnasal endoscopic medial maxillectomy with medial shift of preserved inferior turbinate and nasolacrimal duct. Laryngoscope. 2011;121(11):2399-401.
61. Weber RK, Werner JA, Hildenbrand T. Endonasal endoscopic medial maxillectomy with preservation of the inferior turbinate. Am J Rhinol Allergy. 2010;24(6):132-5.
62. Garth RJ, Cox HJ, Thomas MR. Haemorrhage as a complication of inferior turbinectomy: a comparison of anterior and radical trimming. Clin Otolaryngol Allied Sci. 1995; 20(3):236-8.
63. Nakamaru Y, Furuta Y, Takagi D, et al. Preservation of the nasolacrimal duct during endoscopic medial maxillectomy for sinonasal inverted papilloma. Rhinology. 2010;48(4):452-6.
64. Stamm A, Pignatari S. Transnasal endoscopic-assisted surgery of the skull base. In: Cummings C, Flint P, Harker L (Eds). Otolaryngology Head and Neck Surgery, 4th edition. Philadelphia, PA: Elsevier; 2005. pp. 3855-76.

CHAPTER

3

Maxillectomy

Rosemary B Ojo, Ralph Abi-Hachem, Bradley J Goldstein

INTRODUCTION

The standard operation for cancer involving the maxilla is maxillectomy. Limited operations, such as medial maxillectomy (either via an open or endoscopic approach), may be appropriate for benign or early stage malignant lesions. Extensive maxillectomies, such as total and subtotal maxillectomies, are performed to resect malignant and extensive benign tumors of the maxillary bone and associated soft tissues. Total maxillectomy may also be indicated for resection of invasive fungal disease, such as mucormycosis, in immune compromised patients, especially if there is an ability to correct the underlying medical process, i.e. diabetic ketoacidosis. Multiple surgical approaches have been developed to resect the maxilla over the past several decades, including lateral rhinotomy (LR), Weber-Ferguson extension (WFE), or midface degloving. These approaches are still widely used. Total maxillectomy refers to surgical resection of the entire maxilla. Resection includes the floor and medial wall of the orbit and the ethmoid sinuses. The surgery may be extended to include orbital exenteration and sphenoidectomy, and resection of the pterygoid plates. It is generally indicated for malignancies involving the maxillary sinus, maxillary bone, and/or orbit and ethmoids, especially tumors for which negative margins would not be possible via an endoscopic resection or limited maxillectomy. Total maxillectomy is potentially complicated by injury to the orbital contents, lacrimal drainage apparatus, optic nerve, ethmoidal arteries, intracranial contents, and may be accompanied by brisk bleeding. A comprehensive understanding of the three-dimensional anatomy of the maxilla and the surrounding structures is, therefore, essential.

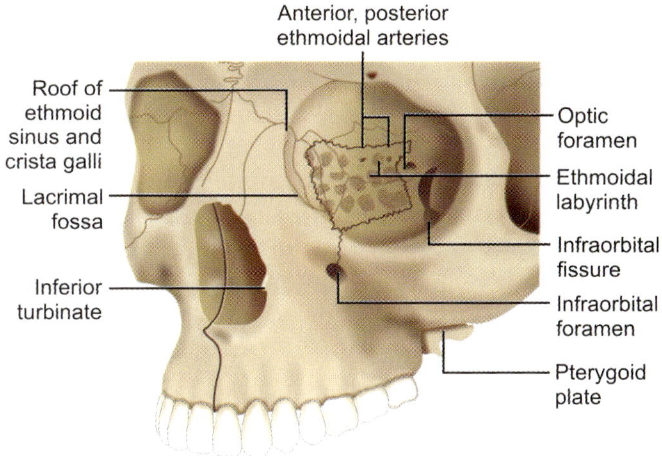

Fig. 3.1: Bony anatomy associated with maxillectomy procedures. Note especially the position of the ethmoidal arteries along the medial orbital wall; this level marks the position of the anterior skull base.

ANATOMY

The bony anatomy involved in maxillectomy procedures is shown in Figure. 3.1.

Critical surgical landmarks include:

- The level of the floor of the anterior cranial fossa (fovea ethmoidalis and cribriform plate), which corresponds with the position of the anterior and posterior ethmoidal foramina located along the frontoethmoidal suture line.
- The proximity of posterior ethmoidal foramen and artery to the optic nerve within the optic foramen.

Another bony structure requiring attention is the palate (Fig. 3.2). In a total maxillectomy, osteotomies will be performed to permit resection of the maxillary floor and hard palate, as indicated. Soft tissue structures of

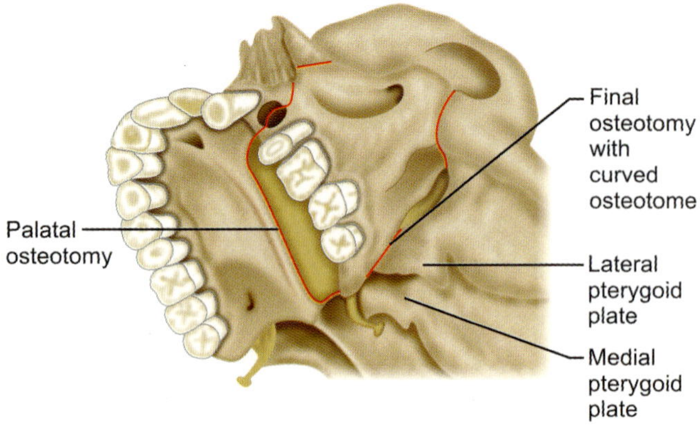

Fig. 3.2: Inferior view of the bony anatomy associated with maxillectomy procedures. Note the typical position of osteotomies used to resect the hard palate.

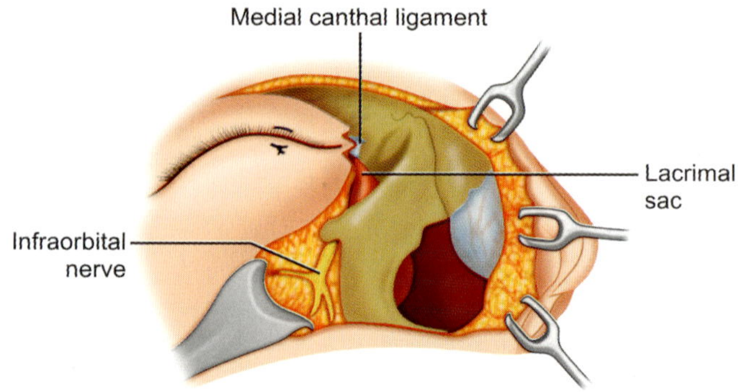

Fig. 3.3: Important soft tissue structures include the lacrimal sac and the infraorbital nerve, depicted here. The lacrimal sac will be transected during maxillectomy.

note include the lacrimal sac and infraorbital nerve. The lacrimal sac is transected at surgery in the lacrimal fossa (Fig. 3.3). Also, the infraorbital nerve is included in the specimen if necessary (Fig. 3.3). Immediately posterior to the maxillary sinus is the pterygopalatine fossa, in which the internal maxillary artery and its branches as well as the sphenopalatine ganglion and its branches are encountered. The pterygopalatine fossa communicates laterally with the infratemporal fossa via the pterygomaxillary fissure, and medially with the nasal cavity via the sphenopalatine foramen.

VASCULATURE

During maxillectomy, blood supplies from both the internal and external carotid systems are encountered.

The *arterial supply* relevant to maxillectomy is as follows:

- External carotid branches include the following:
  - *Facial/external maxillary artery* encountered during soft tissue approach.
  - *Internal maxillary artery* passes through the pterygomaxillary fissure to enter the pterygopalatine fossa. Branches of the internal maxillary artery of surgical significance include:
    - *Greater palatine artery* (descending palatine) that passes inferiorly from the pterygopalatine fossa through the pterygopalatine canal and emerges from the greater palatine foramen of the hard palate. It then runs anteriorly medial to the superior alveolus and enters the incisive foramen.
    - *Infraorbital artery* courses in the infraorbital groove and canal with the infraorbital nerve in the floor of the orbit/roof of antrum and exits anteriorly via the infraorbital foramen to supply the overlying soft tissues of the face.
    - *Sphenopalatine artery* enters the nasal cavity through the sphenopalatine foramen at the back of the superior meatus.
    - *Posterior lateral nasal arteries* are the branches of the sphenopalatine artery.
    - *Posterior septal artery* is a branch of the sphenopalatine artery that crosses the posterior nasal cavity just above the posterior choana to end on the nasal septum; one branch descends in a groove in the vomer to enter the incisive canal and anastomose with the greater palatine artery.
- *Internal carotid branches* include the following:
  - *Anterior ethmoidal artery* originates from the ophthalmic artery and enters the orbit through the anterior ethmoidal foramen located approximately 25 mm from the anterior lacrimal crest.
  - *Posterior ethmoidal artery* originates from the ophthalmic artery and enters the orbit through the posterior ethmoidal foramen. It is located approximately 35 mm from the anterior lacrimal crest and 12 mm (8–19 mm) from the anterior ethmoidal foramen.
  - *Ophthalmic artery* emerges with the optic nerve from the optic foramen, 44 mm from the anterior lacrimal crest and approximately 6 mm (5–11 mm) from the posterior ethmoidal foramen.

- *Veins* encountered during maxillectomy include the *angular vein* at the medial canthus, and a *pterygoid venous plexus* in the pterygopalatine fossa, located in proximity to internal maxillary artery branches. This plexus may be a source of troublesome bleeding following final osteotomies to release the specimen.

NERVES

The maxillary division of cranial nerve V (V2) enters the pterygopalatine fossa via foramen rotundum. The only branch of surgical significance is the infraorbital nerve. It runs in the floor of the orbit/roof of the antrum to exit from the infraorbital foramen (*see* Fig. 3.3). The other cranial nerve that requires consideration during maxillectomy is cranial nerve II (the optic nerve), which is sacrificed during orbital exenteration. Cranial nerve I fibers (the olfactory nerves) are encountered in the cribriform plate region, which is preserved unless craniofacial resection is necessary.

ORBITAL DETAIL

During dissection of the orbit, the following structures are encountered: medial palpebral ligament, orbital septum, lacrimal sac, periosteum, anterior and posterior ethmoidal arteries, and inferior orbital fissure. During orbital exenteration, the superior orbital fissure is also encountered.

The orbital septum is a connective tissue structure that attaches circumferentially to the periosteum of the orbital margin and acts as a diaphragm that retains the orbital contents. Laterally, it is attached to the orbital margin 1.5 mm anterior to the attachment of the lateral palpebral ligament at the lateral orbital tubercle. The medial canthal tendon is a fibrous band that fixes the tarsal plates to the medial orbital wall. It is intimately related to the lacrimal drainage system. It lies anterior to the canaliculi, but a deep head inserts into the posterior lacrimal crest and onto the fascia of the lacrimal sac. The lacrimal sac is located in the lacrimal fossa, which is bound medially by the lacrimal bone and the frontal process of the maxilla. It is related anteriorly, laterally, and posteriorly to the medial canthal tendon. The inferior orbital fissure is situated in the floor of the orbit and separates the sphenoid bone from the maxilla. It transmits the maxillary nerve and a few minor nerves, but no vessels of surgical significance. The superior orbital fissure lies between the lesser and greater wings of

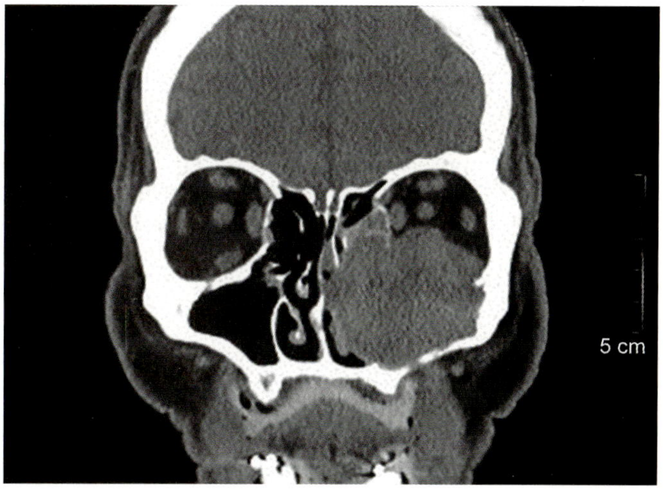

Fig. 3.4: Coronal CT image shows a left sinonasal mass based at the maxillary sinus with orbital involvement. Biopsy confirmed a malignancy, mucosal melanoma. Total maxillectomy with orbital exenteration was performed.

the sphenoid bone. Important anatomical structures that pass through the fissure are cranial nerves III, IV, VI; and the superior and inferior divisions of ophthalmic vein.

SURGICAL PROCEDURES

Indications/Contraindications

Maxillectomy is indicated for malignant neoplasm of the maxilla (Fig. 3.4). It may also be indicated for resection of invasive fungal disease in an immunocompromised setting. Contraindications include comorbidities that would preclude safe general anesthesia, or extensive disease that would preclude an ability to obtain adequate margins of resection.

TOTAL MAXILLECTOMY

Total maxillectomy involves resection of the entire maxilla, including the orbital floor and medial wall of the orbit and the ethmoid sinuses (Figs. 3.5A to C). The surgery may be extended to include resection of the lateral orbital wall and zygoma, exenteration of the orbit, sphenoidectomy, and resection of the pterygoid plates.

Radiological Evaluation

CT scanning is an important means of determining the superior (orbit and roof of ethmoids), posterior (pterygoid plates), lateral (zygoma and infratemporal fossa), and medial extent of the tumor and, therefore, the resection

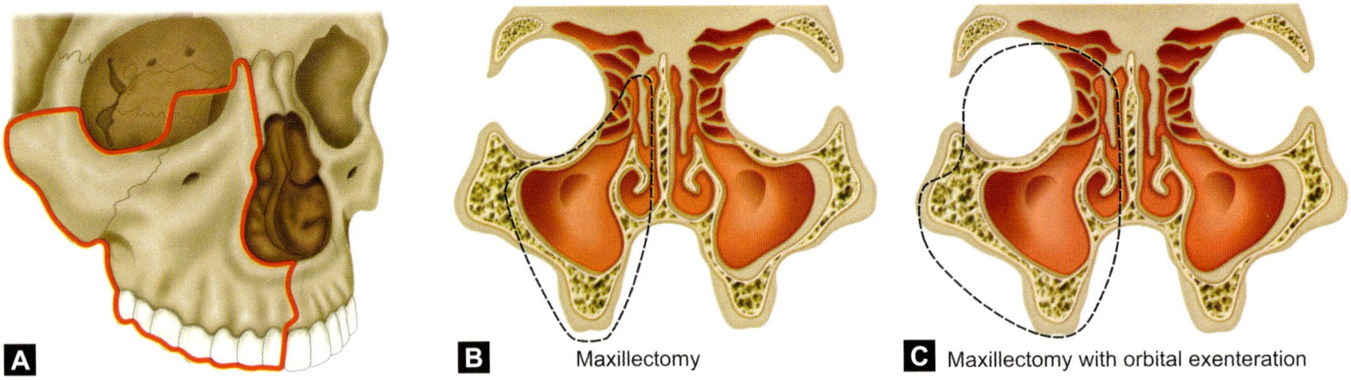

Figs. 3.5A to C: Schematic depiction of the extent of tissue resection in maxillectomy, with or without orbital exenteration.

required. If a tumor involves orbital fat and/or muscle, then orbital exenteration is generally recommended (*see* Fig. 3.4). Tumor extension to involve the pterygoid muscles may preclude maxillectomy, as obtaining clear margins becomes unlikely. Obvious intracranial extension may require neurosurgical involvement or may preclude resection.

Magnetic resonance imaging (MRI) with contrast will help delineate the tumor from the surrounding soft tissue, differentiate between tumor bulk and secretions in obstructed sinuses, and assess for perineural spread as well as extension of malignant tumors into Meckel's cave and the pterygomaxillary and infratemporal fossa.

Angiography with carotid flow study is indicated in patients with tumor surrounding the carotid artery. A balloon occlusion test is recommended to assess the risk of ischemic stroke if sacrifice of the carotid artery is considered.

Preoperative consent includes discussing the need for a tracheostomy, the facial incisions, loss of sensation in the infraorbital nerve distribution, diplopia, epiphora, enophthalmos, telecanthus, potential injury to the optic nerve, and cerebrospinal fluid (CSF) leak.

The operation is done under general anesthesia, with orotracheal intubation. If the eye is to be preserved then tarsorrhaphy should be done. The eyelids are sutured together with 4-0 silk taking care not to invert the eyelashes so as to avoid corneal abrasions, unless an orbital exenteration is planned. A tracheostomy is then done. Perioperative broad-spectrum antibiotics are administered for 24 hours. Lidocaine 1% with 1:100,000 epinephrine is injected along the planned skin incisions. The nasal cavity is decongested with a topical vasoconstrictor such as Afrin or 4% topical cocaine.

SURGICAL STEPS

Approaches

Maxillectomy may be done via LR or midfacial degloving approach (Figs. 3.6A and B). The midfacial degloving approach avoids facial scars and is suited to resections that do not extend above the orbital floor, i.e. do not include resection of the lamina papyracea and ethmoids. If the resection requires removal of the medial wall of the orbit and the ethmoids, LR provides better access. A Weber-Ferguson extension of the LR permits orbital exenteration.

Procedures

Soft Tissue Resection

- A tarsorrhaphy stitch is placed prior to skin prep.
- Midfacial degloving approach requires a sublabial mucosal incision with electrocautery along the gingivobuccal sulcus onto the maxilla and extended to the maxillary tuberosity (Figs. 3.6A and B).
- A LR incision is performed with a #15 blade; with a Weber-Ferguson approach, the lower lid incision is placed close to the palpebral margin so as to avoid edema of the lower lid above the scar following surgery.
- The remainder of the soft tissue dissection may be done with electrocautery. The incision is extended onto the nasal bone and maxilla (Figs. 3.7A and B). The angular vessels will need to be cauterized or ligated adjacent to the medial canthus of the eye. The lower lid skin is elevated down to the inferior orbital rim.
- The soft tissues of the face are elevated off the anterior maxilla using cautery or a freer elevator, remaining hard on bone while performing this dissection. Once

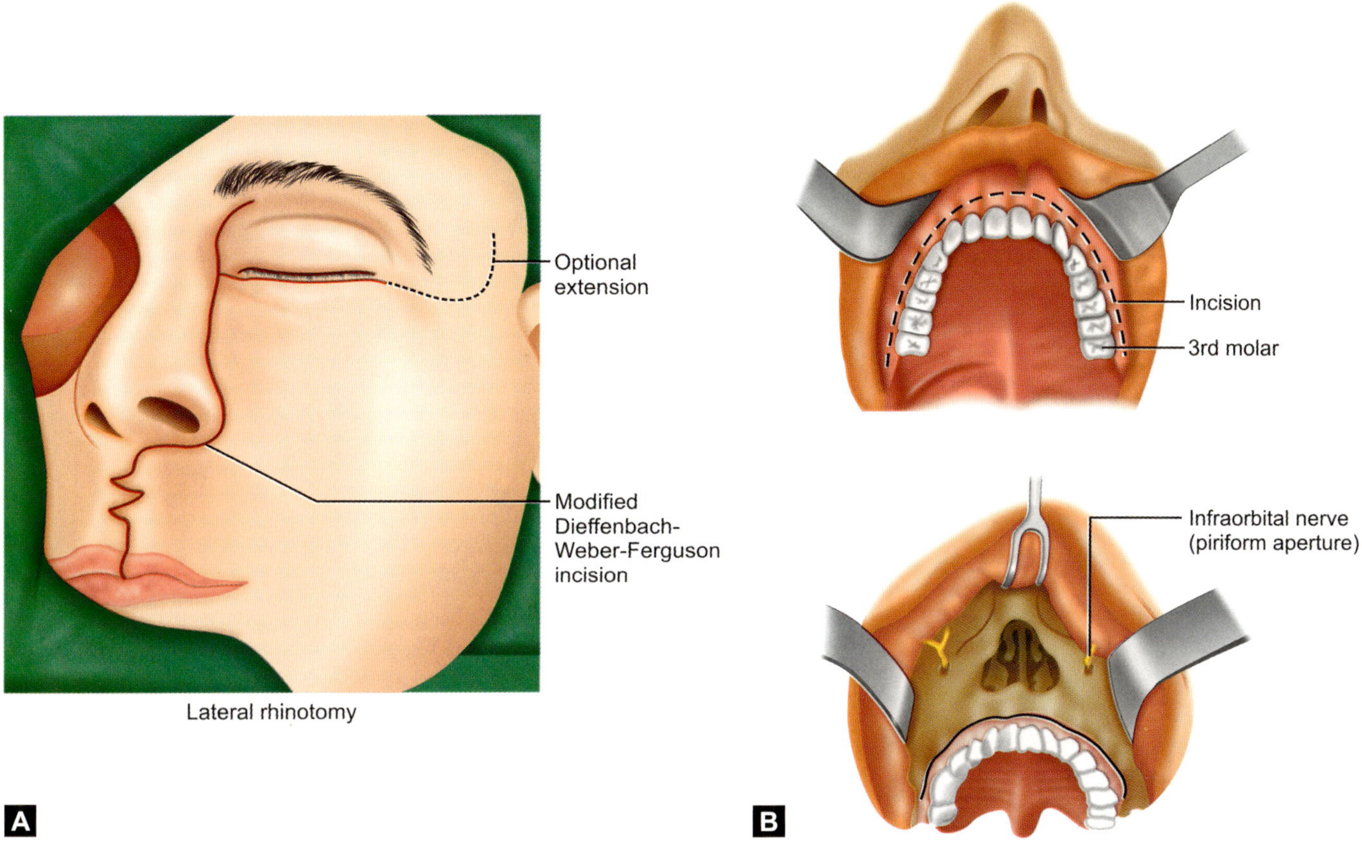

Figs. 3.6A and B: Incisional approaches for maxillectomy. The lateral rhinotomy, with or without extension, provides the best superior exposure and is therefore most useful for total maxillectomy. The dissection involved in the midface degloving exposure is depicted; however, this approach is most suitable for inferior maxillectomies.

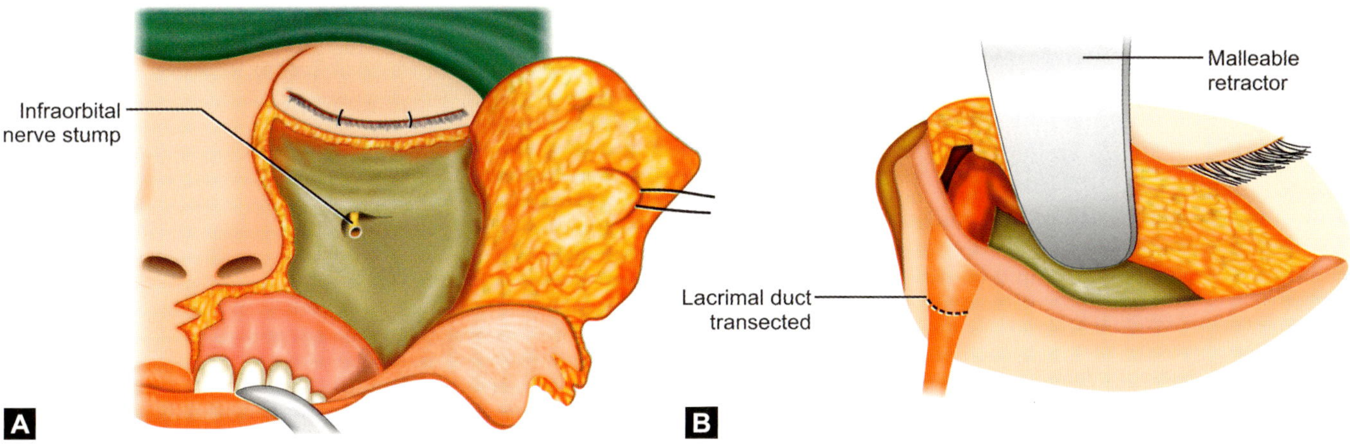

Figs. 3.7A and B: Soft tissue dissection and exposure of the anterior maxilla, infraorbital nerve, and medial orbit. Note transection of the lacrimal sac.

the entire face of the maxilla is exposed, the infraorbital nerve and vessels can be transected with cautery (Figs. 3.7A and B); if there is concern about perineural invasion, the nerve can be sampled with intraoperative frozen pathology sections to ensure clear margins. Dissection is continued around the maxilla up to

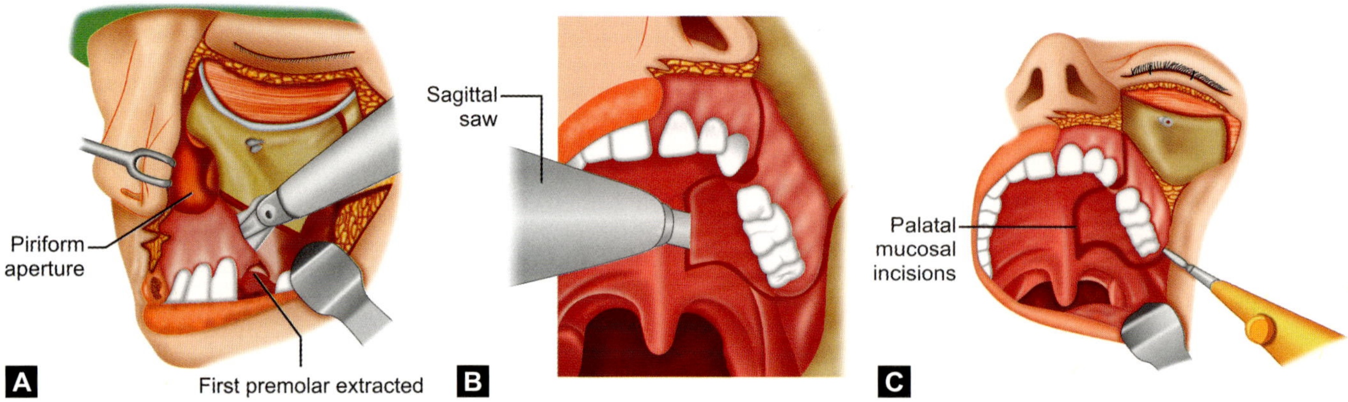

Figs. 3.8A to C: Soft tissue dissection along the nasal aperture and palate. This dissection will permit subsequent performance of osteotomies.

the pterygomaxillary fissure and the zygoma. Sharp dissection beyond the fissure is avoided, to prevent transecting the internal maxillary artery.

- The medial palpebral ligament, anterior lacrimal crest, lacrimal sac in the lacrimal fossa, and posterior lacrimal crest are next identified. The medial palpebral ligament is divided and then the lacrimal sac is elevated from its fossa. The sac is transected as distally as possible to facilitate fashioning a dacryocystorhinostomy (DCR) (*see* Figs. 3.7A and B).
- Next, the medial and inferior orbit is exposed. The orbital contents are elevated in a subperiosteal plane from the lamina papyracea and frontal bone taking care not to fracture or penetrate the paper-thin bone of the lamina papyracea.
- The frontoethmoidal suture must next be identified. This is a crucial surgical landmark, as it corresponds with the level of the cribriform plate and the anterior and posterior ethmoidal foramina. Gently retract the orbital contents laterally and identify the anterior ethmoidal artery as it bridges the divide between the anterior ethmoidal foramen and the periorbita (*see* Fig. 3.1). The anterior ethmoidal artery is ligated and divided, thereby providing access to the posterior ethmoidal artery. It is generally not necessary to divide this vessel.
- The floor of the orbit is stripped in a subperiosteal plane. Care is taken to prevent tearing the periosteum at the inferior orbital margin at the attachment of the orbital septum so as to avoid entering the orbit and causing extrusion of orbital fat.
- The soft tissues from the bone up to the anterior free margin of the nasal aperture are released with bovie electrocautery (Figs. 3.8A to C). The nasal ala is retracted and the lateral wall of the nasal vestibule is incised to expose the ipsilateral nasal cavity and inferior turbinate, taking care not to injure the inferior turbinate or septum, to prevent bleeding.
- Using a sweetheart retractor in the mouth to retract the tongue, the hard and soft palate is visualized. One may then identify the maxillary tuberosity and the bony spines of the pterygoid plates immediately posterior to the tuberosity.
- Using electrocautery, an incision is made in the mucosa of the hard palate along the planned medial resection margin, and the sublabial incision is extended laterally around the maxillary tuberosity, and into the groove between the tuberosity and the pterygoid plates. Removal of a tooth may be helpful. Palpation to define the posterior edge of the hard palate will permit division of the attachment of the soft palate to the hard palate with electrocautery, thereby entering the nasopharynx. Bleeding from branches of the greater and lesser palatine arteries should be anticipated and cauterized. This completes the inferior soft tissue dissection.

Bony Resection

The extent of the bony resection is tailored to the primary tumor and may include the lateral wall of the orbit and zygoma, especially if the antrum is seen to extend into the zygoma on CT imaging. The sequence of the osteotomies is planned to reserve troublesome bleeding to the end of the procedure.

- Osteotomies are shown in Figure 3.9. Osteotomy is made through the inferior orbital rim and along the orbital floor. A sharp osteotome/oscillating sagittal saw is used to cut through the malar buttress/inferior

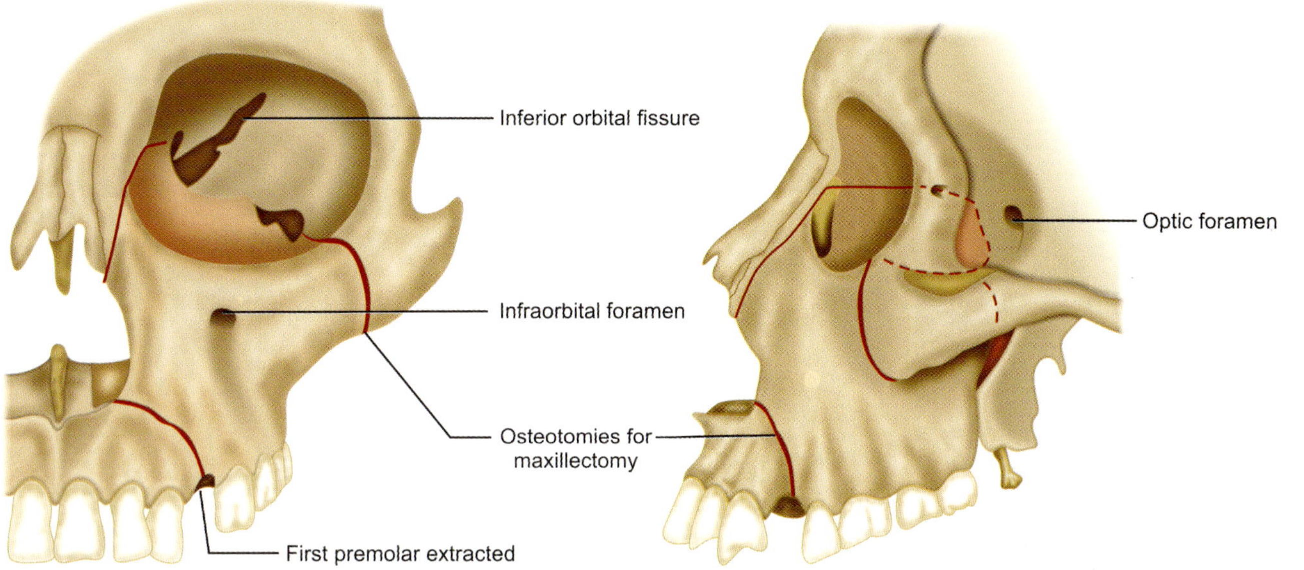

Fig. 3.9: Osteotomies performed in maxillectomy. *See* the text for details regarding each bone cut.

orbital rim. This osteotomy is placed lateral to the antrum as seen on the CT scan so as not to enter the antrum.

- While retracting and protecting the orbital contents with a narrow malleable retractor, osteotomy is then continued posteriorly through the thin bone of the orbital floor/antral roof using a sharp osteotome and aiming for the infraorbital fissure.
- Next is osteotomy through frontal process of maxilla and lacrimal bone. This thick bone is best transected with a Kerrison's rongeur or oscillating saw. There is often persistent minor bleeding from the bone that may be controlled with bone wax or cautery. The osteotomy is directed toward, but kept a few millimeters below, the level of frontoethmoidal suture line.
- Osteotomy is then made through lamina papyracea and anterior ethmoids. This osteotomy is done by gently tapping on an osteotome to enter the ethmoid air cell system while carefully retracting the orbital contents laterally. It is critical that this osteotomy be kept a few millimeters below the level of the frontoethmoidal suture line and the ethmoidal foramina so as to avoid fracturing or penetrating through the cribriform plate resulting in a CSF leak. The osteotomy stops short of the posterior ethmoidal artery and then is directed inferiorly toward the orbital floor so as to safeguard the optic nerve.
- Palatal osteotomy can be performed using a sharp osteotome/power saw is used to cut vertically through the superior alveolus and hard palate. The placement of this osteotomy is dependent on the palatal extent of the tumor. It is often preferable to extract a tooth and to place the osteotomy through the dental socket, rather than to place it between two teeth as this might devitalize the adjacent two teeth and it makes soft tissue closure more difficult. The palatal osteotomy is extended to the posterior margin of the hard palate. Osteotomy of nasal septum is only required when the palatal osteotomy is placed across the midline. The nasal septum is then divided parallel to the nasal floor with an osteotome or heavy scissors.
- Osteotomy to separate maxillary tuberosity from pterygoid plates. This is the final osteotomy, and is done by tapping with a (curved) osteotome in the groove between the maxillary tuberosity and the pterygoid bone. Superiorly this cut ends in the pterygomaxillary fissure and the pterygopalatine fossa. The maxillectomy specimen can now be gently downfractured (Figs. 3.10A and B).
- The internal maxillary artery tethers the specimen laterally, and is clipped and divided where it enters the pterygomaxillary fissure. If the artery is inadvertently transected, it is clipped and ligated. If the artery is not apparent, then it should be specifically looked for as it may have gone into spasm and may bleed later. The specimen is removed and inspected to determine the adequacy of the tumor resection.
- The remnants of the ethmoids are carefully inspected. An external ethmoidectomy may safely be completed

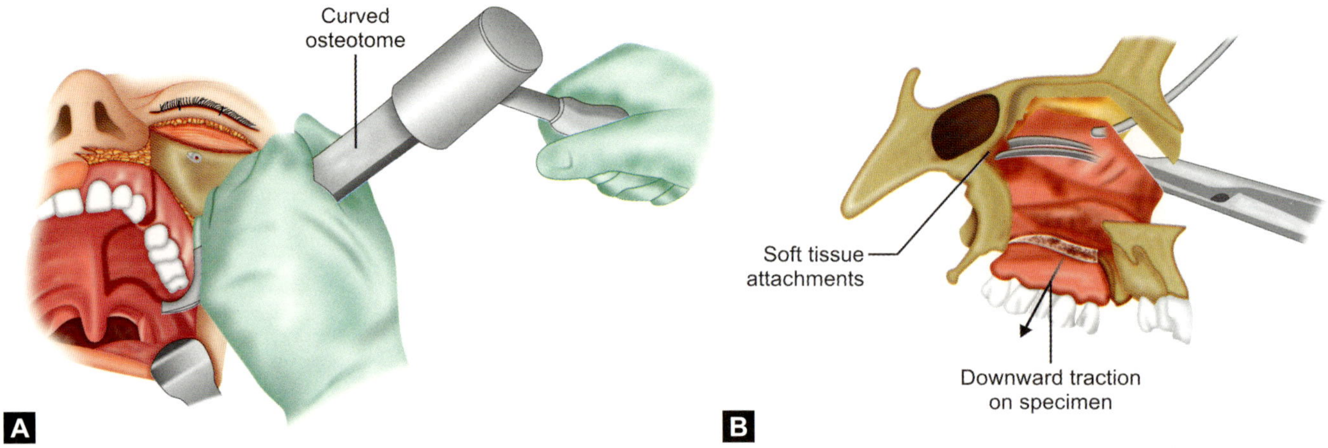

Figs. 3.10A and B: Maxillectomy: posterior osteotomies and specimen delivery.

up to the cribriform plate. The need for external frontoethmoid-ectomy +/- sphenoidectomy is determined, and evidence of a CSF leak is excluded. Arterial and venous bleeding occurs from the pterygoid venous plexus; it may initially be controlled with packing. Meticulous hemostasis is achieved with bipolar cautery, suture ligatures, clips, bone wax, and topical hemostatic agents such as Gelfoam.

ORBIT

Orbital exenteration is generally indicated when tumor has extended through periosteum to involve fat and/or muscle and/or the globe; the eyelids; and the lacrimal apparatus. Involvement limited to the bone or periosteum can be managed by resecting the involved periosteum. The clearest indications for orbital exenteration are those involving malignant tumors with no hope of salvaging vision in the affected eye such as squamous cell carcinoma and other epithelial malignancies. Whenever possible the eyelids are preserved (lid-sparing versus lid-sacrificing exenteration) so they may be sutured together at completion of the surgery by making palpebral incisions just above and below the eyelashes. It gives excellent color match to surrounding skin and heals relatively quickly.

The skin is then elevated from the tarsal plates with monopolar cautery up to the orbital rims circumferentially. The periosteum is incised circumferentially just medial to the orbital rim, exposing the underlying bone. Take care not to injure the supraorbital nerve so as to preserve sensation to the forehead.

The orbital contents are mobilized in the relatively avascular subperiosteal plane inferiorly, laterally, and superiorly. This is achieved by simply stripping the periosteum from the bone with a Freer's dissector, except along the inferior orbital fissure where the tissues are divided with scissors.

Transect the ocular muscles and optic nerve and ophthalmic vessels at the orbital apex. Avoid undue traction on the optic nerve as this can injure the contralateral optic nerve. Exposure may be improved by decompressing the globe with a large bore needle. Use curved scissors to transect the orbital apex and to deliver the orbital contents. Pack the orbit for a few minutes, and then use bipolar cautery or a ligature to control the brisk bleeding from the ophthalmic artery.

Postoperative management of the orbital cavity can be managed in a number of ways. Patients may be left with the orbital cavity exposed +/– an (immobile) ocular prosthesis. When wearing a prosthesis is not an option, patients prefer to have the cavity filled with a flap. Another option is to leave to granulate that requires a skin graft. Suturing the eyelids together and close to the cheek advancement flap is another viable option.

CLOSURE AND RECONSTRUCTION

The simplest option is healing by secondary intention or granulation. The advantages of such healing are shorter operating time, good color match to surrounding tissue, and excellent visibility for monitoring of possible recurrence of disease. However, its disadvantages include a long healing time and the necessity for several painful dressing changes.

Split-thickness skin grafts (Fig. 3.11), most commonly taken from the thigh, are frequently used to line the orbital

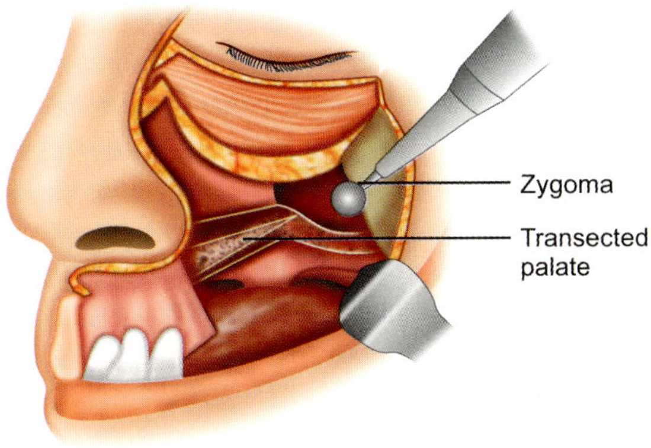

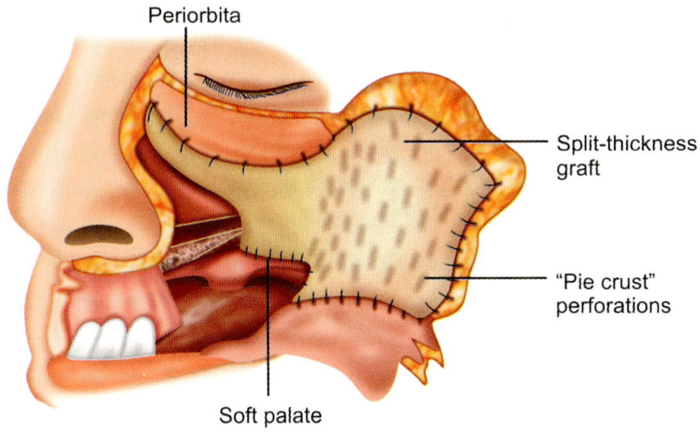

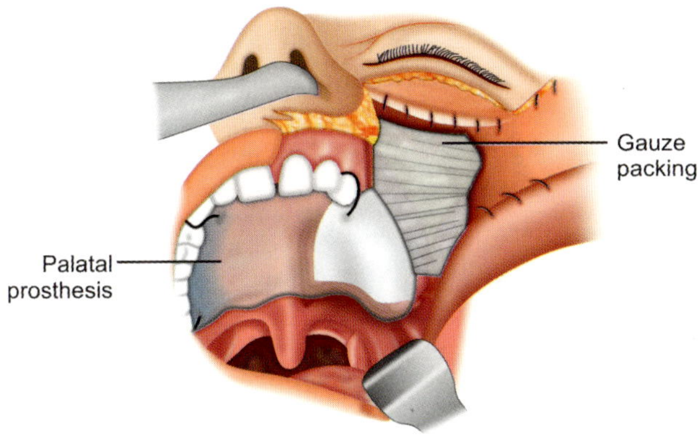

Fig. 3.11: Maxillectomy: defect repair and wound closure.

cavity when total exenteration with removal of periosteum is performed; they assist in faster healing and provide excellent monitoring for recurrence.

Local or free tissue flaps are most commonly performed particularly for defects resulting from concurrent partial or complete maxillectomy. This includes radial forearm free flap, rectus abdominis flap, fibular free flap, and scapula free flap are all excellent options of reconstruction.

These flaps provide good vascularized tissue in the setting of radiation therapy. However, it requires high specialized microsurgical techniques, donor site morbidity, and longer operative time. Prosthesis may be molded by a prosthodontist and affixed with topical adhesive. Prosthesis can be magnetically fixed to osseointegrated dental implant.

POSTOPERATIVE CARE

Oral hygiene is promoted through the use of irrigation with chlorhexidine gluconate in a "swish and spit" technique. Although routine tracheostomy may not be necessary for all total maxillectomy procedures, temporary tracheostomy is often utilized, for instance if a flap reconstruction or obturator and packing may lead to potential airway obstruction. The tracheostomy tube is typically changed by postoperative day 3–5 and capped soon after, with decannulation prior to discharge from the hospital. Arrangements should be made so that the prosthodontist is available on approximately the fifth postoperative day when the surgical splint and packing are removed. After removal of the obturator, the patient should be seen immediately by the prosthodontist for insertion of an interim prosthesis, which will allow the patient to continue with an oral diet as healing continues. When postoperative radiation therapy is deemed necessary, the changes incurred may prevent final modification of the prosthesis until the radiation therapy has been completed and wound contracture has stabilized. The final prosthetic repair should facilitate chewing and help restore appearance when teeth are added to the prosthesis. Monitoring of the vascular anastomosis of a free flap is accomplished with the use of Doppler ultrasonography. The vascularity of the free flap can be assessed clinically by looking for cutaneous blanching. Other standard postoperative care is followed, including deep vein thrombosis prophylaxis, early ambulation, and appropriate nutrition.

COMPLICATIONS

Possible postoperative complications following total maxillectomy can include the following, divided into early or late problems.

Early Complications

- *Orbit/skull base*: Most of the major potential intraoperative complications associated with total maxillectomy have to do with the central nervous system and the orbit. If an osteotomy is performed superior to the level of the anterior ethmoid artery and frontoethmoid suture, it is possible to enter the cranial cavity with resultant leakage of CSF. Extending the dissection medial to the attachment of the middle turbinate will also precipitate CSF leakage. This complication should be recognized and repaired immediately. If an actual defect in the dura is noted, a septal mucosal flap or a flap from the middle turbinate may be used. Most CSF leaks can be controlled when they are encountered.

  The proximity of the orbit puts the eye at risk in all operations involving the lateral nasal wall. Injury to the orbit and the optic nerve is a potentially serious complication. Note that during orbital exenteration, intraoperative bradycardia can occur when the optic nerve is transected.

  If preserving the eye, it is important to not lacerate the periorbita to avoid herniation of fat with the subsequent possibility of enophthalmos. If such lacerations occur, effort should be made to replace the herniated fat within the periorbita to close the laceration. If the periorbita has been removed, it may be replaced with temporalis fascia. Carrying the osteotomies too far posteriorly or not being precise with the soft tissue cuts may result in direct injury to the optic nerve. Preserving the posterior third of the lamina papyracea and being cautious with the osteotomies can prevent inadvertent optic nerve injury.
- *Bleeding*: It may occur from a raw surface area or granulation tissue from the wound. In these instances, it is controlled using silver nitrate or packing of the maxillectomy cavity. However if more severe bleeding occurs, the origin can be arterial from one of the main branches or venous from the pterygoid plexus. In that case, bleeding is temporized by packing the maxillectomy cavity and controlled in the operating room using either an endoscopic or an open approach based on the source of bleeding and the surgeon's preference.
- *Infection*: Cellulitis and infection of the maxillectomy cavity are best treated using culture directed antibiotics, frequent irrigation with nasal saline, and removal of the crust from within the cavity. It can lead to venous retrograde seeding of the infection with subsequent cavernous sinus thrombosis and intracranial abscess.
- *Wound breakdown*: This is seen with reconstruction of the maxillectomy defect using either a skin graft or a free flap. The skin graft should be well bolstered for 5–7 days in order for the graft to heal appropriately.
- Loss of the reconstructive flap: If the surgical defect is reconstructed using a free flap and there is an issue with flap perfusion especially in the first 48 hours, then the microvascular surgeon should be promptly alerted and decide whether or not to re-explore the flap to salvage it.
- *Diplopia*: It can occur in the immediate postoperative period and is due to edema of the orbital soft tissue content or injury to the oculomotor muscle and/or its innervation. It is managed conservatively with steroids. Diplopia may be alleviated by alternating an eye patch.

  Entrapment of the muscle within the osteotomy site can also lead to diplopia. Prompt diagnosis and urgent surgical release are the key steps in order to prevent any long-term sequelae.
- Lower lid edema.

Late Complications

- *Epiphora*: The nasolacrimal duct is transected during total maxillectomy, and subsequent scarring and stenosis of the lacrimal duct will lead to epiphora. Patients should be treated with an open DCR at the time of the maxillectomy or cannulation of the lacrimal canaliculi for 3–6 months in order to prevent epiphora. Endoscopic endonasal DCR at a later stage also has a high success rate in this patient population.
- *Paresthesia of the cheek*: It occurs due to injury or sacrifice of the infraorbital nerve. Infraorbital sensation should be assessed preoperatively to determine if the nerve is involved by the tumor.

- *Atrophic rhinitis*: It will lead to nasal crusting and overgrowth of bacteria. Frequent irrigation using saline solution and debridement during clinic visit help maintain nasal hygiene.
- *Enophthalmos/hypophthalmos*: It is caused by loss of support at the inferior and/or medial orbital walls.
- Ectropion, diplopia
- Dystopia, facial contracture, other cosmetic deformity
- Oral incompetence
- *Speech dysfunction*: If the reconstruction using either an obturator or a free flap is not sealing the nasal cavity from the oral cavity then speech might be unintelligible and will require further reconstructive consideration.
- *Eustachian tube dysfunction*: If the posterior limit of the resection is involving the tensor veli palatine, there is an increased risk of eustachian tube dysfunction with subsequent middle ear effusion, which is treated with a ventilation tube.

FURTHER READING

1. Brickman DS, Reh DD, Schneider DS, et al. Airway management after maxillectomy with free flap reconstruction. Head Neck. 2013;35:1061-5.
2. Brown JS, Shaw RJ. Reconstruction of the maxilla and midface: introducing a new classification. Lancet Oncol. 2010; 11(10):1001-8.
3. Clark RK, Chow TW, Luc HW, et al. Prosthodontic aspects of a new method for functional reconstruction following maxillectomy. J Prosthet Dent. 1995;73(6):559-62.
4. Cordeiro PG, Santamaria E, Kraus DH, et al. Reconstruction of total maxillectomy defects with preservation of the orbital contents. Plast Reconstr Surg. 1998;102(6):1874-84.
5. Cordeiro PG, Santamaria E. A classification system and algorithm for reconstruction of maxillectomy and midfacial defects. Plast Reconstr Surg. 2000;105:2331-46.
6. Essig GF, Newman SA, Levine PA. Sparing the eye in craniofacial surgery for superior nasal vault malignant neoplasms: analysis of benefit. Arch Facial Plast Surg. 2007;9(6):406-11.
7. Hanna EY, Westfall CT, Myers EN, et al. Cancer of the nasal cavity, paranasal sinuses, and orbit. In: Myers EN, Suen JY, Myers JN, (Eds). Cancer of the Head and Neck. Philadelphia, PA: Saunders; 2003. pp. 155-206.
8. Kazaoka Y, Shinohara A, Yokou K, et al. Functional reconstruction after a total maxillectomy using a fibula osteocutaneous flap with osseointegrated implants. Plast Reconstr Surg. 1999;103:1244-6.
9. Keyf F. Obturator prostheses for hemimaxillectomy patients. J Oral Rehabil. 2001;28:821-9.
10. Lin HS, Wang D, Fee WE, et al. Airway management after maxillectomy: routine tracheostomy is unnecessary. Laryngoscope. 2003;113:929-32.
11. Martin JW, Austin JR, Chambers MS, et al. Postoperative care of the maxillectomy patient. ORL Head Neck Nurs. 1994;12:15-20.
12. Muneuchi G, Miyabe K, Hoshikawa H, et al. Postoperative complications and long-term prognosis of microsurgical reconstruction after total maxillectomy. Microsurgery. 2006;26:171-6.
13. Myers E. Operative Otolaryngology Head and Neck Surgery, 2nd edition. Philadelphia, PA: Elsevier-Saunders. 2008.
14. Myers EN, Aramany MA. Rehabilitation of the oral cavity following resection of the hard and soft palate. Trans Am Acad Ophthalmol Otolaryngol. 1977;84:941-8.
15. Triana RJ, Uglesic V, Virag M, et al. Microvascular free flap reconstructive options in patients with partial and total maxillectomy defects. Arch Facial Plast Surg. 2000;2(2): 91-101.

CHAPTER

4 Anterior Craniofacial Resection

Francis Hall, Ian Lee

INTRODUCTION

Anterior craniofacial (ACF) resection is a term used to describe a group of operations designed to remove tumors involving the anterior skull base. The operation can also be adapted to nonneoplastic pathologies involving the anterior skull base. The anterior skull base includes the cribriform plates, the fovea ethmoidalis, roof of the orbits, and the planum sphenoidale. The operation is done through either an open approach, an endoscopic approach, or through a combination of the two. This chapter concentrates on the open approach and includes patient selection, the type of open approach, the extent of resection, reconstruction of the anterior skull base, complications, and their management and prognosis.

Tumors involving the anterior skull base usually arise from the nose or paranasal sinuses but may arise from within the cranial cavity, orbit, or skin. Table 4.1 lists some of the more common tumors seen in this area. Most tumors arise for unknown reasons; some tumors arise following exposure to a known carcinogen, usually in the setting of occupational exposure.[1-3] Table 4.2 lists some of the carcinogens and occupations associated with sinonasal tumors. An important concept in the surgical management of malignancy with curative intent is the complete resection of the cancer. This involves resection of the cancer with a margin of normal tissue. What constitutes an adequate margin? Although in some areas, for example, the oral tongue, the surgeon often aims to excise the cancer with a 1-cm margin, such a margin is frequently not achievable for cancers involving the anterior skull base. Rather than a dimension, the concept of the next anatomical plane is more relevant. So if the lamina papyracea is involved with cancer then the periorbita is resected. If the periorbita is involved then the contents of the orbit are removed. If the dura is involved with cancer then the dura is resected. The concept of 'en bloc' resection is neither relevant nor practical in this location or some other locations in the head and neck. Transoral laser surgery frequently involves cutting right through the cancer to assess the depth of the cancer. In ACF resections tumors are usually carefully removed piece by piece, clearing each area in turn. This is done because the size of the tumor limits exposure, this is especially true for endoscopic approaches but also applies to open approaches.

Table 4.1: Some neoplasms that may involve the anterior skull base.
Benign tumors
Angiofibroma
Inverting papilloma
Meningioma
Malignant tumors
Squamous cell carcinoma
Adenocarcinoma
Adenoid cystic carcinoma
Sinonasal undifferentiated carcinoma (SNUC)
Mucosal melanoma
Ethesioneuroblastoma
Skin cancer (BCC, SCC, melanoma)

Table 4.2: Carcinogens/occupations associated with sinonasal tumors.

Ultraviolet light, UVb	Cutaneous SCC, BCC, melanoma
Hard woods	Adenocarcinoma of the ethmoid sinuses
Soft woods	Squamous cell carcinoma of the ethmoid sinuses
Chromates	
Nickel	
Leather tanning	
Soldering and welding	
Radium	
Isopropyl oils	
HPV 6, 11, 18	Inverting papilloma
Aflatoxin	
Mustard gas	
Polycyclic hydrocarbons	
Mesothorium (Thorotrast)	

Table 4.3: Symptoms of patients with tumors involving the anterior skull base.

Nasal symptoms
Nasal obstruction
Epistaxis
Anosmia
Sinus pain
Nasal deformity—widening of the nasal dorsum
Orbital symptoms
Change in vision
Diplopia
Epiphora
Eye pain
Intracranial symptoms
Head ache
Change in personality, behavior, routines
Other symptoms
Patient may notice a neck lump
B symptoms—fever, weight loss, night sweats

PRESENTATION AND INVESTIGATION

Patients with tumors involving the anterior skull base usually present late with progressive symptoms. Small tumors involving the anterior skull base are usually asymptomatic but may be detected coincidentally when a patient has a computed tomography (CT) or magnetic resonance imaging a (MRI) scan for investigation of another condition. Symptoms of tumors of the anterior skull base are usually nasal, orbital, intracranial, or other (Table 4.3). Diplopia may be due to either direct extension into one of the extraocular muscles or to cranial nerves 3, 4, or 6. The chemical formula-[LR6(SO_4)]3 is a useful way of remembering which cranial nerves supply which extraocular muscles. LR= lateral rectus supplied by the sixth cranial nerve, SO= superior oblique supplied by the fourth cranial nerve, all the other extraocular muscles are supplied by the third cranial nerve. A change in a patient's usual routine, personality, behavior, or judgment may indicate frontal lobe involvement.

On examination a nasal mass is usually detected. Sometimes an orbital mass and diplopia are detected. It is important to do a full head and neck examination including fiberoptic examination of the nasal cavities and nasopharynx and palpation of the neck for any associated lymphadenopathy. Orbital examination, including assessment of visual acuity, range of eye movements, and detection of diplopia are routinely tested. Testing of sensation in the area of distribution of the infraorbital, supratrochlear, and supraorbital nerves is important.

Imaging studies requested usually include both a CT scan and an MRI scan. The CT scan is useful to determine the presence and extent of any bony erosion. The MRI scan helps detect the extent of soft tissue involvement including brain, dura, orbit, optic nerve, infraorbital nerve, internal carotid artery, and cavernous sinus. Tumors enhance on T1-weighted images, whereas sinonasal secretions are bright on T2-weighted images and do not enhance with contrast. Tumors frequently block the ostia of paranasal sinuses, resulting in retained secretions. Comparison of T1- and T2-weighted images will help differentiate between tumor and retained secretions within a sinus. A CT scan of the chest is usually requested to help exclude

Table 4.4: T staging of nasal cavity and ethmoid carcinoma.[4]

T1	Tumor is confined to the ethmoid sinus with or without bone erosion.
T2	Tumor invades two subsites in a single region or extends to involve an adjacent region within the nasoethmoid complex with or without bony erosion.
T3	Tumor extends to invade the medial wall or floor of the orbit, maxillary sinus, palate or cribriform plate.
T4a	Tumor invades any of the following: anterior orbital contents, skin of nose or cheek, minimal extension to anterior cranial fossa, pterygoid plates, sphenoid or frontal sinuses.
T4b	Tumor invades any of the following: orbital apex, dura, brain, middle cranial fossa, cranial nerves other than (V2), nasopharynx, or clivus.

Subsites within the nasal cavity include the septum; superior, middle and inferior turbinates; and olfactory region of the cribriform plate.

distant metastases. Occasionally additional studies such as positron emission tomography/CT scan, carotid angiogram, or carotid balloon test occlusion are requested. Preoperative cerebral angiogram with intent to embolize tumor vessels can be quite helpful in decreasing blood loss during tumor removal as well as to "soften" the tumor due to necrosis.

For staging of carcinoma of the nasal cavity and ethmoid sinuses, *see* Table 4.4.

PATIENT SELECTION

The axiom, "choose well, cut well, get well" applies to all head and neck cancer patients. In advanced cancers, salvage surgery and skull base surgery careful patient selection is very important. The surgery itself is merely a technical exercise, be it a very important one. All patients with tumors of the anterior skull base should be discussed in a head and neck tumor board. Patients are also often discussed in a brain tumor board and skull base tumor board. Patients with benign tumors are usually treated just with surgery. Patients with previously untreated cancers are usually treated with both surgery and radiotherapy and sometimes with chemotherapy as well. Patients with recurrent tumors are usually treated just with surgery. Some centers treat certain pathologies, for example, advanced sinonasal undifferentiated carcinoma with chemoradiotherapy with surgery reserved for salvage if appropriate.

Some patients do not make good surgical candidates, and such patients are usually obvious. Patients who do not consent for surgery, patients with very poor social supports, patients with significant comorbidities such as very poor cardiac or respiratory function make poor surgical candidates. Occasionally, such factors can be corrected but usually this is not the case.

There is no doubt that tumors that were previously thought to be unresectable are now resectable with modern surgical techniques. However, just because a tumor is resectable does not mean that a surgeon should resect the tumor. Controversy exists as to what tumors should be resected with some surgeons being a lot more aggressive than others. Relative contraindications to surgery include bilateral optic nerve involvement, cavernous sinus involvement by cancer, internal carotid artery involvement, and extensive frontal lobe involvement. Good judgment comes with experience and senior colleagues may help guide a younger surgeon in the decision-making process.

PLANNING FOR SURGERY

The patient and their family need to be informed about the diagnosis, the natural history of the disease, the proposed intervention, the side effects, potential complications, alternative treatments, and the prognosis. When the surgeon and the patient have similar expectations this usually results in a happier outcome. Details of the proposed operation need to be discussed with the patient.

The surgeon needs to decide on three main aspects of the surgery:

1. Incisions and approach (Fig. 4.1).
2. What is going to be resected (Fig. 4.2).
3. What reconstruction is going to be performed.

Usually, a head and neck surgeon and a neurosurgeon are involved and it is important that each understands what his or her role is. Discussion between surgeons is important and each needs to have a clear idea about what portion of the operation he or she is expected to do. Who is going to do the reconstruction? Sometimes a third surgeon may be asked to do the reconstruction depending on the extent of the resection and the skill set of the head and neck surgeon.

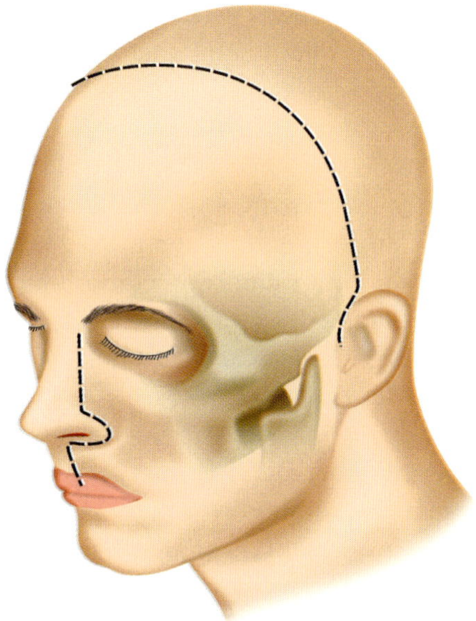

Fig. 4.1: Open approach requires bicoronal skin incision with a midface approach, in this case a modified Weber-Ferguson incision. The bicoronal incision is made at posterior hairline and extends from the tragus on one side to the tragus on the other side. The modified Weber-Ferguson incision is created at the naso-orbital and nasomedial region.

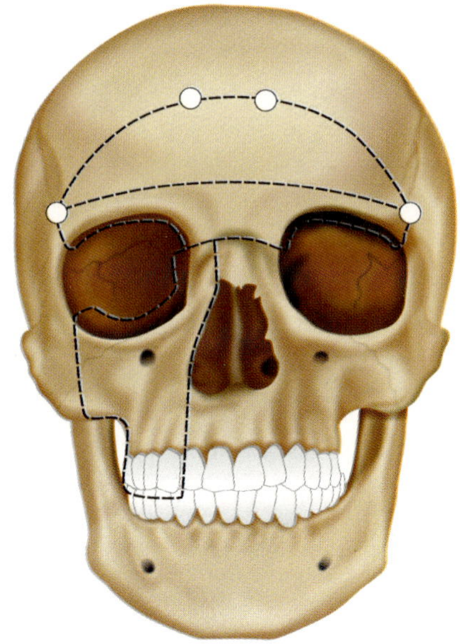

Fig. 4.2: The outline of osteotomies for anterior craniofacial resection includes a bifrontal craniotomy and some form of maxillectomy—in this case a total maxillectomy. Exposure of the cranial base can be further increased through a subfrontal approach.

Preparation for Surgery

Surgery is done under general anesthesia with an oral endotracheal tube. Some surgeons have a preference for tracheostomy in the belief that this reduces the rate of pneumocephalus. Intravenous antibiotics are given. Kraus et al. advocate a three-drug broad-spectrum antibiotic regime of ceftazidime, metronidazole, and vancomycin.[5] Subcutaneous heparin to prevent deep venous thrombosis is avoided as it may increase the risk of intracranial hemorrhage. A sequential pneumatic calf compression apparatus is applied. A lumbar drain is placed. The patient is in a supine position. Many neurosurgeons prefer the head in a Mayfield frame so that there is no movement of the head whatsoever thereby eliminating head movement as a cause of complications. In addition, use of the Mayfield frame allows for the bicoronal incision to be placed more posteriorly, thus providing exposure for a large pericranial flap. The reconstructive surgeon may need the head in an extended position and rotated to the opposite side so as to gain access to vessels. Most surgeons shave the anterior portion of the head. A line is drawn from the root of the helix on one side to the root of the helix on the other side. Local anesthetic with epinephrine is infiltrated into the scalp. Bilateral temporary tarsorrhaphies are performed. If an orbital exenteration is being performed then a unilateral tarsorrhaphy is performed. The patient is prepped with an aqueous solution of povidone-iodine taking care not to let any iodine pool around the eyes. The patient is draped so that the surgeon has full exposure to the oral and nasal cavities.

The Operation

The incision and approach work consists of two parts—the cranial part and the facial part. It can be done in either order—either the facial part first or the facial part second.

The Incisions and Approach Work

Step 1: A bicoronal incision is made from the root of the helix on one side to the root of the helix on the opposite side. The incision goes through the skin, subcutaneous fat, connective tissue, aponeurosis, and stops within the loose areolar tissue immediately superficial to the pericranium. The pericranium is simply the periosteum on the outside of the skull (Fig. 4.3). Hemostasis is secured with the bovie and Raney clips.

Step 2: A scalp flap is raised in the subgaleal plane down to the level of the supraorbital ridge. This is easily done within the loose areolar tissue. Laterally, over the

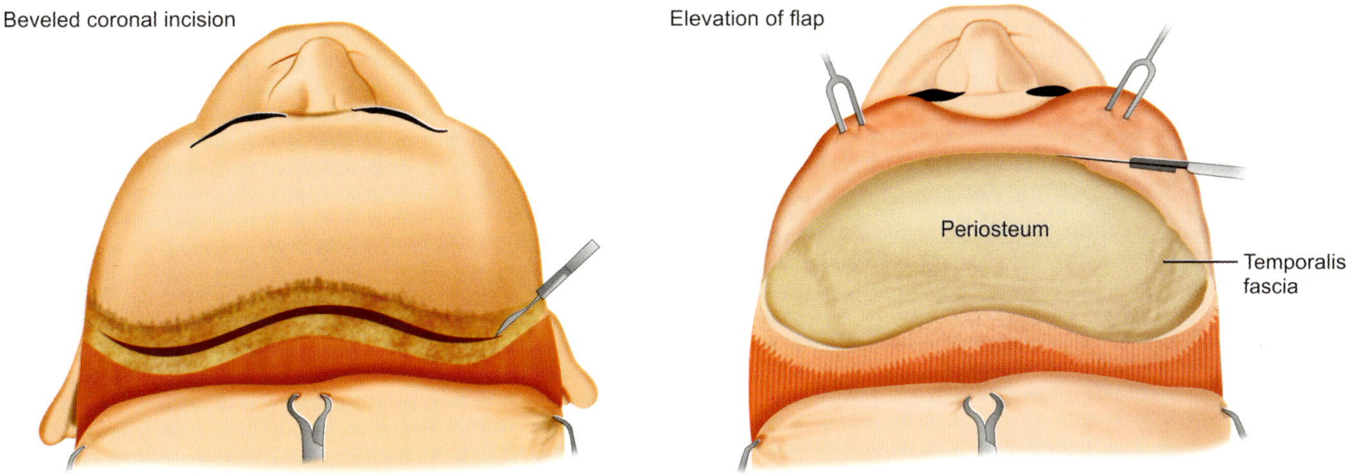

Fig. 4.3: The coronal flap provides a panoramic view of the upper third of the face. The incision begins at the root of one helix and ends at the root of the other helix. To preserve the hair follicles and prevent alopecia, one should bevel the incision parallel to the hair follicles. The design is of a lazy "S" or sinusoidal pattern to camouflage its outline. Dissection is in the relatively avascular, loose areolar tissue in the subgaleal plane. This level of dissection preserves the pericranium to be required for reconstruction of the skull base deficit.

temporalis muscle, as the hairline is approached, incise the temporalis fascia and raise the flap deep to the temporalis. This avoids injury to the temporal branch of the facial nerve as this nerve lies in a superficial plane (Fig. 4.4). Based on surgeon's preference, it is also possible to perform an interfascial dissection of the temporalis, which also serves to protect the facial nerve. Care is taken to avoid injury to the supratrochlear and supraorbital nerves. If a subcranial approach is being performed, then the supraorbital nerve is freed from the supraorbital foramen by carefully osteotimizing the canal. Alternatively, a small rongeur can be used to open the foramen. This frees up the nerve and allows it to be retracted with the bicoronal flap.

Step 3: A pericranial flap is raised. The pericranium is incised posteriorly and the flap elevated with a periosteal elevator up to the orbits. Care is taken to maintain the integrity of the pericranium, taking special care at the coronal suture as the pericranium tends to be adherent there. Another option is to raise the pericranial flap along with the scalp flap. The pericranium can then be dissected from the scalp flap at the time of anterior cranial base reconstruction. This prevents dehydration and devitalization of the pericranial flap during the approach and tumor resection (Figs. 4.5A and B).

Step 4: A frontal craniotomy is performed (Figs. 4.6A to C). The neurosurgeon frees up the anterior portion of the temporalis muscle elevating it off the underlying skull,

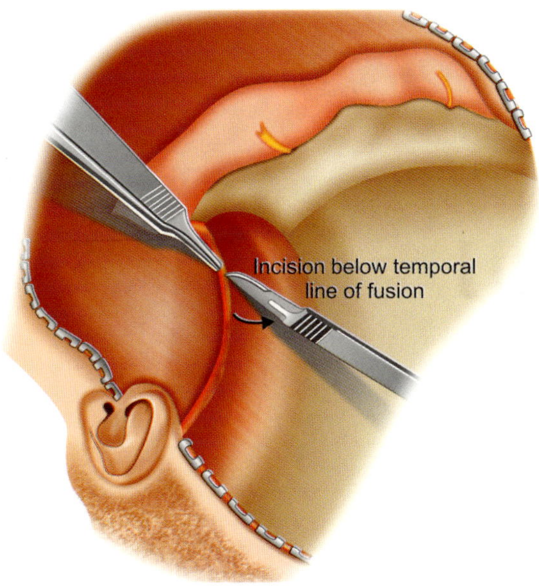

Fig. 4.4: When elevating the lateral aspect of the bicoronal flap, it is imperative to preserve the temporal branch of the facial nerve. It normally lies just deep to the SMAS as it crosses the zygomatic arch and innervates the undersurface of the frontalis muscle. To protect the nerve, dissection is carried out on or just deep to the superficial layer of the deep temporal fascia. Dissection into or below the temporal fat pads affords an extra layer of protection.

thus exposing the "keyholes," at the junction of the supraorbital ridge and the superior temporal line. The neurosurgeon drills several bur holes—one under the temporalis muscle on each side that is freed up and several either side

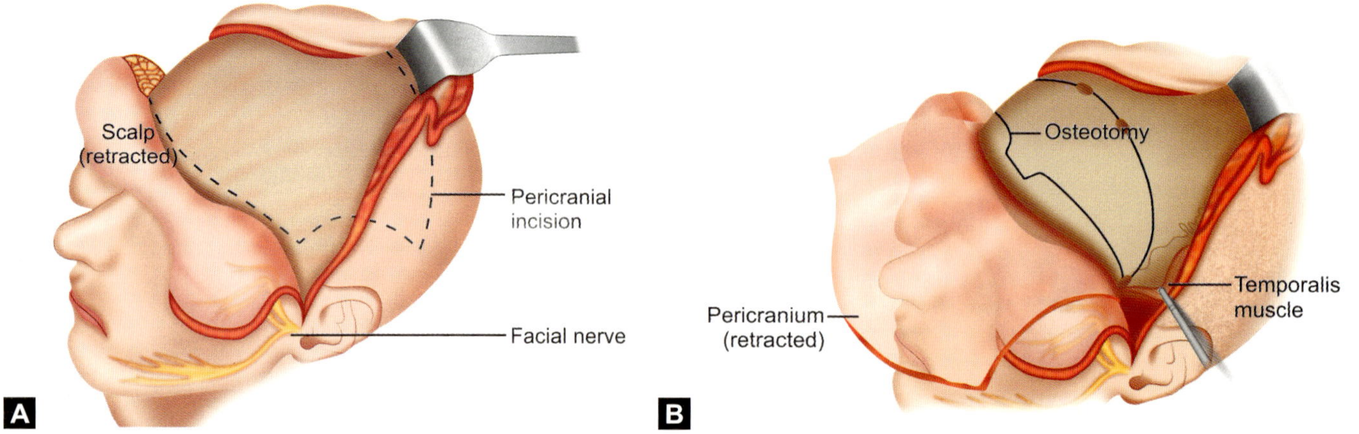

Figs. 4.5A and B: The pericranial flap is dissected free from the underlying bone and reflected anteriorly with the use of periosteal elevators.

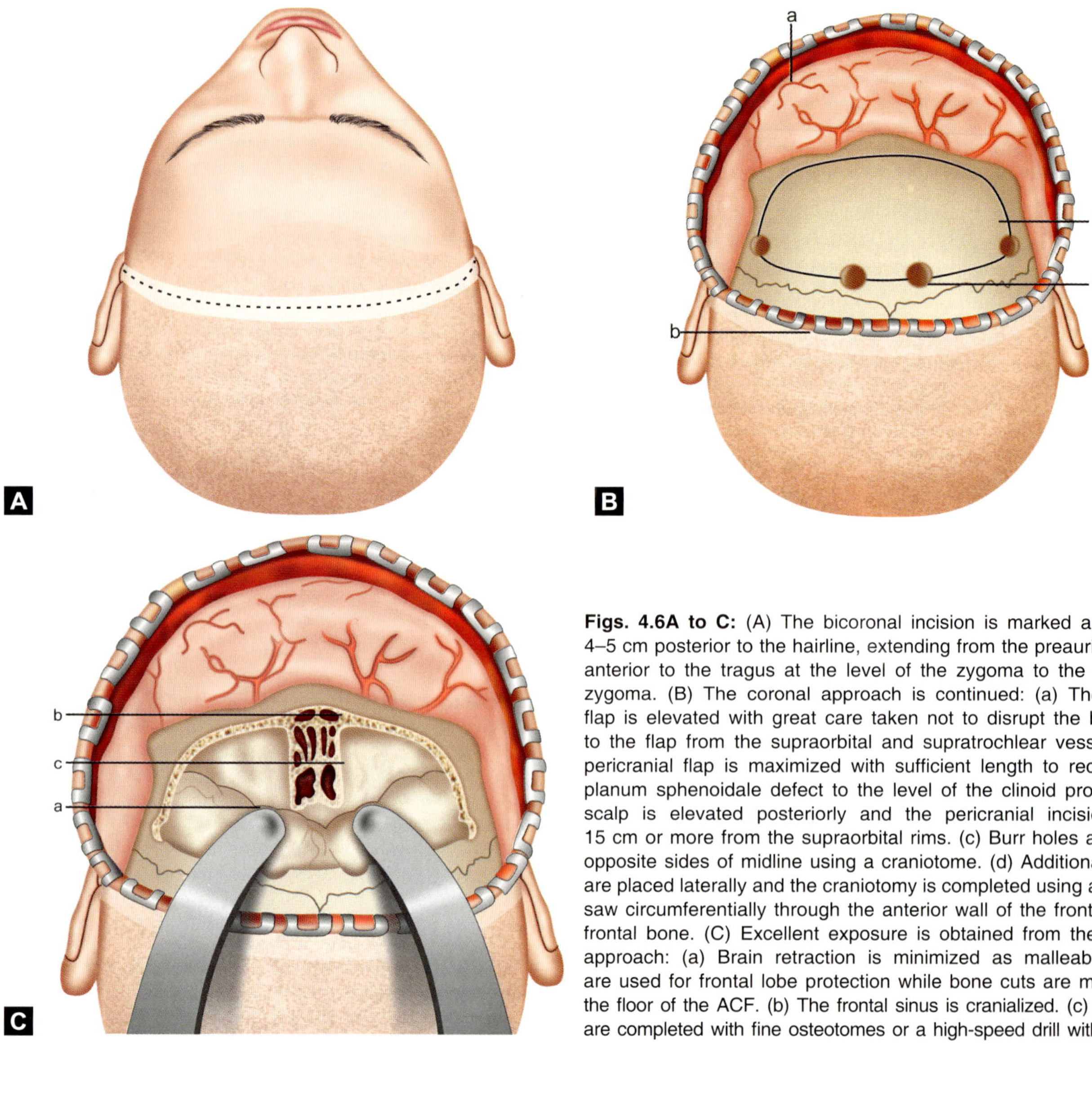

Figs. 4.6A to C: (A) The bicoronal incision is marked approximately 4–5 cm posterior to the hairline, extending from the preauricular crease anterior to the tragus at the level of the zygoma to the contralateral zygoma. (B) The coronal approach is continued: (a) The pericranial flap is elevated with great care taken not to disrupt the blood supply to the flap from the supraorbital and supratrochlear vessels. (b) The pericranial flap is maximized with sufficient length to reconstruct the planum sphenoidale defect to the level of the clinoid processes. The scalp is elevated posteriorly and the pericranial incision is made 15 cm or more from the supraorbital rims. (c) Burr holes are placed at opposite sides of midline using a craniotome. (d) Additional burr holes are placed laterally and the craniotomy is completed using a Midas–Rex saw circumferentially through the anterior wall of the frontal sinus and frontal bone. (C) Excellent exposure is obtained from the intracranial approach: (a) Brain retraction is minimized as malleable retractors are used for frontal lobe protection while bone cuts are made through the floor of the ACF. (b) The frontal sinus is cranialized. (c) Osteotomies are completed with fine osteotomes or a high-speed drill with a fine burr.

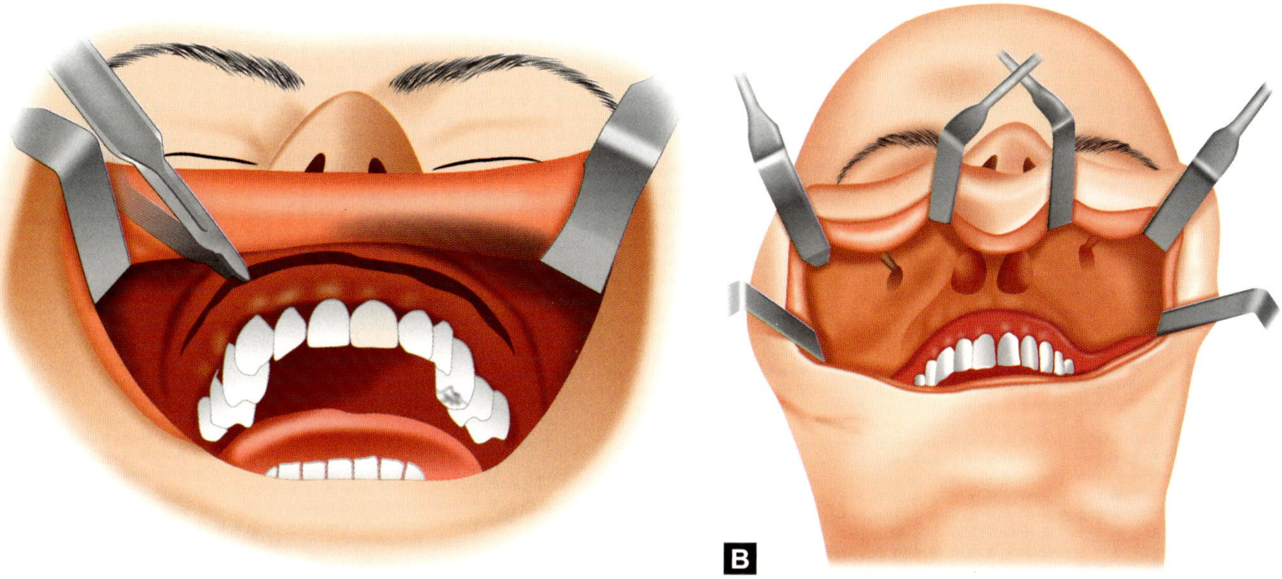

A B

Figs. 4.7A and B: Midfacial degloving permits wide access to the middle third of the face. The incision is in the gingivobuccal sulcus from first molar to first molar. It is important to leave a 1-cm cuff of mucosa to facilitate closure. Degloving may be performed with the gingivobuccal incision alone or with a full transfixion incision plus bilateral intercartilaginous incisions to improve access to the pyriform aperture and the nasal sidewalls. The plane of dissection is in the subperiosteal plane. Midface tissue is elevated to the infraorbital rims taking care to avoid injury to the infraorbital neurovascular structures. Laterally, the dissection is carried to the zygoma.

of the midline at two levels. Using an elevator the dura is elevated away from the bone. A craniotomy saw is used to cut the skull connecting one bur hole with the next. The osteomized skull is carefully elevated from the underlying dura taking care to free the dura. Typically, the skull flap is taken in two pieces divided at the midline to prevent injury to the superior sagittal sinus, although this varies according to surgeon's preference. After the skull flap has been removed, the lumbar drain is opened to allow for brain relaxation. If needed, the orbital ridge can now be removed by osteotomizing the supraorbital ridge. By performing this maneuver, less brain retraction is needed for the tumor resection.

Step 5: The facial portion of the procedure can be approached endoscopically or through a midface degloving approach or through a transfacial approach depending on the extent of the tumor, the degree of involvement of the soft tissues of the nose, eye, forehead and cheek, and the preference of the surgeon.

A sublabial incision is performed from just short of one maxillary tuberosity to the corresponding position on the other side (Figs. 4.7A and B). A full transfixion incision is made through the membranous septum and continued anteriorly into intercartilagenous incisions on both sides.

A transfacial approach is a good choice if there is involvement of the soft tissues of the nose, eye, cheek, or forehead. It is also an acceptable option for many patients with no soft tissue involvement. A lateral rhinotomy or Weber-Ferguson incision is used depending on the extent of the tumor. For small tumors a lateral rhinotomy incision is frequently used. For larger tumors a Weber-Ferguson incision is used (Figs. 4.8 and 4.9). The incision is adapted to encompass any soft tissue involvement with a margin of usually 1 cm.

The skin is marked with a marking pen and infiltrated with about 3–4 mL of 1% lignocaine with 1:100,000 epinephrine. An incision is made with a number 15 blade from just inferior to the medial aspect of the eyebrow in a curved fashion down to the junction of the lateral nasal subunit and the medial cheek subunit. It continues around the ala in the nasoalar fold. It is easily extended through the midline of the lip into a sublabial incision. The angular vein is encountered and either ligated or cauterized. Dissection continues down onto the underlying bone. The periosteum is elevated off the bone and dissection proceeds along the medial orbital wall as outlined below.

Step 6: Using an elevator the soft tissues are elevated off the anterior wall of each maxilla and off the cartilaginous dorsum. If required the soft tissues can be elevated off the nasal dorsum, in this way it is possible to elevate the tissues of the nose all the way up to the bicoronal flap.

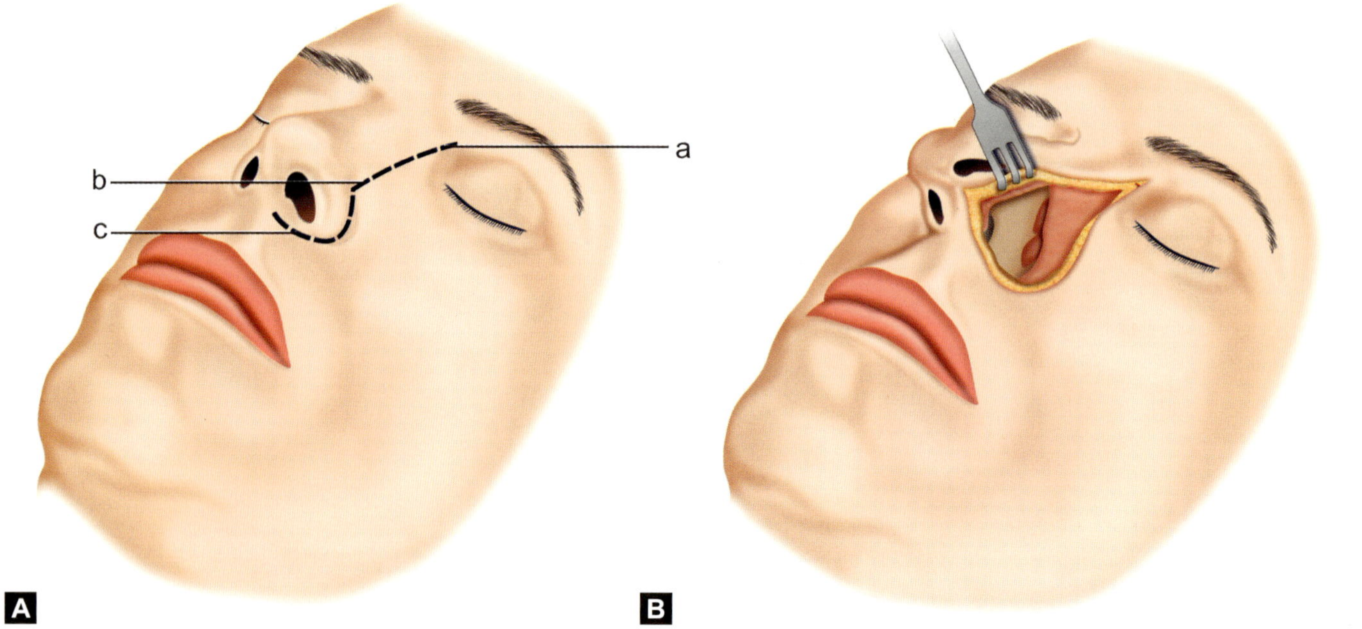

Figs. 4.8A and B: (A) The lateral rhinotomy incision. (a) The incision starts at a point 1 cm lateral to the medial-most aspect of the eyebrow. (b) The incision extends inferiorly at the junction of the lateral nasal wall and the cheek to the alar crease, where it changes direction acutely to parallel the crease. We prefer to stay 1–2 mm away from the alar crease to prevent dimpling in this region. (c) The incision extends around the alar crease medially to the philtrum, terminating where the crease blends with the skin of the nasal tip. (B) The exposure provided by the lateral rhinotomy approach includes access to the nasal cavity, lateral nasal wall, nasal septum, nasal roof, maxillary sinus, pterygopalatine fossa, pterygoid plates, ethmoid sinuses, medial and inferior orbital walls, sphenoid sinus, nasopharynx, clivus, and medial aspect of the infratemporal fossa.

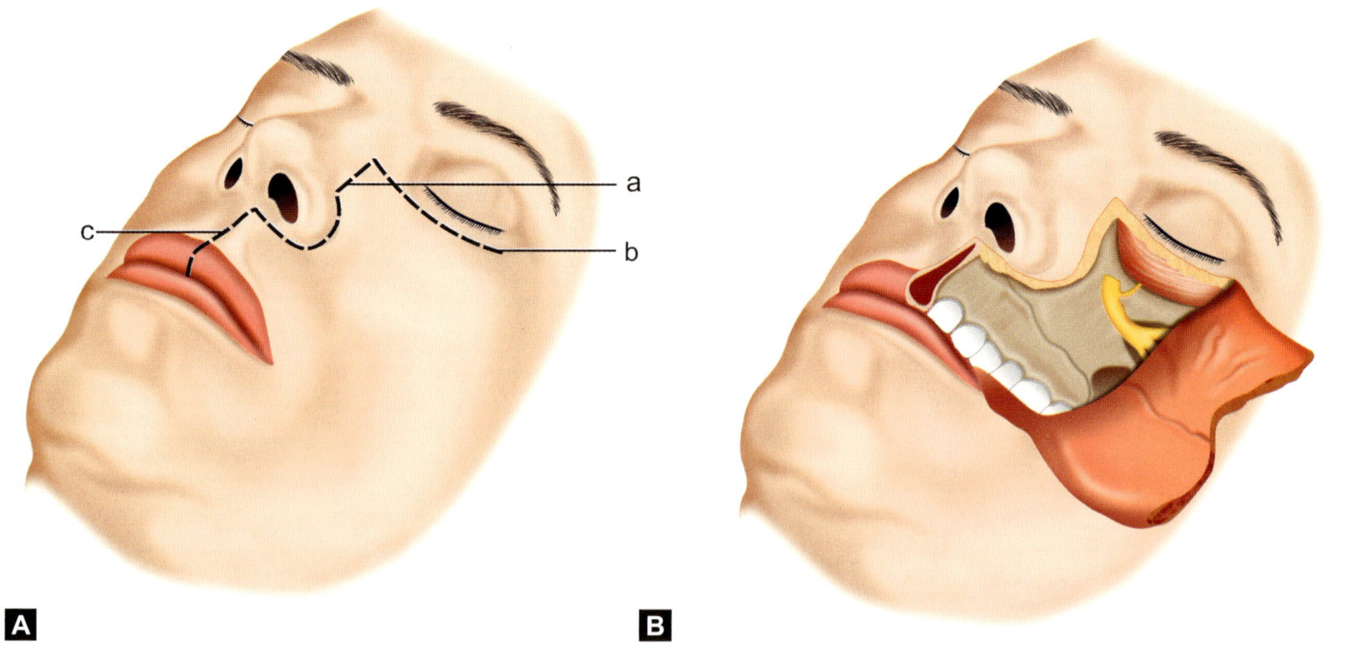

Figs. 4.9A and B: (A) The Weber-Ferguson incision. (a) The lateral rhinotomy incision is incorporated in this approach. (b) The incision is extended inferiorly to include (if needed) a splitting of the upper lip in the midline with sublabialgingivobuccal and palatal extensions. (c) Superiorly, the incision may be extended in a subciliary fashion or may include a contralateral Lynch extension to provide adequate access to the orbit. (B) The Weber-Ferguson incision provides excellent access to the hard palate, lower half of the nasal cavity, maxilla, maxillary sinus, and infratemporal fossa, and allows adequate exposure if orbital exeneration is indicated.

Tumor Resection

Although this varies according to the specific tumor characteristics, for tumors with intracranial extension, the intracranial portion is usually excised first. This then provides exposure for removal of the more inferior portion of the tumor through the anterior cranial base. In addition, the dura is also reconstructed prior to the nasal cavity tumor removal, providing a layer of tissue to prevent brain injury during resection. After sufficient relaxation of the brain with the lumbar drain along with medicines, such as dexamethasone, mannitol, and furosemide, the tumor can be exposed. It may also be advisable to resect some frontal lobe. The brain can swell quite impressively postoperatively, thus judicious frontal lobe resection can prevent malignant cerebral edema. The intracranial tumor resection can now be undertaken in a piecemeal fashion. For harder tumors, use of a cavitating ultrasonic aspirator or morsellating device may aid with removal. Care must be taken not to injure the normal intracranial vasculature, thus preoperative cerebral angiogram may be useful in these situations to delineate the location of important vessels. For tumors, which have infiltrated the dura, it is important to leave a cuff of dura of at least 5 mm anterior and medial to the optic chiasm and nerves, respectively. This may mean that some tumor is left behind, but watertight dural reconstruction is of paramount importance in these cases.

Step 7: Under direct vision the septum is incised a suitable distance, usually 1 cm, from the tumor. The tumor usually involves the superoposterior portion of the nasal septum. It is often possible to preserve the anteroinferior portion of the nasal septum, including the dorsal and caudal cartilaginous nasal septum. This provides essential support to the nasal tip. To give a good view of the nasal septum it may be necessary to remove some of the tumor from the nasal cavities.

Step 8: If the tumor is involving the lateral nasal wall, then this is included in the resection. A fenestra is made inferior to the inferior turbinate into the maxillary sinus with an osteotome. Using a large Mayo scissor, one blade is placed into the maxillary sinus and one blade is placed within the nasal cavity. The scissors are closed thereby making an incision inferior to the inferior turbinate. Care is taken not to divide the sphenopalatine artery, which lies posterior to the middle turbinate.

Step 9: Often, the tumor is involving the ethmoid sinuses on at least one side. Through the bicoronal incision the orbital periosteum is elevated off the underlying medial orbital bony wall on the involved side. Care is taken to elevate the lacrimal duct out of the lacrimal fossa before dividing it with sharp dissection usually with tenotomy scissors. The anterior and posterior ethmoidal arteries are ligated either with a small vascular titanium clip or with bipolar. Monopolar is avoided in this area owing to the proximity of the optic nerve and the possibility of inadvertent damage.

If the periorbita is involved with cancer then orbital exenteration is required.

Step 10: The tumor is identified and dissected free from the dura. If the dura is involved it is excised. The tumor is freed from adjacent areas, taking care to identify and avoid important structures like the optic chiasma. The olfactory tracts are divided with sharp dissection.

Step 11: The superior medial orbital dissection is continued through the anterior skull base into the anterior cranial fossa under direct vision from above. A malleable retractor should be placed between the anterior skull base and the dura overlying the frontal lobe to protect the dura and frontal lobe from inadvertent damage. Alternatively, the orbit can be entered from the anterior cranial fossa through the anterior skull base. Again care is taken to prevent inadvertent injury to the orbit.

Step 12: The natural ostia of the sphenoid sinus are identified. The anatomy of the sphenoid sinus is analyzed by studying the CT scan in all three planes preoperatively. In most cases, it is safe to enlarge the ostia in an inferior then lateral direction. The neurosurgeon identifies the optic chiasma. The sphenoid sinus is entered anterior to the optic chiasma through the planum sphenoidale.

Step 13: It should now be possible to drop the anterior skull base inferiorly and remove it through the nose. The surgical defect is carefully inspected and any remaining tumor is removed. The resection specimen is also carefully inspected and any close margins addressed by taking additional tissue in that area. The surgeon examines the specimen with the pathologist and together they decide on which margins to examine with frozen section. If there is tumor at any margin then additional tissue is taken from that area. Hemostasis is secured.

Reconstruction and Closure

Step 14: The type of reconstruction required varies depending on the extent of the surgical defect. The main goal

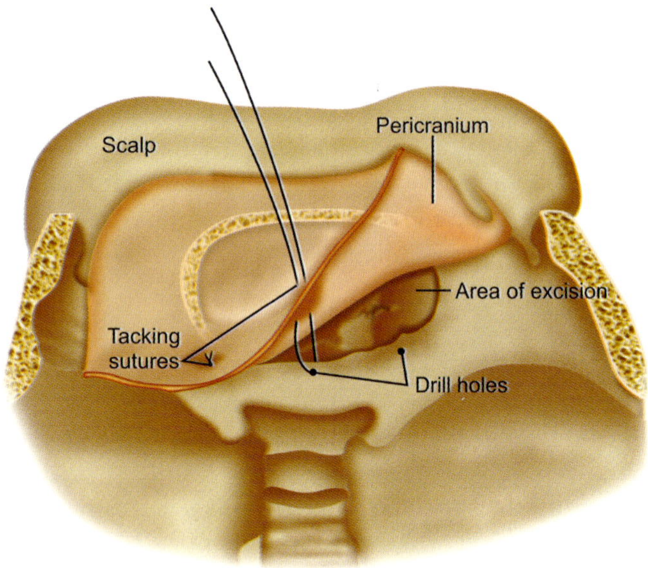

Fig. 4.10: Reconstruction of the anterior skull base with a pericranial flap.

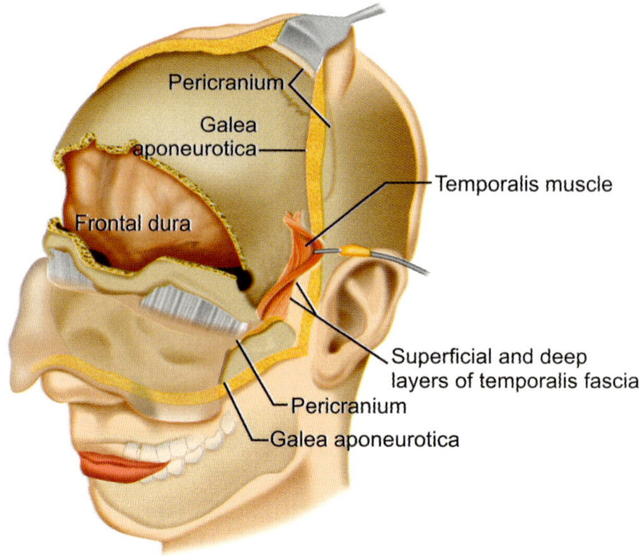

Fig. 4.11: Bifrontal approach for anterior craniofacial resection. The pericranial graft has been elevated and a low midline craniotomy has been performed.

of reconstruction of skull base defects is to separate the cranial cavity from the nose and sinuses. If only the cribriform plate has been resected then reconstruction usually involves placing tensor fascia lata across the defect and placing the pericranial flap immediately superior to this (Figs. 4.10 and 4.11).

If the dura has been taken, then the dura needs to be meticulously repaired so that there is a watertight repair. There are a variety of methods, which many surgeons have used successfully to reconstruct the dura. It should be noted, however, that the pericranial flap is usually too thin and delicate to provide for a robust dural reconstruction. In our center, a three layer closure is used. The tensor fascia lata graft is approximated to the posterior edge of the dura leaving a cuff of tensor fascia lata graft than can be folded inferiorly and anteriorly. The pericranial graft can then be layed in between the layers of the tensor fascia lata graft. After dural reconstruction is completed, its integrity can be tested by performing a Valsalva maneuver. Any egress of cerebrospinal fluid (CSF) must be found and meticulously closed. Fibrin sealant or Duraseal can serve as a buttress for the dural closure but cannot be intended to serve as the primary closure. Also, it is important that the dural graft be relatively redundant to give enough space for the brain to reexpand to occupy the anterior cranial fossa. If the medial bony walls of both orbits have been taken, then reconstruction with mini-plates and/or calvarial bone graft is indicated. Suturing the medial canthal tendons to either each other, miniplates or calvarial bone graft prevents telecanthus. Intercanthal wiring with 26 gauge wire over buttons is a useful technique. If the anterior skull base and roof of the orbits have been resected, then free flap reconstruction is indicated. A radial forearm free flap that has been de epithelialized works well (the dermis side faces the nose and the pedicle is brought out through a lateral bur hole). If the contents and bony walls of the orbit have been taken, the patient will have a large skull base deficit that will need to be reconstructed. In most cases this is best achieved with a free flap, frequently an anterolateral thigh flap or a rectus abdominis flap. Similarly, if there is extensive soft tissue loss of either the forehead, periocular or nasal skin, then an anterolateral or rectus abdominis free flap is a good option for reconstruction.

Step 15: On the back table the posterior wall of the frontal sinus is removed and discarded. All the mucosa of the anterior wall of the frontal sinus is removed. Using a 4–6 mm cutting bur the anterior wall of the frontal sinus is burred to remove any tiny invaginations of mucosa. Mucosa is removed from the frontal duct and soft tissue, temporalis muscle and temporalis fascia or left over tensor fascia lata is placed in the frontal duct. The frontal bone and orbital bar are replaced and held in placed with titanium screws and plates. Titanium plates are placed over the bur holes to hide the bur holes. If bone has been resected, split calvarial bone graft can be harvested from the frontal bones on the back table and used to fill in the bony defect.

Step 16: The bicoronal flap is returned to its native position. The bicoronal incision is closed in two layers with 3/0 braided absorbable suture and either staples or 3/0 nylon to skin. We usually do not use either epidural or subgaleal drains (especially on suction), as they can lead to tension pneumocephalus or development of CSF fistula. The intercartilagenous and full transfixion incision are closed with 4/0 braided absorbable suture. The sublabial incision is closed with 3/0 braided absorbable suture. The lateral rhinotomy incision is closed in two layers with 3/0 braided absorbable suture and 5/0 nylon. The authors prefer not to use a head bandage. The temporary tarsorrhaphy sutures are removed. The patient is extubated and transferred to the neurosurgical intensive care unit.

POSTOPERATIVE CARE

The patient is nursed at 30–45°. Care is taken to maintain an adequate blood pressure to ensure good cerebral perfusion. Likewise, oxygen is administered to assist adequate supply of oxygen to the brain. Regular neurological observations are performed. The Glasgow coma scale is recorded (Table 4.5). This scale is used to allocate a number to a patient's overall neurological state. If a free flap has been used to reconstruct then regular flap observations are performed. If a tracheostomy has been performed then routine tracheostomy care is required. A CT scan is done on the night of surgery to assess any acute changes and as a new baseline to compare any subsequent scans. The patient is advised not to blow their nose in the immediate postoperative period. Antibiotics are continued for 24–48 hours or if nasal packing is used until the packing has been removed. Anticonvulsants are given for 3 months. The indwelling urethral catheter is removed on the first postoperative day, and the patient is mobilized. The CSF drain is removed either in the operating room or in the first 5 days at the direction of the neurosurgeon (usually, the lumbar drain is removed immediately after the operation to prevent tension pneumocephalus and downward herniation). The patient rests on their bed for 12 hours after CSF drain removal to prevent headache. The indwelling urethral catheter is removed on the first postoperative day and the patient is mobilized. Chest physical therapy and incentive spirometry help prevent atelectasis and pneumonia. Facial sutures are removed in 5 days, scalp sutures are removed in 7–14 days. Any wound drains are removed when there is <25 mL over 24 hours.

Table 4.5: Glasgow coma scale.

Eyes	
Open	
Spontaneously	4
To command	3
To pain	2
No response	1
Motor	
To verbal command	6
To painful stimulus	
Localizes pain	5
Flexion-withdrawal	4
Flexion-abnormal	3
Extension	2
No response	1
Verbal	
Orientated and converses	5
Disorientated and converses	4
Inappropriate words	3
Incomprehensible sounds	2
No response	1
Total	**3-15**

COMPLICATIONS

Cerebrospinal Fluid Leak

Cerebrospinal fluid leak should be suspected if there is leakage of clear fluid from the nose or through an incision site, especially the bicoronal incision. A history of leakage of clear fluid from the nose when bending over is characteristic of CSF leak. The fluid should be collected in a container and testing for beta-2-transferrin. Management of CSF leakage should start before laboratory confirmation. Bed rest with the head elevated, stool softeners, and avoidance of straining are appropriate management for a small leak. A lumbar CSF drain may help in the management of a small leak. Antibiotic use in the treatment of uncomplicated CSF is controversial, and many surgeons with hold antibiotics in this setting unless there are signs of sepsis. Patients with moderate and large leaks or small persistent leaks should be taken back to the operating room. The nose should be thoroughly examined with an endoscope. Intrathecal fluorescein and/or a CT cisternogram may help locate the leak. Small to moderate size leaks can be managed endoscopically. A fat plug technique is suitable for small leaks. Endoscopic repair of the skull base with a layered approach: fascia, fibrin glue, fascia, Gelfoam, and packing is appropriate for moderate size leaks. Massive leaks may occur as the result of failure of a free flap and require salvage or replacement of the free flap.

Tension Pneumocephalus

Tension pneumocephalus is suspected if there is a rapid deterioration in the neurological status or vital signs of a skull base patient in the early postoperative period. A ball valve mechanism may occur as a result of straining, coughing, or grunting respiration. The immediate management of tension pneumocephalus is aspiration of air through a burr hole. The defect in the dura must be sealed. Stool softeners, avoidance of straining, and a tracheostomy help prevent recurrence of the pneumocephalus.

Bleeding

Bleeding in the postoperative period is broadly divided into intracranial or extracranial. Extracranial bleeding can present as epistaxis. Epistaxis may occur especially after packing is removed. It usually responds to bed rest with the head elevated and sedation. If prolonged then nasal endoscopy with local measures including silver nitrate cautery and dissolvable nasal packing may be required. Heavy nasal bleeding is uncommon but may require return to the operating room with ligation of the offending vessel. Bleeding from the pterygoid venous plexus is characterized by low pressure bleeding, which can be heavy and persistent. It is best controlled with epinephrine soaked pledgets, following by judicious use of bipolar diathermy, Gelfoam, and hemostatic agents. If all else fails it will respond to packing. Sites of arterial bleeding include the sphenopalatine artery and the maxillary artery. Free flaps can also be a source of bleeding, especially the pedicle of the flap, the anastomosis or the edges of the flap.

Significant intracranial bleeding usually presents as a sudden change of consciousness in the early postoperative period. An urgent CT scan and a return to the operating room is required.

Meningitis

Meningitis is suspected in any skull base patient with any of the following: fever, headache, nuchal rigidity, a positive Kernig sign, or change in neurological status. CT scan and/or MRI should be performed. If safe, a lumbar puncture should be performed and sent for urgent Gram stain and culture. Microbiology specimens should be taken from the nasal cavity and from the wounds. Intravenous antibiotics that cross the blood-brain barrier should be commenced after urgent consultation with an infectious disease specialist.

Brain Abscess

Brain abscess can occur following meningitis or can occur as a result of an area of necrotic tissue. Treatment involves intravenous antibiotics and if it does not settle then may require surgical evacuation. Necrotic material should be removed at the time of surgical drainage.

Diplopia

Diplopia indicates injury to the orbital contents, cranial nerves 3, 4 or 6, or changes in the position of the orbital walls. Early consultation by an ophthalmologist is advised with treatment directed toward the cause.

Wound Infection

Wound infections occur at two distinct time periods—early, usually between the 5 and 10 days and late, often about 3 weeks later. Microbiology specimens of any pus should be taken and sent for Gram stain and culture. Consultation with an infectious disease specialist is recommended.

Seroma

A seroma is common after a bicoronal flap. It is best observed unless it is very large or there is overlying wound breakdown.

Wound Healing Problems

Wound healing problems are more common and more severe in patients who have had prior irradiation to the operative site. In these patients microvascular reconstruction brings healthy vascular tissue to the area.

The best high volume microvascular surgical units have a 2% free-flap failure rate with an additional 2%

of flaps being successfully salvaged. In patients taken back to the operating room with occlusion of a vascular anastomosis—90% of cases—there is venous compromise and in only 10% of cases is there a problem with the arterial anastomosis. The design of the flap and the vessel geometry are paramount to good outcomes.

Occasionally, osteomyelitis may occur, it is best treated with long-term intravenous antibiotics in consultation with infectious diseases. Necrotic bone will need to be resected. Replacement with split calvarial bone is usually best deferred for 12 months.

RESULTS

When comparing the results of large series of patients who have undergone ACF resection the reader needs to appreciate that the mix of pathologies, the stage of disease, and tumors that have been previously treated all influence the survival results. In a series of 166 patients over a period of 27 years who underwent ACF resection Bentz et al.[6] reported 5-year disease-specific survival (DSS) of 57%. In this series, 24% of patients had squamous cell carcinoma, 12% adenocarcinoma, and 12% esthesioneuroblastoma. Cantu et al.[7] reported a 10-year DSS of 53% in a series of 366 patients who underwent anterior skull base surgery over a period of 20 years. In this series, 49% had adenocarcinoma, 12% squamous cell carcinoma, and 10% esthesioneuroblastoma. Dura or brain involvement was noted in 25% and orbital spread was noted in 30%. In an international collaborative study,[8] 334 patients from 17 institutions with tumors arising in the paranasal sinuses were evaluated. Patients with esthesioneuroblastomas were excluded. The most common tumor was adenocarcinoma (32%), closely followed by squamous cell carcinoma (30%). Most of the patients (56%) had been previously treated. The 5-year DSS was 53%.

Breheret et al.[9] reported 5-year DSS of 44% in a retrospective study of 41 patients with adenocarcinoma of the ethmoid sinus, with most (78%) treated with surgery followed by radiotherapy.

Several authors report a statistically significant difference in survival in patients undergoing ACF resection for esthesioneuroblastoma compared with patients undergoing ACF for other pathologies. Patients with esthesioneuroblastoma had a 5-year DSS of 90% compared with a 5-year DSS of 59% for other pathologies in the paper by Levine.[10] A number of studies have looked at very long-term survival rates. de Gabory et al.[11] have reported 20-year DSS of 60% in a group of 28 patients with esthesioneuroblastoma. Loy et al.[12] reported 15-year DSS of 83% in a group of 50 patients with esthesioneuroblastoma. In an analysis of the SEER database (Platek et al.[13]) over a period of 33 years, 511 patients with esthesioneuroblastoma were identified. Overall survival at 5 years was 73% for surgery combined with radiotherapy, 68% for surgery alone and 35% for radiotherapy alone. In this paper, there was no significant difference in survival for the group treated with surgery and radiotherapy compared with the group treated with surgery alone. Most institutions treat esthesioneuroblastoma with surgery followed by radiotherapy. There is considerable debate in the literature regarding treatment of the neck in the elective setting. Gore and Zanation[14] reported a rate of cervical metastases of 20% in 678 patients with esthesioneuroblastoma in a meta-analysis of 33 articles. In patients who developed late neck metastases, defined as occurring 6 months or more after the initial diagnosis, they advocated neck dissection followed by radiotherapy with a successful salvage rate of 31%. Howell et al.[15] reported a similar incidence of cervical lymph node involvement in a series of 48 patients with esthesioneuroblastoma. In this series 29% developed lymph node metastases with 36% having lymph node metastases at initial presentation and 64% developing lymph node metastases subsequently. With such a high incidence of neck disease, Monroe et al.[16] have advocated elective neck irradiation, showing no neck recurrences in 11 patients treated in such a manner. In contrast, surgeons usually do not advocate elective neck dissection for patients with esthesioneuroblastoma.

KEY POINTS

- Select patients carefully
- Refer patients to multidisciplinary clinic (tumor board)
- Surgery-head and neck surgeon, neurosurgeon, +/– reconstructive surgeon
- Reconstruction—separate nasal cavity from cranial cavity

REFERENCES

1. Acheson ED, Hadfield EH, Macbeth RG. Carcinoma of the nasal cavity and accessory sinuses in woodworkers. Lancet. 1967;1(7485):311-2.
2. Voss R, Stenersen T, Roald Oppedal B, et al. Sinonasal cancer and exposure to softwood. ActaOto-Laryngologica. 1985;99(1-2):172-8.

3. Leclerc A, Luce D, Demers PA, et al. Sinonasal cancer and occupation. Results from the reanalysis of twelve case-control studies. Am J Industrial. 1997;31(2):153-65.
4. Sobin LH, Gospodarowicz MK, Wittekind C. TNM classification of malignant tumors, 7th edition. Oxford: Wiley-Blackwell UICC; 2009. pp. 46-50.
5. Kraus DH, Gonen M, Mener D, et al. A standardized regimen of antibiotics prevents infectious complications in skull base surgery. Laryngoscope. 2005;115:1347-57.
6. Bentz BG, Bilsky MH, Shah JP, et al. Anterior skull base surgery for malignant tumors: a multivariate analysis of 27 years experience. Head Neck 2003;25:515-20.
7. Cantu G, Solero CL, Miceli R, et al. Anterior craniofacial resection for malignant paranasal tumors: a monoinstitutional experience of 366 cases. Head Neck 2012;34:78-87.
8. Ganly I, Patel SG, Singh B, et al. Craniofacial resection for malignant paranasal sinus tumors: report of an international collaborative study. Head Neck. 2005;27:575-84.
9. Breheret R, Laccourreye L, Jeufroy C, et al. Adenocarcinoma of the ethmoid sinus: retrospective study of 42 cases. Eur. Annals Otorhino Head Neck Dis. 2011;128(5):211-7.
10. Levine PA, Debo RF, Meredith SD, et al. Craniofacial resection at the University of Virginia (1976-1992): survival analysis. Head Neck 1994;16:574-77.
11. de Gabory L, Abdulkhaleq H, Darrouzet V, et al. Long-term results of 28 esthesioneuroblastomas managed over 35 years. Head Neck. 2011;33:82-6.
12. Loy A, Reibel J, Read P, et al. Esthesioneuroblastoma. Continued follow-up of a single institution's experience. Arch Otolaryngol Head Neck Surg. 2006;132:134-8.
13. Platek ME, Merzianu M, Mashtare T, et al. Improved survival following surgery and radiation therapy for olfactory neuroblastoma: analysis of the SEER database. Rad Onc. 2011;6:41. http://www.ro-journal.com/content/6/1/41. Last accessed 2/06/2015.
14. Gore M, Zanation AM. Salvage treatment of late neck metastasis in esthesioneuroblastoma. A meta-analysis. Arch Otolaryngol Head Neck Surg. 2009;135:1030-34.
15. Howell MC, Branstetter BF, Snyderman CH. Patterns of regional spread for esthesioneuroblastoma. Am J Neuroradiol. 2011;32:929-33.
16. Monroe AT, Hinerman RW, Amdur RJ, et al. Radiation therapy for esthesioneuroblastoma: rationale for elective neck irradiation. Head Neck. 2003;25:529-34.

CHAPTER 5

Endoscopic Anterior Skull Base Resection and Endoscopic Repair of Skull Base Defects

Liat Shama, Francis Hall

ENDOSCOPIC ANTERIOR SKULL BASE RESECTION

Evolution

As with many techniques involving the paranasal sinus, the resection of anterior skull base tumors has followed a path from an open to an endoscopic approach. For selected tumors, it has been shown that endoscopic resection is as safe and as effective as open resection. Given the significant morbidity often associated with open approaches, this has improved patient care and satisfaction. Initially, there was concern regarding the difficulty of performing an en bloc resection endoscopically; this has been shown not to have a detrimental effect on patient outcomes. The importance of patient selection cannot be overestimated nor can careful review of preoperative imaging. The initial chance for cure for a tumor lies with the initial surgery; determination of the best approach should take this into account.[1] For tumors of the midline and paramidline anterior and middle skull base, endoscopic resection has been shown to be feasible, safe, and is associated with outcomes better than if not comparable to open approaches. It is evolving into the gold standard for selected anterior and middle skull base tumors, both benign and malignant.

Indications

Endoscopic anterior skull base resection is indicated for both benign and malignant tumors that can be fully accessed and resected endoscopically. Some instances may utilize endoscopic resection as part of palliation; this is not specifically discussed as part of this chapter, although the same techniques and approaches can be used for palliation. In addition, endoscopic procedures may be performed in combination with open approaches.[2-4] Several approaches for evaluating anterior and middle skull base lesions have been proposed. Fokkens et al. discuss the skull base in the sagittal plane, dividing the approaches by regions into transcribriform, transplanum, and transtuberculum.[5] Another widely described classification of approaches to the same region of the skull divides the skull base into the following regions: transfrontal, transcribriform, transplanum, trans-sellar, transclival, and transodontoid (Fig. 5.1).[6-9]

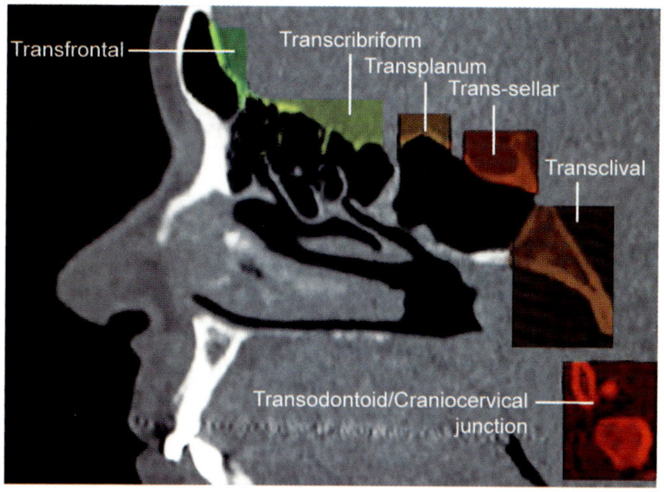

Fig. 5.1: Skull base.

Open versus Endoscopic Approach

The safety and feasibility of endoscopic anterior skull base resection has been examined. It has been shown to be comparable to open anterior skull base resection in selected cases and with selected pathology such as meningioma or esthesioneuroblastoma.[5,10-17] Additionally, morbidity, mortality, and local recurrent rates have been shown to be similar for open and endoscopic anterior skull base resection. Cosmesis may be improved with the endoscopic approach.[18-22]

Endoscopic approaches to the anterior skull base for tumor resection involve extending approaches often used for endoscopic sinus surgery. The limits of access of the endoscopic skull base resection are defined by the regions accessible by this method. The limits of anterior skull base resection are the posteromedial wall of the frontal sinus, planum sphenoidale, bilateral superomedial orbital walls, bilateral ethmoid roof, crista galli, and anterior and posterior ethmoid arteries.[2]

This approach is best for midline tumors and those that do not extend lateral to the internal carotid artery, lateral to the orbit and/or the optic nerve, and those tumors that do not involve the facial skin or scalp or encase the internal carotid artery.[5,11,14,23-26]

Review of cases at a Multidisciplinary Head and Neck Tumor Board is recommended for all tumors prior to determination of a treatment plan as many head and neck malignancies will require associated chemotherapy and/or radiation therapy either in neoadjuvant or adjuvant fashion.[27,28]

Imaging

Patient selection is critical as is preoperative review of preoperative imaging. Both CT and MRI are necessary. CT evaluates the bony anatomy and landmarks; MRI is essential for identifying soft tissue involvement of the tumor as well as its boundaries. MRI may also provide helpful information in differentiating benign from malignant features of tumors and differentiating neoplasms from inflammatory disease. It is essential for surgical planning. Image guidance is recommended for these cases. PET scan may be appropriate in selected cases depending on pathology. A team approach between otolaryngology and neurosurgery is essential.

Equipment and Setup

Equipment and room setup for endoscopic medial maxillectomy uses the standard setup for endoscopic sinus surgery. As with most surgical cases, routinizing the setup and flow of events leads to a controlled environment that provides for a smooth flow of events, setting the stage for minimizing errors. Surgical technicians and scrub nurses should be familiar with the equipment and room setup. Instruments normally used for endoscopic sinus surgery are used for this procedure, including angled endoscopes, bipolar suction forceps, and a drill as needed. Endoscopic clip appliers may be advantageous as well in cases of vascular tumors.

Endoscopic anterior skull base resection should utilize image guidance. Image guidance, or computer-assisted navigation, has evolved over many years to the current devices, which are versatile and accurate to within 2 mm.[29] Although these devices are not a substitute for thorough knowledge of sinonasal anatomy, there is a possibility for more complete surgery with the use of these devices as additional information is available to the surgeon. The main limitation of image guidance is that the images are obtained preoperatively and are therefore not an accurate reflection of any changes applied during surgery. Intraoperative imaging is available and although it has yet to be widely incorporated into the realm of endoscopic sinus surgery, it has become increasingly used in endoscopic skull base cases and may be useful in select cases.

Operative Steps

A spinal drain may be placed in some cases; this would be performed by the neurosurgeon at the beginning of the case.

The nasal cavities are topically anesthetized and decongested with various agents on cottonoid pledgets. Diluted 4% cocaine, high concentration epinephrine (1:1,000), and Afrin have all been used to improve hemostasis. Thereafter, intranasal injections are undertaken with a mixture usually of 1–2% lidocaine with 1:80,000–100,000 of epinephrine. Often, especially with extended maxillary sinus procedures, pterygopalatine fossa block is performed transorally through the greater palatine canal usually with 1% lidocaine with 1:100,000 of epinephrine.

The tumor is debulked as necessary. This allows for exposure of landmarks as well as the limits of dissection and, more importantly, the site of origin of the tumor.[2] It is recommended that frozen sections be sent as needed to confirm diagnosis and/or to evaluate margins. If closure of a large defect is anticipated, harvest of a nasoseptal flap at this point may be indicated and is discussed in the section on endoscopic skull base reconstruction.[30-32]

For anterior skull base resection to be feasible, the entire skull base should be exposed. This entails complete sphenoethmoidectomy as well as exposure of the frontal

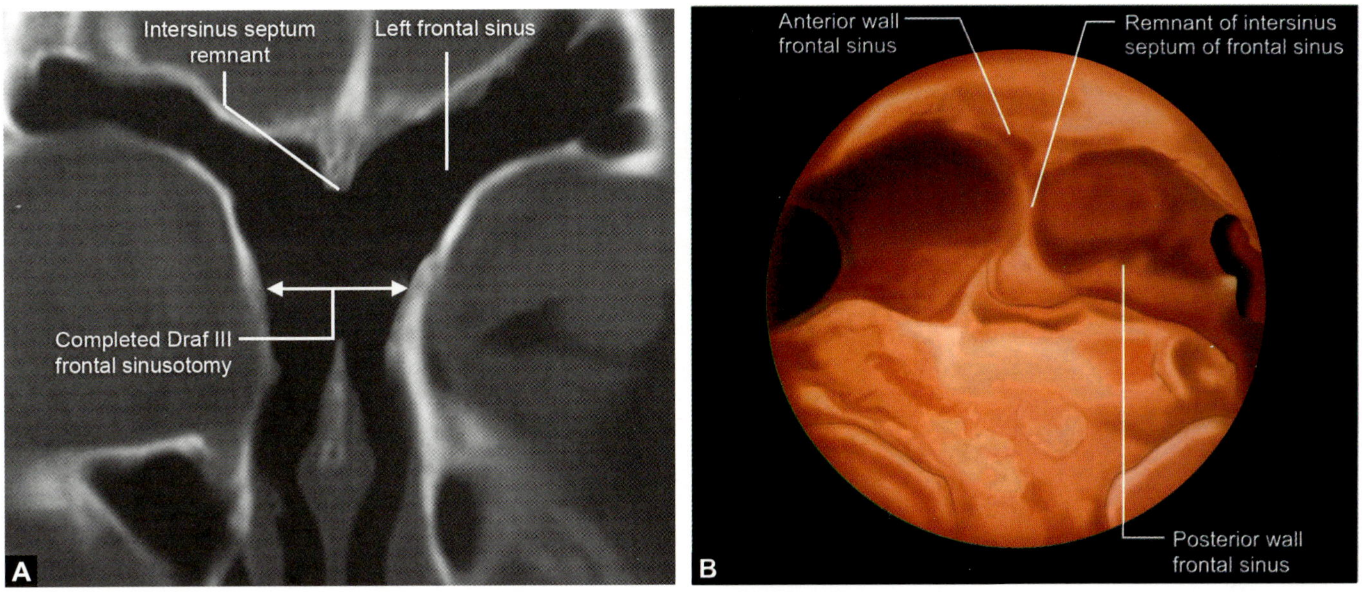

Figs. 5.2A and B: Endoscopic modified Lothrop procedure.

sinus ostia. The remainder of the anterior skull base is exposed with an endoscopic modified Lothrop procedure (Figs. 5.2A and B).[22] For tumors involving the ethmoid sinus, endoscopic medial maxillectomy is performed. This is discussed in detail in Chapter 2. For some tumors, bilateral resection is necessary. Regardless, bilateral exposure will allow for manipulation of instruments through both nares simultaneously.

A complete sphenoethmoidectomy is performed. This is often done bilaterally, but may be modified in select cases requiring only unilateral exposure. The sphenoidotomy is performed with wide exposure inferiorly, laterally, and superiorly. In certain cases, this is followed by exposure and removal of the sphenoid rostrum. This generally requires the use of rongeurs as well as a high-speed drill. Next, the intersinus septum of the sphenoid sinus is removed sharply. Extreme care is exercised at this point, as the intersinus septum generally inserts along the carotid canal on one side. Removal of the sphenoid rostrum as well as the intersinus septum exposes the entire sella and also allows for bilateral access to the entire skull base. At this point, if indicated, the planum sphenoidale is drilled to allow for access to the tumor. For transtubercular and suprasellar lesions, the planum sphenoidale should be drilled. Once the bony portions of the sella and planum sphenoidale are removed, the dura is exposed. In cases of small tumors without bilateral dural involvement, the resection may be done unilaterally, provided uninvolved dura can be resected around the tumor.[22]

For tumors along the anterior skull base, a modified Lothrop procedure is performed to expose the anterior limit of dissection. Traditionally, this procedure begins with identification of the frontal sinus recess on one side and then the other. Thereafter, a superior septectomy anterior to the middle turbinate is performed. In some cases, the middle turbinate may be removed. The frontal process of the maxilla is then drilled above the axilla of the middle turbinate. The frontal sinus is then entered through the natural ostium. Next, the cavity is opened medially, including the intersinus septum. A crescent-shaped opening is formed at this point and further opened to a large oval. Angled endoscopes and angled burs are used.

An outside-in approach to the modified endoscopic Lothrop procedure has been described and has been shown to be both feasible and safe. Additionally, it has been shown to be faster than the traditional modified endoscopic Lothrop procedure. This method involves removal of mucosa over the frontal process of the maxilla, followed by creation of a septal window. The bony septum is removed and periosteum identified on each side. The bone is removed between the lateral limits of dissection, including bone anterior to frontal process followed by removal of the bone between the created cavity and true frontal recess.[33]

Next, if it has not already performed, the bony septum is separated from the skull base, usually done sharply with forceps or an osteotome. At this point, the entire skull base should be accessible and attention is turned to removing the bony portion of the skull base. This is generally thinned with a high-speed drill to expose the dura circumferentially. This includes the fovea ethmoidalis, planum sphenoidale, and laterally the lamina papyracea as indicated (Fig. 5.3).

At this point, the dura is fully exposed without residual bony covering except for the crista galli. For some lesions, ligation of the anterior and/or posterior ethmoid arteries is indicated to improve hemostasis and decrease vascularity of the tumor, especially those along the anterior skull base.

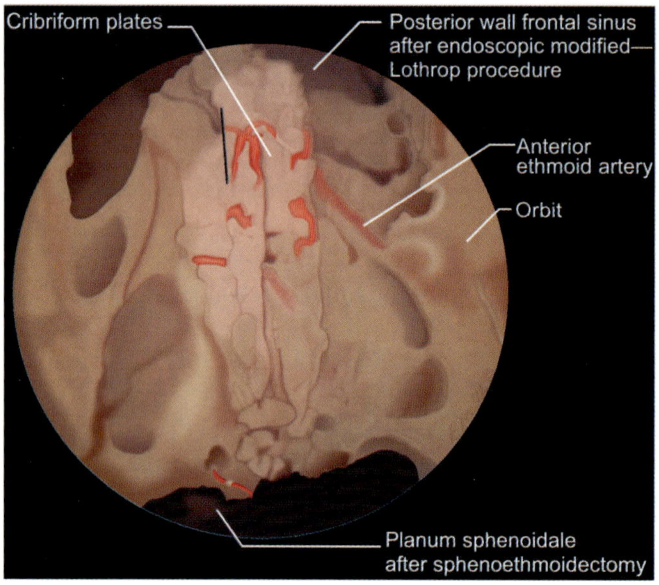

Fig. 5.3: Exposure of skull base.

This is generally not indicated for removal of sellar lesions and pituitary tumors. However, for some lesions along the planum sphenoidale, the posterior ethmoid artery is along the anterior margin and is therefore ligated or cauterized after exposure. The dura is incised sharply with a margin of uninvolved dura, followed by incision of the falx cerebri to fully release the skull base and tumor. The specimen will include the dura, cribriform plate and olfactory bulbs, superior aspect of septum and crista galli. This can be done en bloc. The resection is generally bilateral; for some isolated unilateral lesions, the contralateral nasal cavity may be spared. Given the generally aggressive nature of anterior skull base malignancies, aggressive resection has been advocated, despite a possibly decreased quality of life with resection of both olfactory bulbs.

The remainder of the dissection from the now exposed anterior skull base is extremely meticulous (Fig. 5.4). Bipolar cautery is essential in cauterizing vessels feeding the tumor; the remaining vessels should be carefully dissected and preserved.[22]

Transcribriform access will allow for removal of lesions in involving the frontal sinus and the crista galli. This requires removal of the anterior/superior septum with sacrifice of olfaction, which may have already been compromised depending on the tumor. A complete ethmoidectomy is performed with endoscopic ligation of the anterior and posterior ethmoid arteries. If the tumor extends laterally or involves the lamina papyracea, it is removed. Otherwise, it is skeletonized. In selected cases,

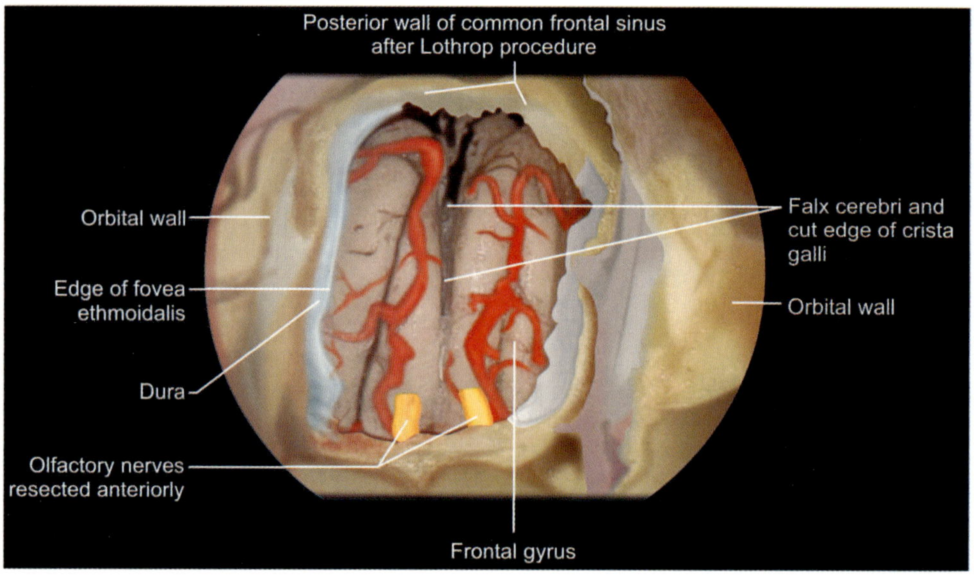

Fig. 5.4: Endoscopic anterior skull base resection.

a modified endoscopic Lothrop procedure is necessary and is performed. A drill is used to thin and allow for fracture of the crista galli. Microdissection with neurosurgery proceeds at this point, usually involving capsular bipolar as well as internal debulking and capsular dissection. Removal in non-en bloc fashion has been shown to be equivalent to en bloc removal; the safest method is undertaken.

For lesions involving the middle skull base, sphenoidotomy is indicated to allow for access to the planum sphenoidale. This may be indicated for lesions involving the sella, especially if there is suprasellar extension.

ENDOSCOPIC REPAIR OF SKULL BASE DEFECTS

Endoscopic reconstruction of skull base defects was previously a limiting factor in the growth of endoscopic techniques for removal of tumors of the anterior and middle skull base. Improvement in these techniques has made endoscopic reconstruction an accepted part of the treatment paradigm for skull base defects. This is important because separation between the extracranial sinonasal and intracranial cavities is necessary to prevent complications stemming from the lack of such a barrier, including cerebrospinal fluid leaks, meningitis, abscesses, and tension pneumocephalus.[5]

Several factors should be considered when determining the type of reconstruction to be used for the defect created during tumor resection. These factors should be considered prior to the procedure because flaps for reconstruction may need to be harvested prior to the tumor resection as the blood supply to some pedicled flaps may be disrupted, making flap harvest after tumor resection either difficult or impossible. The pathology of the tumor should be considered, including the need for postoperative radiation therapy. Whether the patient has had prior surgery is important as well. For example, patients with prior endoscopic trans-sphenoidal tumor resection, usually with resection of the sphenoid rostrum, may not have intact blood supply for a nasoseptal flap. Patients with prior endoscopic sinus surgery and/or septoplasty may have had disruption of normal landmarks and blood supply to possible pedicled flaps. The experience and comfort level of the surgical team is important both in tumor resection and reconstruction of the skull base defect. The goal of care for any patient is to first not cause harm, and therefore the best option in the particular surgical team's hands is the safest option. Much as with any surgical technique, there is a role for cadaveric dissection, both in the laboratory and as part of surgical dissection courses. Smaller defects can be repaired with free tissue grafts, either mucosa, acellular dermal grafts (Alloderm) or Duragen. However, larger defects require a more complex and layered reconstruction. In cases of malignancies, the need for postoperative radiation therapy should be considered, as this will impact the healing process.

Endoscopic anterior skull base resection necessitates closure of a defect of varying sizes. Watertight closure with multiple layers of reconstruction is paramount. For some smaller defects, such as those from a pituitary tumor resection, use of nonpedicled-free mucosal grafts may be sufficient. Larger defects with higher flow cerebrospinal fluid leakage require a robust closure, often with vascularized tissue.[30,32,34,35] For some larger defects, a nasoseptal flap (Hadad-Bassagasteguy flap) may be used.

Free tissue grafts, such as nasal mucosa or acellular dermal grafts, should be placed as part of a layered reconstruction. Free autograft tissue may be harvested from the nasal septum, middle turbinate, or inferior turbinate. Adherence followed by serum imbibition over the first week of healing of these grafts allows for the process of revascularization, which requires tissue contact without intervening fluid such as a hematoma, seroma, or cerebrospinal fluid. Free tissue followed by fibrin glue and possibly packing, such as Merocel packs or Foley catheter balloon, helps prevent disruption of this process. Harvested fat graft may be placed in a large spatial defect as well, usually deep to mucosal reconstruction and fibrin glue. This type of reconstruction works well for smaller defects without cerebrospinal fluid leak or small, low-flow cerebrospinal fluid leakage with excellent success rate.[5,36-43]

The Hadad-Bassagasteguy flap is pedicled on the posterior septal branch of the sphenopalatine artery (Figs. 5.5A and B).[30] It should generally be harvested early in the case as the sphenoidotomy and resection of the sphenoid rostrum may disrupt the blood supply and removal of the superior aspect of the nasal septum will disrupt some of the mucosa. It is placed in the nasopharynx or maxillary sinus if antrostomy is performed during the rest of the procedure. The flap is generally harvested with monopolar cautery, although it may be done sharply in some portions as well. The superior cut is made posterior to the basal lamella and taken superiorly along the inferior aspect of the sphenoid sinus ostium and initially

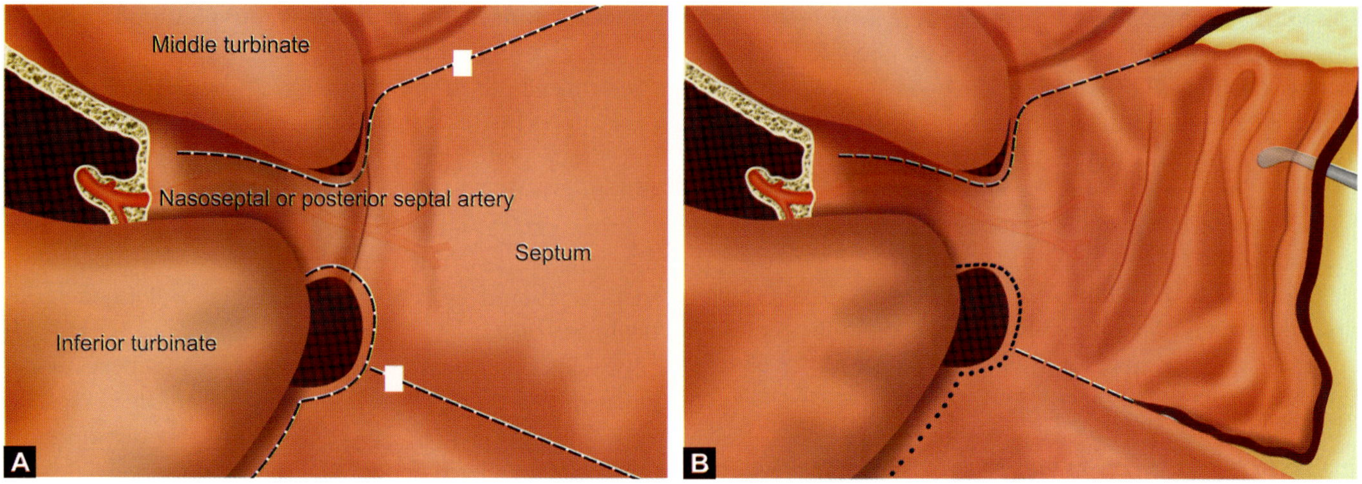

Figs. 5.5A and B: Hadad-Bassagasteguy or nasoseptal flap.

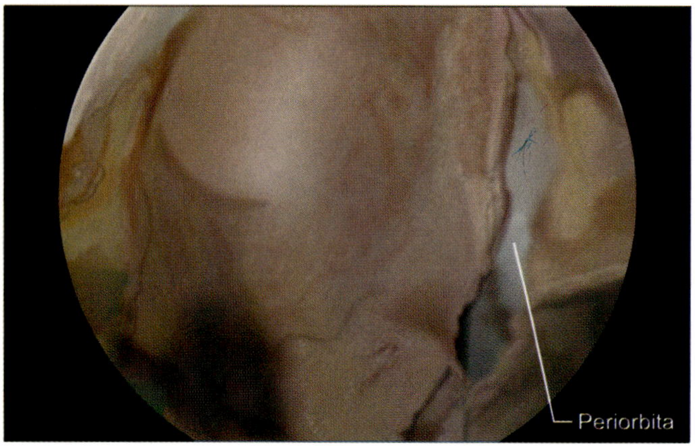

Fig. 5.6: Endoscopic anterior skull base reconstruction, with nasoseptal flap reconstruction.

inferiorly along the septum to preserve olfactory mucosa. As it courses anteriorly along the septum anterior to the middle turbinate, the cut is extended superiorly. The inferior cut is taken along the most inferior aspect of the sphenoid rostrum and anteriorly along the inferior aspect of the septum; it may incorporate the floor of the nasal cavity if necessary. The anterior vertical cut is made as far anteriorly as the mucocutaneous junction of the septum with the columella. The flap is then elevated in a submucoperichondrial and submucoperiosteal plane until it is fully elevated and then stored for later use.[28,31,32] This flap is widely versatile and provides tissue with a surface area up to 25 cm (Fig. 5.6).[43-45] It is also very successful with minimal postoperative cerebrospinal fluid leak.[31,32] As the need for such a flap is not always foreseen, it has been proposed that during cases involving sphenoidotomy, the mucosa along the anterior face of the sphenoid and along the rostrum be preserved so that a rescue flap can be harvested if necessary. This involves the initial steps of the nasoseptal flap by making the posterior incisions, allowing for preservation of the blood supply for a rescue flap should the need arise.

For larger defects such as those encountered in endoscopic anterior skull base resection, layered materials are necessary. The closure materials often retract, so the amount of tissue necessary to reconstruct the defect is larger than the actual defect. Tensor fascia lata from the thigh has been used successfully.[22] Acellular dermal allograft, or Alloderm, has also been used successfully in the repair of large anterior skull base defects.[46] The first layer of materials used to reconstruct the skull base should be placed extradurally, intracranially as an underlay graft if possible. The graft layer may be sutured to the dura anteriorly if there is sufficient dura. The next layer of graft material (or first layer if underlay graft is not possible), fascia lata or possibly Alloderm or pedicled graft, is placed as an overlay graft extracranially. Care should be taken to ensure that the material lies flat without any redundancy or gaps. Fibrin glue or DuraSeal is applied at this point to ensure a watertight seal. Nasal packing is then placed. Several types of packing have been proposed, including gauze soaked in various preparations including bismuth iodoform paraffin paste.[22] Care must be taken not to place the packing too tightly along the skull base or the lamina papyracea. Deep extubation is recommended. Packing is removed after 1 week. Antibiotics are given for toxic shock syndrome prophylaxis during that time.

Other vascularized flaps have been proposed and used for closure of endoscopic skull base defects; the most commonly used flaps have been described thus far and have the advantage of not requiring additional incisions (tensor fascia lata is the exception). Additional intranasal pedicled flaps include the posterior pedicled inferior and middle turbinate flaps, both with relatively small surface area and pedicled on branches of the spheno-palatine artery. For larger defects, pericranial flap may be used. This requires a bicoronal incision for harvest and may be indicated in certain cases with very large defects. Temporoparietal fascial flap may be used as well via transpterygoid transposition. This is pedicled on the superficial temporal artery and will require an external incision.[35] From review of the literature, the Hadad-Bassagasteguy flap has been the choice for vascularized pedicled flaps in endoscopic skull base reconstruction, especially for pathologies requiring adjuvant therapy. Use of acellular dermal graft such as Alloderm has also been shown to be successful in large skull base defects with cerebrospinal fluid leakage.[46]

SUMMARY

Overall, great progress has been made in the use of endoscopic techniques for resection of skull base tumors. This has improved both morbidity and mortality of surgical resection of the tumors. The ability to close these defects as well as evidence that the endoscopic route provides at least comparable rates of recurrence and tumor removal with open techniques has validated it as part of the treatment paradigm for benign and malignant neoplasms of the skull base.

REFERENCES

1. Stammberger H, Anderhuber W, Walch C, et al. Possibilities and limitations of endoscopic management of nasal and paranasal sinus malignancies. Acta Otorhinolaryngol Belgica. 1999;53(3):199-205.
2. Casiano R, Herzallah I, Anstead A, et al. Advanced endoscopic sinonasal dissection. In: Casiano R (Ed). Endoscopic Sinonasal Dissection Guide. New York: Thieme Medical Publishers, Inc; 2012. pp. 59-99.
3. Thaler ER, Kotapka M, Lanza DC, et al. Endoscopically assisted anterior cranial skull base resection of sinonasal tumors. Am J Rhinol. 1999;13(4):303-10.
4. Yuen AP, Fung CF, Hung KN. Endoscopic cranionasal resection of anterior skull base tumor. Am J Otolaryngol. 1997;18(6):431-3.
5. McLaughlin N, Prevedello D, Ditzel Filho l, et al. Anterior skull base tumors and approaches: transtuberculum, transplanum, and transcribriform. In: Georgalas C, Fokkens W (Eds). Rhinology and Skull Base Surgery. Stuttgart: Thieme Medical Publishers, Inc; 2013. pp. 772-90.
6. Kassam A, Snyderman CH, Mintz A, et al. Expanded endonasal approach: the rostrocaudal axis. Part I. Crista galli to the sella turcica. Neurosurg Focus. 2005;19(1):E3.
7. Kassam A, Snyderman CH, Mintz A, et al. Expanded endonasal approach: the rostrocaudal axis. Part II. Posterior clinoids to the foramen magnum. Neurosurg Focus. 2005;19(1):E4.
8. Nogueira JF, Stamm A, Vellutini E. Evolution of endoscopic skull base surgery, current concepts, and future perspectives. Otolaryngol Clin North Am. 2010;43(3):639-52, x-xi.
9. Snyderman CH, Pant H, Carrau RL, et al. What are the limits of endoscopic sinus surgery?: the expanded endonasal approach to the skull base. Keio J Med. 2009;58(3):152-60.
10. Carrabba G, Dehdashti AR, Gentili F. Surgery for clival lesions: open resection versus the expanded endoscopic endonasal approach. Neurosurg Focus. 2008;25(6):E7.
11. Dehdashti AR, Ganna A, Witterick I, et al. Expanded endoscopic endonasal approach for anterior cranial base and suprasellar lesions: indications and limitations. Neurosurgery. 2009;64(4):677-87; discussion 87-9.
12. Fraser JF, Nyquist GG, Moore N, et al. Endoscopic endonasal transclival resection of chordomas: operative technique, clinical outcome, and review of the literature. J Neurosurg. 2010;112(5):1061-9.
13. Gardner PA, Kassam AB, Snyderman CH, et al. Outcomes following endoscopic, expanded endonasal resection of suprasellar craniopharyngiomas: a case series. J Neurosurg. 2008;109(1):6-16.
14. Gardner PA, Kassam AB, Thomas A, et al. Endoscopic endonasal resection of anterior cranial base meningiomas. Neurosurgery. 2008;63(1):36-52; discussion 52-4.
15. O'Malley BW, Jr, Grady MS, Gabel BC, et al. Comparison of endoscopic and microscopic removal of pituitary adenomas: single-surgeon experience and the learning curve. Neurosurg Focus. 2008;25(6):E10.
16. Snyderman CH, Carrau RL, Kassam AB, et al. Endoscopic skull base surgery: principles of endonasal oncological surgery. J Surg Oncol. 2008;97(8):658-64.
17. Tabaee A, Anand VK, Barron Y, et al. Endoscopic pituitary surgery: a systematic review and meta-analysis. J Neurosurg. 2009;111(3):545-54.
18. Batra PS, Citardi MJ, Worley S, et al. Resection of anterior skull base tumors: comparison of combined traditional and endoscopic techniques. Am J Rhinol. 2005;19(5):521-8.
19. Buchmann L, Larsen C, Pollack A, et al. Endoscopic techniques in resection of anterior skull base/paranasal sinus malignancies. Laryngoscope. 2006;116(10):1749-54.
20. Castelnuovo PG, Belli E, Bignami M, et al. Endoscopic nasal and anterior craniotomy resection for malignant naso-ethmoid tumors involving the anterior skull base. Skull Base. 2006;16(1):15-8.
21. Leong JL, Citardi MJ, Batra PS. Reconstruction of skull base defects after minimally invasive endoscopic resection of anterior skull base neoplasms. Am J Rhinol. 2006;20(5):476-82.

22. Wormald PJ. Endoscopic sinus surgery: anatomy, three-dimensional reconstruction, and surgical technique, 2nd edition. New York: Thieme Medical Pulishers, Inc; 2008.
23. de Divitiis E, Cavallo LM, Esposito F, et al. Extended endoscopic transsphenoidal approach for tuberculum sellae meningiomas. Neurosurgery. 2007;61(5 Suppl 2):229-37; discussion 37-8.
24. Eloy JA, Vivero RJ, Hoang K, et al. Comparison of transnasal endoscopic and open craniofacial resection for malignant tumors of the anterior skull base. Laryngoscope. 2009;119(5):834-40.
25. Folbe A, Herzallah I, Duvvuri U, et al. Endoscopic endonasal resection of esthesioneuroblastoma: a multicenter study. Am J Rhinol Allergy. 2009;23(1):91-4.
26. Solares CA, Ong YK, Snyderman CH. Transnasal endoscopic skull base surgery: what are the limits? Curr Opin Otolaryngol Head Neck Surg. 2010;18(1):1-7.
27. Harvey RJ, Dalgorf DM. Chapter 10: Sinonasal malignancies. Am J Rhinol Allergy. 2013;27(Suppl 1):S35-8.
28. Jardeleza C, Seiberling K, Floreani S, et al. Surgical outcomes of endoscopic management of adenocarcinoma of the sinonasal cavity. Rhinology. 2009;47(4):354-61.
29. Kennedy DW, Ramakrishnan V. Functional endoscopic sinus surgery: concepts, surgical indications, and techniques. In: Kennedy DW, Hwang PH (Eds). Rhinology: Diseases of the Nose, Sinuses, Skull Base. New York: Thieme Medical Publishers, Inc; 2012. pp. 306-35.
30. Hadad G, Bassagasteguy L, Carrau RL, et al. A novel reconstructive technique after endoscopic expanded endonasal approaches: vascular pedicle nasoseptal flap. Laryngoscope. 2006;116(10):1882-6.
31. Kassam AB, Thomas A, Carrau RL, et al. Endoscopic reconstruction of the cranial base using a pedicled nasoseptal flap. Neurosurgery. 2008;63(1 Suppl 1):ONS44-52; discussion ONS-3.
32. Zanation AM, Carrau RL, Snyderman CH, et al. Nasoseptal flap reconstruction of high flow intraoperative cerebral spinal fluid leaks during endoscopic skull base surgery. Am J Rhinol Allergy. 2009;23(5):518-21.
33. Chin D, Snidvongs K, Kalish L, et al. The outside-in approach to the modified endoscopic Lothrop procedure. Laryngoscope. 2012;122(8):1661-9.
34. Esposito F, Dusick JR, Fatemi N, et al. Graded repair of cranial base defects and cerebrospinal fluid leaks in transsphenoidal surgery. Neurosurgery. 2007;60(4 Suppl 2): 295-303; discussion 303-4.
35. McLaughlin N, Carrau RL, Kassam A, et al. Reconstruction of the Skull base and management of skull base surgery complications. In: Georgalas C, Fokkens W (Eds). Rhinology and Skull Base Surgery. Stuttgart: Thieme Medical Publishers, Inc; 2013. pp. 791-809.
36. Carrau RL, Snyderman CH, Kassam AB. The management of cerebrospinal fluid leaks in patients at risk for high-pressure hydrocephalus. Laryngoscope. 2005;115(2):205-12.
37. Castelnuovo P, Dallan I, Bignami M, et al. Endoscopic endonasal management of petroclival cerebrospinal fluid leaks: anatomical study and preliminary clinical experience. Minim Invasive Neurosur. 2008;51(6):336-9.
38. Castelnuovo PG, Delu G, Locatelli D, et al. Endonasal endoscopic duraplasty: our experience. Skull Base. 2006;16(1): 19-24. PubMed PMID: 16880897.
39. Hegazy HM, Carrau RL, Snyderman CH, et al. Transnasal endoscopic repair of cerebrospinal fluid rhinorrhea: a meta-analysis. Laryngoscope. 2000;110(7):1166-72.
40. Kassam A, Carrau RL, Snyderman CH, et al. Evolution of reconstructive techniques following endoscopic expanded endonasal approaches. Neurosurg Focus. 2005;19(1):E8.
41. Locatelli D, Rampa F, Acchiardi I, et al. Endoscopic endonasal approaches for repair of cerebrospinal fluid leaks: nine-year experience. Neurosurgery. 2006;58(4 Suppl 2): ONS-246-56; discussiom ONS-56-7.
42. Schick B, Ibing R, Brors D, et al. Long-term study of endonasal duraplasty and review of the literature. Ann Otol Rhinol Laryngol. 2001;110(2):142-7.
43. Zweig JL, Carrau RL, Celin SE, et al. Endoscopic repair of cerebrospinal fluid leaks to the sinonasal tract: predictors of success. Otolaryngol Head Neck Surg. 2000;123(3):195-201.
44. Cappabianca P, Cavallo LM, Colao A, et al. Surgical complications associated with the endoscopic endonasal transsphenoidal approach for pituitary adenomas. J Neurosurg. 2002;97(2):293-8.
45. Pinheiro-Neto CD, Prevedello DM, Carrau RL, et al. Improving the design of the pedicled nasoseptal flap for skull base reconstruction: a radioanatomic study. Laryngoscope. 2007;117(9):1560-9.
46. Germani RM, Vivero R, Herzallah IR, et al. Endoscopic reconstruction of large anterior skull base defects using acellular dermal allograft. Am J Rhinol. 2007;21(5):615-8.

Section 2

Oral Cavity and Oropharynx

Section Editor: ***Steven S Chang***

Chapters

CHAPTER

6

Surgical Management of Lip Cancer

Theresa Guo, Steven S Chang

BACKGROUND

The lip is classified as a subsite of the oral cavity. Despite this classification, cancers of the lip hold many similarities to skin-based malignancies. Like skin cancers, UV sun exposure is the most established risk factor for the development of lip cancer.[1] Patients with chronic immunosuppression such as HIV and renal transplant patients are also at higher risk for development of lip malignancies. Other proposed risk factors include tobacco and alcohol use.

Cancers of the lip are the most common of all oral malignancies with an incidence of approximately 12–13.5/100,000 person-years.[1] Demographics of lip cancers are similar to those of skin cancer with a strong white male predominance, with prevalence peaking in the sixth and seventh decades of life.[1] They are rare in Black and Asian individuals. Lip cancers are predominately well-differentiated squamous cell carcinomas (>90%). In addition, the vast majority (>90%) of lip cancers occur in the lower lip. Basal cell carcinomas also occur and are more common on the upper lip and in females.[2]

While lip cancers bear many similarities to skin cancers in epidemiology, the importance of the lip as an oral cavity site is seen in its prognosis, staging, and likelihood of spread. Staging of lip cancers is similar to that of other oral cavity tumors (Table 6.1). Lymphatic spread of lip cancers follow patterns similar to other oral cavity tumors with spread into the submental and upper jugulodigastric nodes. Risk of nodal metastasis increases with T stage, with 5–10% risk in T1 lesions, 20–50% in T2 lesions, and 50–70% in T3/T4 lesions.[3,4] Risk of nodal metastasis also increases in patients with perineural invasion,[3] history of immunosuppression, and lesions involving the oral commissure.[5]

Table 6.1: TNM staging of lip cancer (NCCN guidelines).[6]

T staging	
T0	No evidence of primary tumor
Tis	Carcinoma in situ
T1	≤ 2 cm
T2	>2 cm but ≤ 4 cm
T3	>4 cm
T4a	Local invasion through cortical bone, inferior alveolar nerve, floor of mouth, extending to skin of face (chin or nose)
T4b	Extension to masticator space, pterygoid plates, skull base, encasement of internal carotid artery
N staging	
Nx	N stage not evaluated
N0	No regional lymph nodes
N1	Single, ipsilateral ≤ 3 cm
N2a	Single ipsilateral >3 cm but ≤ 6 cm
N2b	Multiple ipsilateral, none >6 cm
N2c	Bilateral/contralateral, none >6 cm
N3	Any lymph nodes >6 cm
M staging	
Mx	Metastasis not evaluated
M0	No distant metastasis
M1	Distant metastasis present

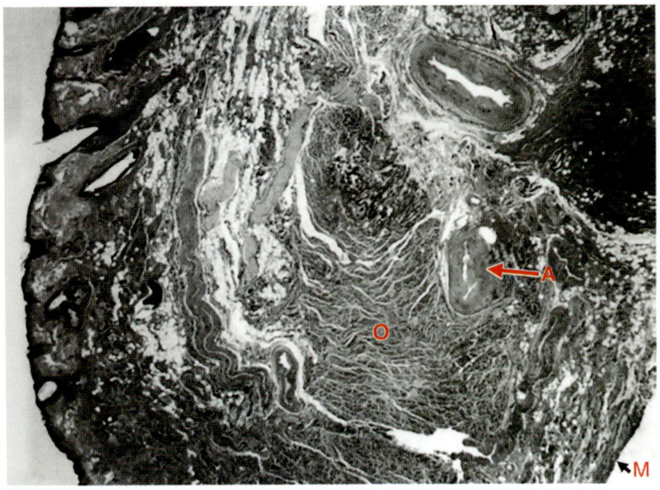

Fig. 6.1: H&E stain of upper lip cross section demonstrating relationship of labial artery (A), which travels in the layer between the orbicularis oris (O) and mucosa (M).
Source: Reproduced from Schulte et al.[8]

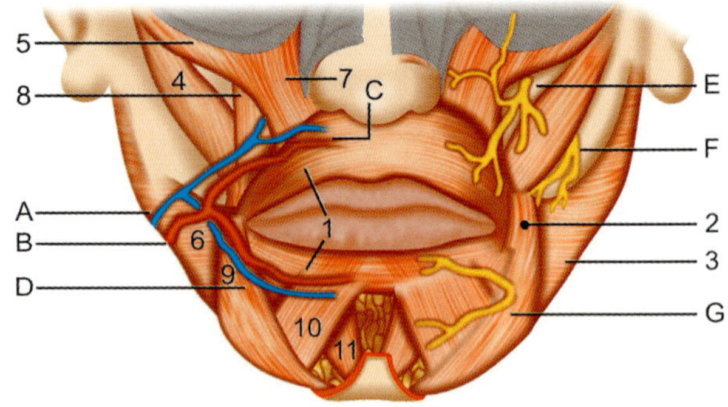

Fig. 6.2: Vessels, nerves, and muscles of the lip. VESSELS: A. Facial vein. B. Facial artery. C. Superior labial artery and vein. D. Inferior labial artery and vein. (The labial vessels run circumferentially around the lip.) NERVES: E. Infraorbital nerve (V2, sensation). F. Buccal nerve (V3, sensation). G. Mental nerve (V3, sensation). MUSCLES: 1. Orbicularis oris. 2. Modiolus. 3. Platysma. 4. Zygomaticus major. 5. Zygomaticus minor. 6. Risorius. 7. Levator labii superioris. 8. Levator anguli oris. 9. Depressor anguli oris. 10. Depressor labii inferioris. 11. Mentalis.
Source: Redrawn friom Platzer.[9]

As lip lesions are highly visible, malignancies are often diagnosed at an early T1 stage.[7] Lesions are present as nonhealing ulcers that may be painful and may also bleed intermittently. Pertinent history may include occupation, sun exposure, chronic immunosuppression, and history of other skin cancers. Evaluation of these lesions should include measurement of size, location (medial, lateral, crossing vermillion border, or involving the lateral commissure), palpation (tenderness, mobility to assess deep invasion), mental nerve sensation, and evaluation of any cervical lymphadenopathy. Further imaging (CT scan) may be obtained if there is strong suspicion for nodal metastasis, including the presence of perineural invasion (loss of sensation in V3), palpable lymphadenopathy, or chronic immunosuppression.

ANATOMY

The lip is defined by the vermillion. The outer limit is the vermillion border at the junction of the facial skin, and inner border at the junction of the buccal mucosa. The upper lip has a unique shape with two peaks, often referred to as "cupid's bow." The two peaks connect to the philtral columns, between which there is a midline depression known as the philtrum. The vermillion is composed of nonkeratinized squamous epithelium with high capillary density that gives the vermillion its red color. Below the epithelium lies, from superficial to deep, the epidermis, subcutaneous tissue, orbicularis oris, and buccal mucosa. The blood supply of the lip is provided by branches of the facial artery. The superior labial artery supplies the upper lip and the inferior labial artery supplies the lower lip. It should be noted that these arteries lie in the layer between the muscle (orbicularis oris) and mucosa (Fig. 6.1).

The orbicularis oris is the main muscle of the lip, which lies in a circumferential fashion around the lips (Fig. 6.2). It provides both functions for facial expression as well as contribution to swallowing and speech. In addition to the orbicularis oris, several muscles attach to the lip allowing for fine motor control.

At the lateral oral commissure there is a thickening known as the modiolus that anchors several facial muscles including the orbicularis oris, buccinators (lines the mouth medially), levator anguli oris, depressor anguli oris, zygomaticus major, and risorius (Fig. 6.2). Muscles that also insert into the upper lip include the levator labii superioris and zygomaticus minor. Those that insert into the lower lip include the depressor labii inferioris, mentalis, and platysma.

Innervation of the lip is provided by the trigeminal and facial nerves. Motor control is provided by the buccal and marginal mandibular branches of the facial nerve. Sensation is provided by the trigeminal nerve (Fig. 6.2). The infraorbital (V2) nerve provides sensation to the upper lip and the mental (V3) nerve provides sensation to the lower lip with some contribution of the buccal nerve as well (V3). Blocks of these nerves may be performed to provide local anesthesia.

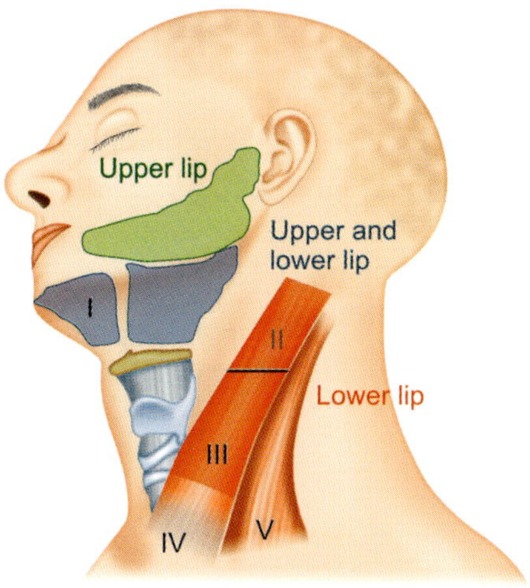

Fig. 6.3: Lymphatic drainage of the lip. The lip primarily drains to the ipsilateral submandibular region (I). The upper lip may also drain into preauricular, periparotid, or perifacial lymph nodes. The lower lip may also drain to submental nodes (I) or upper jugulodigastric nodes (II, III).

Lymphatic drainage of the lips is primarily to the ipsilateral submandibular lymph nodes. The midline lower lip is additionally drained by the submental nodes and upper juglodigastric nodes and may also drain to contralateral nodes. The midline upper lip is also drained by the preauricular, periparotid, and perifacial nodes (Fig. 6.3).[3]

TREATMENT

Surgical resection is the mainstay of treatment for lip malignancies and will be the primary focus of the remainder of this chapter. The primary goal of surgical resection should be full resection with the goal of cure. Following adequate resection, the next considerations should be focused on maintenance of lip function: speech, oral competence, maximizing mouth opening, and satisfactory cosmetic outcome. Lesions should be removed with a margin of at least 5 mm. Frozen sections may be sent intraoperatively to ensure complete resection. Squamous cell carcinoma and basal cell carcinoma should be removed with a margin of at least 5 mm and margins may be to be assessed on frozen section.[10] Melanoma cannot be assessed with frozen section and requires a staged procedure for reconstruction. Surgical margins must be clear before proceeding with any reconstruction or rotational flap. Reexcision of positive margins after reconstruction is considerably problematic.

As noted previously, lip cancers have a propensity for local metastasis to the neck similar to other oral cavity malignancies. Elective neck dissection is not recommended for T1 or T2 lesions. For T3 and T4 lesions with N0 disease, ipsilateral or bilateral (for midline lesions) selective neck dissection (at least levels I-III) should be performed. Presence of any lymphadenopathy (either palpable or on imaging) necessitates neck dissection with or without contralateral neck dissection based on the location of the primary lesion.

Surgery is the preferred treatment modality for lip malignancies, but for poor surgical candidates radiation treatment is an alternative. Lesions that fail primary radiation treatment are recommended for salvage surgery. Adjuvant radiation can be used in the postoperative setting for adverse characteristics identified on the surgical pathology. These include primary lesions with positive margins, perineural or lymphovascular invasion, nodal disease with adverse features including multiple positive nodes, and perineural or lymphovascular invasion. Nodal disease with extracapsular spread is recommended for adjuvant chemoradiation treatment.[6] For patients with a single positive node without other adverse features, adjuvant radiation is optional.

Surveillance after treatment should follow standard National Comprehensive Cancer Network guidelines for oral cavity lesions.[6] This includes close follow-up for the first 5 years. Clinical examination should occur at least every 3 months in the first year, 4 months in the 2nd year, 6 months in years 3–5, and annually thereafter. Post-treatment imaging may be obtained as a baseline; additional surveillance imaging is not indicated unless there is clinical suspicion for recurrence.

Surgical Resection

Surgical planning for resection of lip lesions and reconstruction depends on both of the location and the size of the lesion. For any malignant lesion, the first priority is adequate oncologic resection. Margins of 5 mm are recommended for squamous and basal cell lesions. Melanoma lesions may require wider margins based on depth of invasion. Surgical planning is started preoperatively, but positive margins may necessitate more extensive resection than anticipated. Decisions for reconstruction are generally separated between upper lip and lower lip defects (Fig. 6.4). Within these categories, lesions can be divided into less than half of the width of the lip, one half to two thirds and greater than two

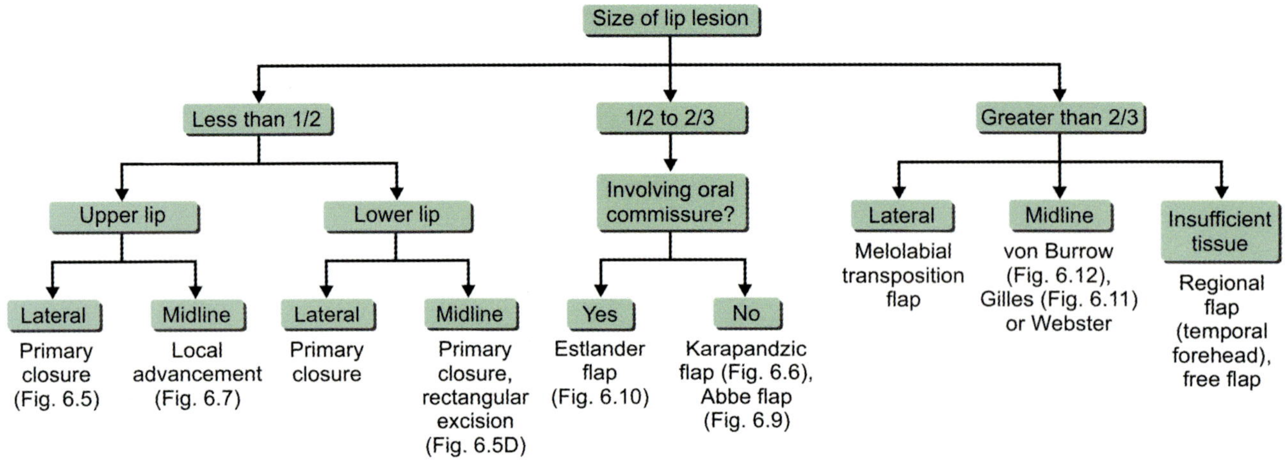

Fig. 6.4: Surgical reconstruction of lip lesions based on location and size.
Source: Adapted from Baker.[11]

thirds. For lesions less than one half of the lip width, generally primary closure can be performed. For lesions that are one half to two thirds, transposition flaps should be considered. Estlander flap for defects involving the commissure and Abbe flaps for those that do not. Larger defects usually require local advancement flaps, with variations depending on location. Similar principles can be applied for reconstruction of other lip deformities such as congenital lesions or traumatic defects.

Primary Closure

In the case of lesions that are less than half the width of the lip (excluding midline upper lip lesions), primary closure can be performed. This can be performed under sedation with local anesthesia. If general anesthesia is used, nasotracheal intubation should be considered to prevent distortion of the lip by pulling of the tube. This also allows freedom of manipulation of the lip without having an endotracheal tube secured around the lip. Perioperative antibiotics should be administered.

Incision planning should be performed prior to any local injection. Margins of 5 mm should be measured and marked. Melanoma lesions may require larger margins (0.5 cm for in situ, 1.0 cm for Breslow depth <2.0 mm, 2.0 cm for Breslow depth >2.0 mm).[6] Small lesions can be excised using a V wedge excision that will allow for simple primary closure (Fig. 6.5A). For lateral lesions, angling the lateral V incision can help reduce height mismatch when reapproximating midline and lateral vermillion (Fig. 6.5C). For wider lesions, a W wedge excision (Fig. 6.5B) is an option that reduces the length of normal tissue excised while still maintaining the width for adequate margins. A rectangular excision can also be performed for slightly larger lesions with relaxing incision laterally (Fig. 6.5D). Before incision and local injection, the vermillion border can be marked either with methylene blue or scored with a scalpel to assist with exact closure. This is extremely important for a satisfactory cosmetic result as even 1 mm misalignment of the vermillion border will be noticeable to the eye. Next local anesthesia can be applied; this should contain epinephrine to assist with hemostasis. The face and lip is prepped with betadine. The surgical field is draped such that the whole lip and philtrum are visible.

Excision should be made full thickness from the skin to the mucosa. Note that the labial artery runs circumferentially between the muscle (orbicularis oris) and the mucosa (*see* Fig. 6.1). After the specimen is removed, frozen sections should be taken of the margins. The margins on the specimens should be marked as well and oriented with at least two stitches.

Once margins are negative, a four-layer closure is performed. The key components of closure are a good multilayer closure and careful attention to the vermillion border for exact approximation. The four layers are the mucosa, muscle, subcutaneous layer, and skin. Chromic gut may be used on the mucosa, Vicryl for the muscle and subcutaneous tissue and interrupted 5-0 Prolene on the lip and skin. When addressing the vermillion border, it may be easiest to approximate the border first, using previous guide marks, before the rest of the lip or skin closure.

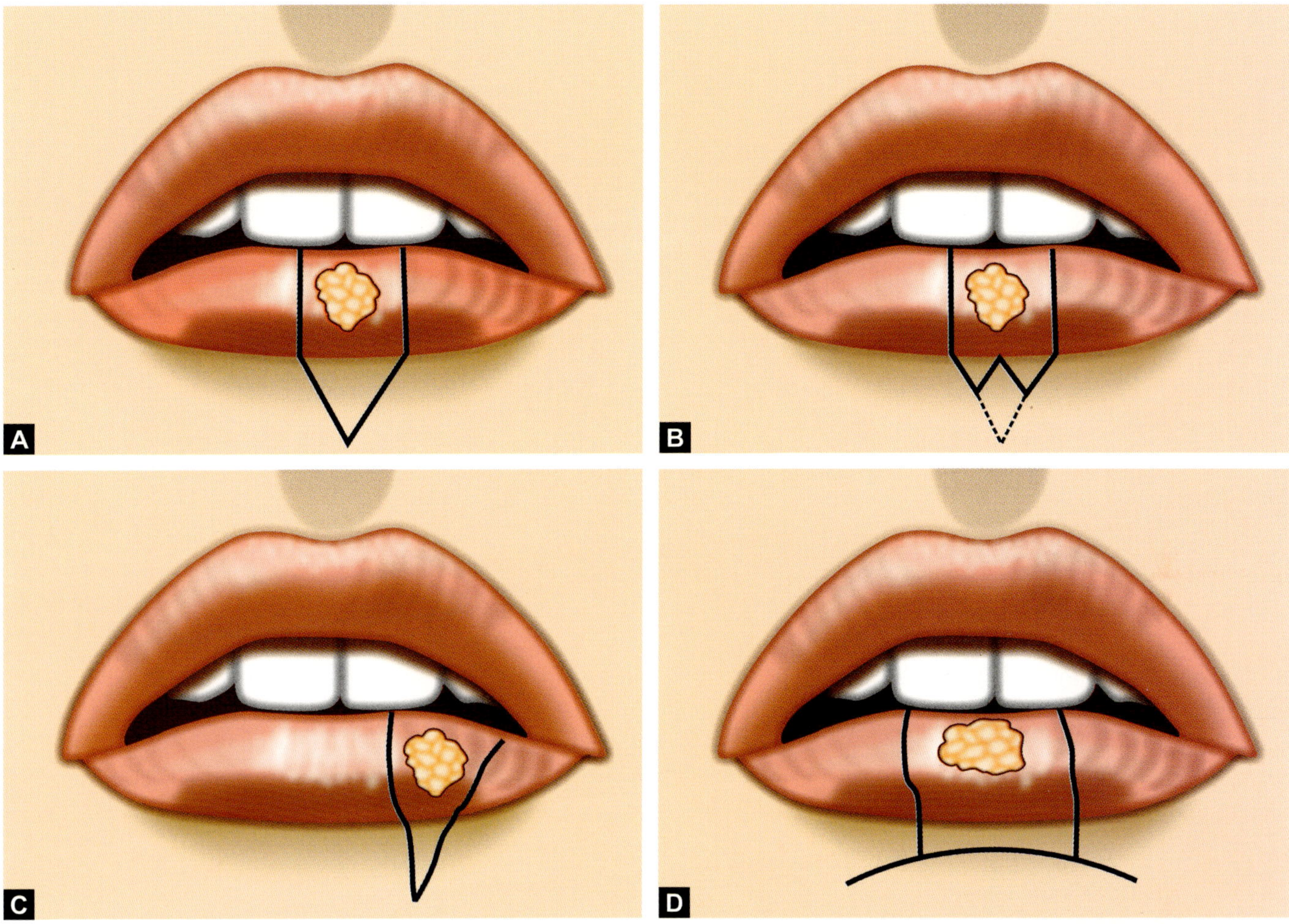

Figs. 6.5A to D: Primary closure incisions. (A) V excision. (B) W excision and reduction in tissue excised (shown in dotted lines). (C) For V excisions that are lateral, angling the lateral incision can correct for the height mismatch of the vermillion to allow better approximation. (D) For lower midline lesions, a rectangular excision may also be considered for large defects with relaxing cuts for closure. The inferior incision should lie along the labiomental crease.

Local Advancement

Local advancement can be considered for the closure of large midline lesions, particularly of the upper lip to prevent distortion of the nose. Bilateral advancement of tissue from the cheek can be performed to allow for adequate closure without tension.

For midline lesions of the lower lip, a rectangular incision is planned (Fig. 6.5D). Margins are marked and two incisions are planned perpendicular to the lip line and extended to the labiomental crease. A horizontal incision is planned along the labiomental crease. This incision should extend laterally on both sides with relaxing incisions to allow for advancement of the tissue for decreased tension on closure. In addition, Burrow's triangles can be created to assist with closure.

If more extensive advancement is required, this can be advanced from the cheek tissue using a Karapandzic flap (Figs. 6.6A to C). After rectangular excision of the lesion is made, the inferior incision is continued around along the nasolabial fold bilaterally. These skin incisions will cross over the labial vessels as they come in from the facial artery. It is important to stay superficial in the subcutaneous tissue to preserve these vessels (*see* Figs. 6.2 and 6.6B) as well as any facial nerve branches such as the buccal branch. One advantage of this flap is that it preserves both motor and sensation to the flap. However, there is a risk for microstomia (small mouth opening).

For large midline lesions of the upper lip, plan two parallel incisions at the excision margin defined by the oncologic resection up to the inferior border of the nose

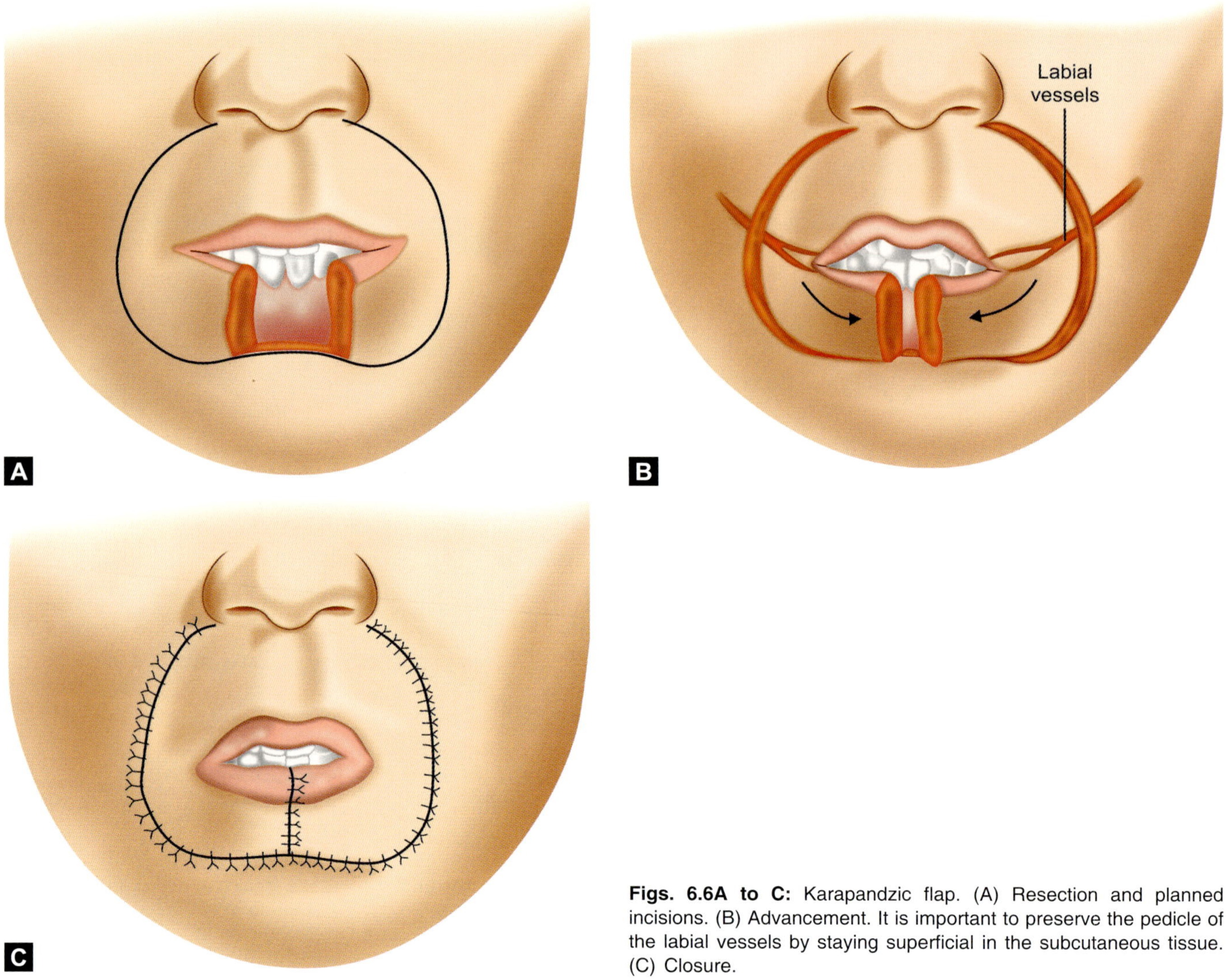

Figs. 6.6A to C: Karapandzic flap. (A) Resection and planned incisions. (B) Advancement. It is important to preserve the pedicle of the labial vessels by staying superficial in the subcutaneous tissue. (C) Closure.

(Figs. 6.7A to C). These are full thickness cuts down to mucosa. Then, an incision is placed across the inferior border of the nose; this step is important to prevent distortion of the nose. This is a variation of the rectangular excision. Next, perialar incisions are performed bilaterally. Tissue should be excised laterally in an arc shape or as a burrow's triangle. Excess tissue that needs to be excised can be estimated by pulling the remaining lip together. Undermining can be performed of the skin and subcutaneous tissue to allow for greater movement of tissue. Once adequate hemostasis is achieved, closure is performed with Burow's triangles or other tissue removed lateral to the ala on both sides to allow advancement and closure. Again four-layer closure should be performed. A similar technique can also be used to address lesions on or near the philtrum.

Lesions One-Half to Two-Thirds of the Lip: Abbe and Estlander Flaps

For lesions in which one-half to two-thirds the length of the lip width (generally up to 2 cm) needs to be resected, an Abbe or Estlander flap may be considered. The Estlander flap is for lesions involving the oral commissure and the Abbe flap for resections that do not extend to the oral commissure. These flaps are often referred to as "lip switch" flaps as they transpose tissue from one lip to the other. These are planned so that the borrowed flap is half the width of the resected lip defect, so that when the flap is switched over, upper and lower lip widths will be equal. These flaps can be used for both upper and lower lip defects.

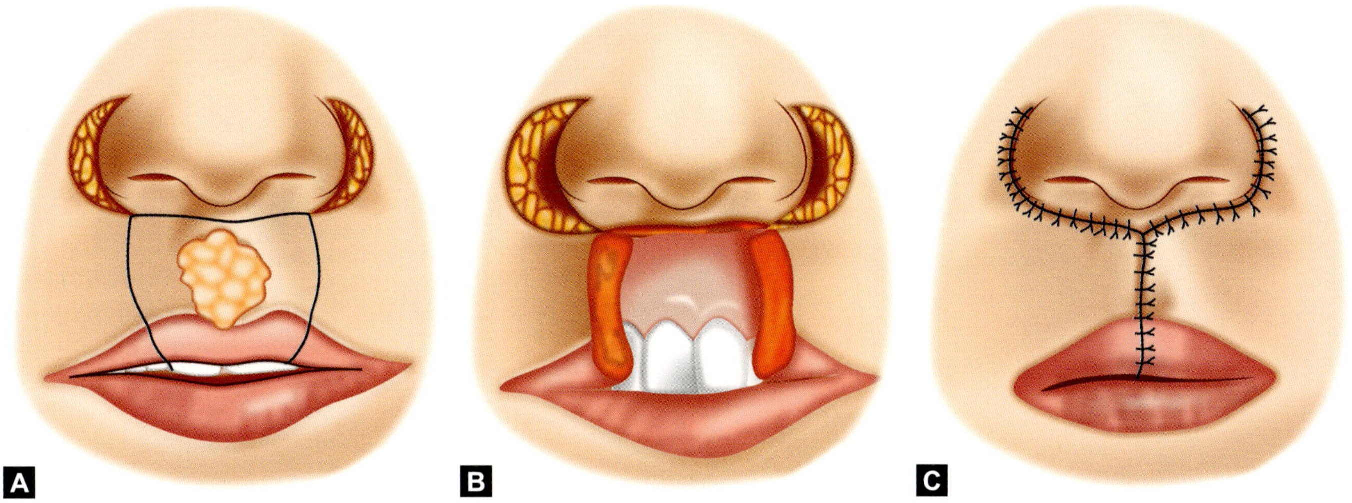

Figs. 6.7A to C: Local advancement flap for excision of midline upper lip lesions.
Source: Redrawn from Cupp et al.[12]

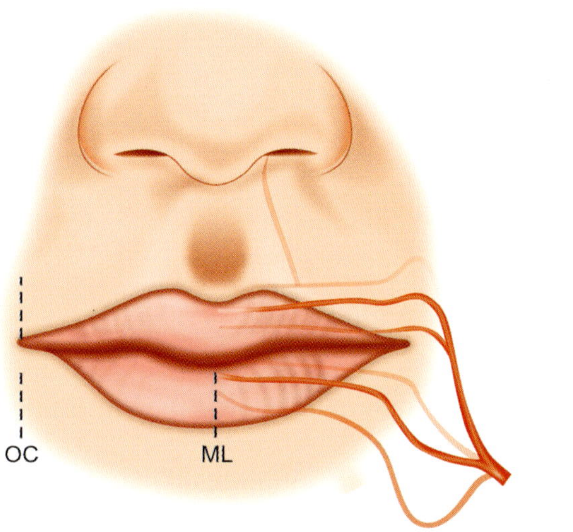

Fig. 6.8: Anatomic basis of Abbe and Estlander flaps. Path of superior and inferior labial arteries. Solid line shows average position with lightened line showing range with relation to the oral commissure (OC) and midline (ML).
Source: Redrawn from Schulte et al.[8]

These are local transposition flaps based off of the superior or inferior labial arteries (Fig. 6.8). Preservation of these arteries is very important for these procedures. Some surgeons use Doppler intraoperatively to confirm presence of the artery within the pedicle. Recall that the labial arteries branch off of the facial artery and generally lie in the plane between the mucosa and muscle. The superior labial artery may occasionally be found within the orbicularis oris muscle, but it is never superficial to the muscle. The labial arteries run within 1 cm of the vermilion border of the lip and tend to be closer (3–5 mm from the edge) toward the midline. These arteries usually run within the red lip and this can be an easy landmark to use, but laterally near the oral commissure the superior labial artery can lie outside the red lip.[8]

The Abbe flap was first described in 1898. It is for reconstruction of lip defects approximately one half to two thirds of the total lip width that do not involve the oral commissure (Figs. 6.9A to D). Margins are marked and planned for the excision of the lesion. A wide-based V wedge is planned for resection of the defect. Directly on the opposite lip, the lateral incision should be planned to extend across to the other lip to form the lateral edge of the donor flap. The donor flap should be designed so that it is half the width of the resected defect (Fig. 6.9A). The height of the donor flap should be slightly longer (1–2 mm) than the resected defect to allow for lengthening of the defect as its width is decreased. Once the lesion and margins are excised and margins are confirmed to be negative, incisions can be made for the donor flap. Full-thickness incisions are made through one side of the donor flap. On the other side, the flap should be freed until about 1 cm from the free edge of the lip. Care should be taken to avoid injury to the labial artery. On this edge of the flap, the skin of the red lip can be incised, but this incision should not go beyond the muscle. Mucosa can be divided as well, but this should be performed carefully as the labial arteries usually run just deep to the mucosa. Once the donor flap is freed, it can be inset by rotating the flap to the opposite lip defect (Fig. 6.9B). The donor flap site is closed primarily.

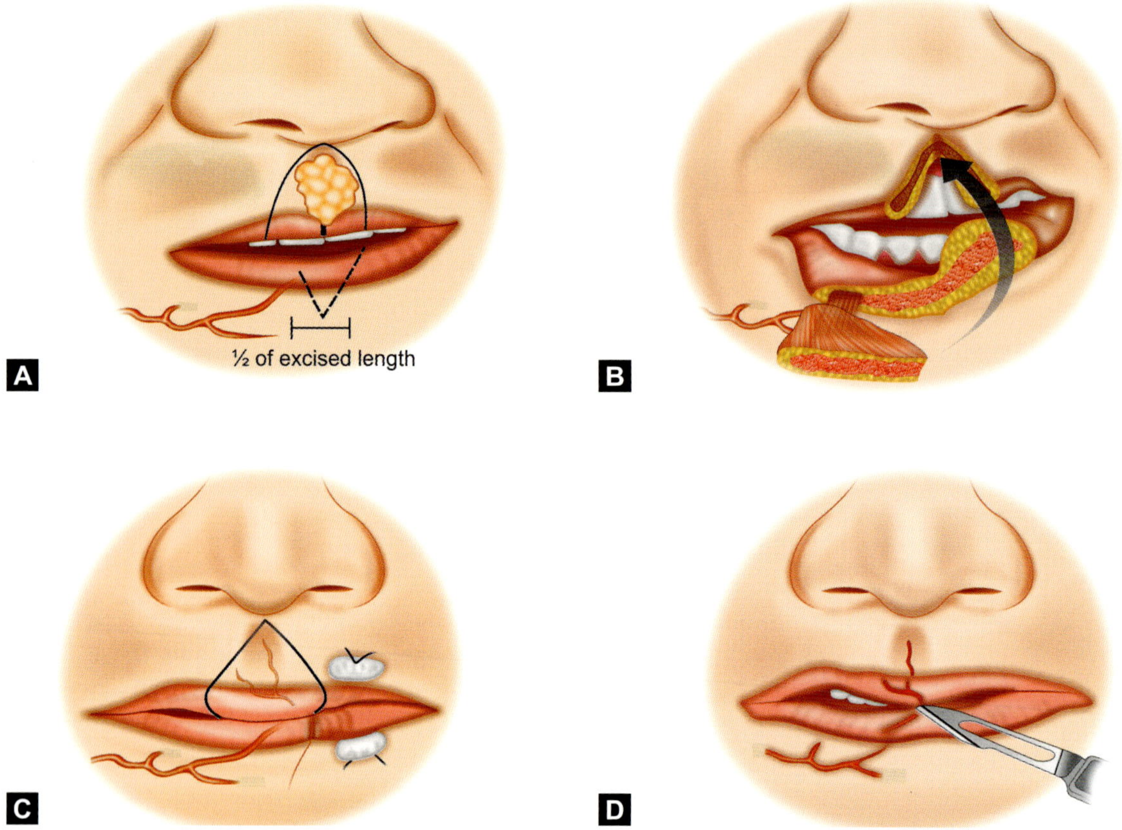

Figs. 6.9A to D: Abbe lip switch flap. (A) Marked excision of lesion with margins. Note opposite lip wedge is half the length of the excised defect. (B) The wedge is partially excised while preserving the vascular pedicle containing labial artery. (C) Wedge is inset into the opposite lip defect with primary closure of donor site. (D) Take down of vascular pedicle, at 2–3 weeks.

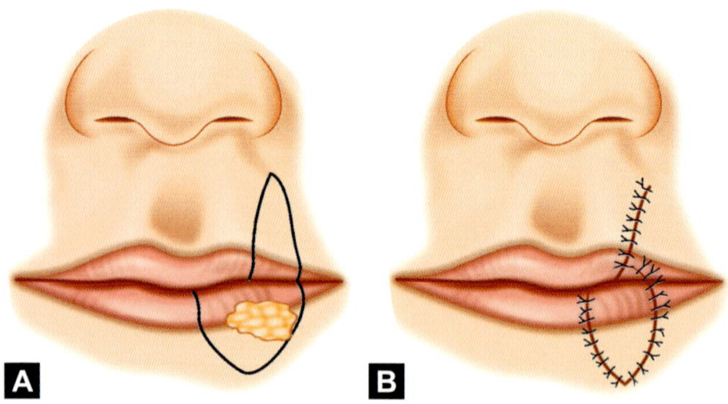

Figs. 6.10A and B: Estlander flap. (A) Planned incisions: donor wedge is half the width of resected defect and slightly taller in length. Incision crosses the oral commissure. (B) After closure.
Source: Redrawn from Cupp et al.[12]

Again layered closure and meticulous approximation of the vermillion border are performed. After the procedure, the patient's lips are tethered together. After 2-3 weeks, the pedicle may be taken down, and the lips are separated (Fig. 6.9D).

The Estlander flap is a variation of the Abbe flap for lesions near or involving the oral commissure. In this case, the lateral incision is made at the oral commissure (Figs. 6.10A and B). Again the lesion is removed with adequate margins and resected with a wide V excision. The donor flap is designed with a line continuing above the oral commissure. The flap again is designed to be half the width of the defect and with 1-2 mm more height (Fig. 6.10A). Incisions made in the skin and mucosa are made with care to preserve the labial artery blood supply to the pedicle. The pedicle is based off of the medial edge of the donor flap. Laterally, or near the oral commissure the labial arteries are not always within the red lip and may lie slightly farther from the lip edge (*see* Fig. 6.8). The flap is inset. No take down is required for this flap, but revision procedures may be performed as the newly formed oral commissure is usually blunted.

Other flaps may be considered for larger lesions that are greater than two thirds of the lip. These include the Gilles flap (Figs. 6.11A and B) and Burrow-Webster

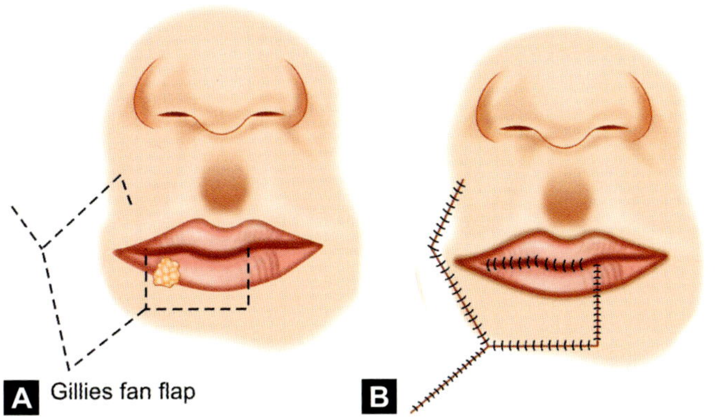

Figs. 6.11A and B: Gilles flap. This is a rhomboid nasolabial transposition flap.[13]

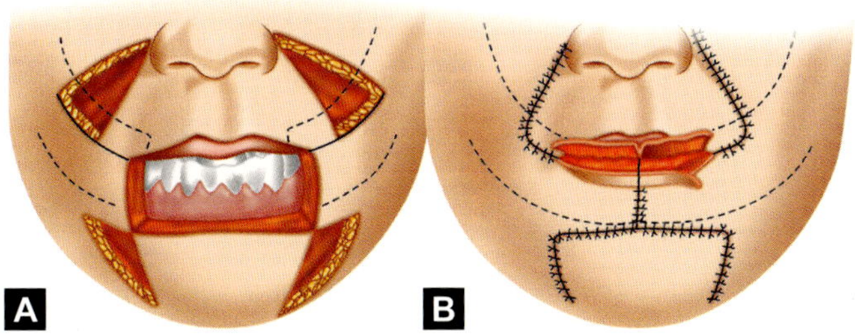

Figs. 6.12A and B: von Burrow flap with Webster modification. (A) This flap allows for nasolabial cheek advancement bilaterally for closure of a large lip lesion. Care should be taken to stay superficial and preserve the labial vessel pedicle from the facial artery, as in the Karapandzic flap (Fig. 6.6). (B) Closure with mucosal advancement flap for recreation of the vermillion.

(Figs. 6.12A and B). Larger lesions may require mucosal advancement flap (advancing mucosa of the vestibule to create a new vermillion) or free tissue transfer.

POSTOPERATIVE CARE

Postoperatively, care of the incisions as well as decreasing movement and tension on the lip help promote healing. Perioperative antibiotics are given for up to 1 week to prevent infection. Incision line should be cleansed with half strength hydrogen peroxide 2–3 times daily and moisturized with vasoline or antibiotic ointment. Sutures should be removed within 7–10 days but may be kept in longer for patients who are immunocompromised or have predictors of poor wound healing (such as diabetes, smoking). Postoperative diet should be liquid diet for at least 48 hours, then advanced to soft diet for one week to decrease tension on the lip by decreasing chewing and lip movement. Patients with pedicled flaps such as Abbe flap will have limited mouth opening and will require liquid diet through a straw until staged division of the pedicle at 2-3 weeks.

Some reconstructions will require staged procedures, such as those for melanoma as frozen sections cannot adequately diagnose negative margins. These wounds can be covered with xeroform or xeroform bolster and kept moist until staged reconstruction.

REFERENCES

1. Moore S, Johnson N, Pierce A, et al. The epidemiology of lip cancer: a review of global incidence and aetiology. Oral Dis. 1999;5(3):185-95.
2. Papadopoulos O Konofaos P, Tsantoulas Z, et al. Lip defects due to tumor excision: apropos of 899 cases. Oral Oncol. 2007;43(2):204-12.
3. Ferris RL, Gillman GS. Cancer of the lip. Myers Operative Otolaryngology: Head and Neck Surgery, 2nd edition, vol 1. Philadelphia: Saunders, Chapter 24;2008:183-93.
4. Vanderlei JP, Pereira-Filho FJ, da Cruz FA, et al. Management of neck metastases in T2N0 lip squamous cell carcinoma. Am J Otolaryngol. 2013; 34(2):103-6.
5. Vartanian JG, Carvalho AL, de Arujo Filho MJ, et al. Predictive factors and distribution of lymph node metastasis in lip cancer patients and their implications on the treatment of the neck. Oral Oncol. 2004;40(2):223-7.
6. Head and Neck Cancer; Oral Cavity (Version 2.2013). National Comprehensive Cancer Network Clinical Practice Guidelines. http://www.nccn.org/professionals/physician_gls/pdf/head-and-neck.pdf. Accessed July 14, 2014.
7. Casal D, Carmo L, Melancia T, et al. Lip cancer: A 5-year review in tertiary referral center. J Plast Reconstr Aesthet Surg. 2010;63 (12):2040-45.
8. Schulte DL, Sherris DA, Kasperbauer JL. The anatomical basis of the Abbe flap. Laryngoscope. 2001;111(3):382-6.
9. Platzer W. Section 5: Head and Neck. In: Color Atlas of Human Anatomy: Volume 1 - Locomotor System, 6th ed, Stuttgart, Germany: Thieme; 2009: 334-367.
10. Gooris PJ, Vermey B, de Visscher JG, et al. Frozen section examination of the margins for resection of squamous cell carcinoma of the lower lip. J Oral Maxillofac Surg. 2003; 61(8):890-4.
11. Baker SR. Chapter 24: Reconstruction of Facial Defects. In: Flint PW, Haughey BH, Niparko JK et al. Cummings Otolaryngology Head and Neck Surgery, 5th ed, Philadelphia, PA: Mosby/Elsevier; 2010: 342-63.
12. Cupp CL, Larrabee WF. Reconstruction of the lips. Oper Techn Otolaryngol Head Neck Surg. 1993;4(2):46-53.
13. Sajjadian A, Stadelmann WK, Tobin GR et al. Lip reconstruction Procedures Treatment and Management. Medscape; 2013.

CHAPTER

7

Floor of Mouth Resection

Sun M Ahn, Steven S Chang

RELEVANT ANATOMY

The floor of mouth is one of the many anatomical components that make up the oral cavity. The oral cavity is defined as the region bordered by the skin-vermilion junction of the lips anteriorly and the junction of the hard and soft palate as well as the line of the circumvallate papillae posteriorly. Along with the floor of mouth, the lips, the buccal mucosa, the alveolar ridges, the retromolar trigone, the anterior two thirds of the tongue, and the hard palate make up the oral cavity.

The floor of mouth is the mucosal surface located between the mandibular alveolus, the oral tongue, and the anterior tonsillar pillar posteriorly. In the midline is the lingual frenulum with Wharton duct orifices on either side. Deep to the floor of mouth mucosa lie a few critical structures in the space between the mylohyoid and the hyoglossus muscles. These include the sublingual gland, the Wharton duct, the lingual nerve superiorly, and the hypoglossal nerve deep (Fig. 7.1).

The lingual artery serves as the main blood supply, while the mandibular branch (V3) of cranial nerve V (the trigeminal nerve) gives sensory innervations through the lingual nerve. The superficial and anterior lymphatic plexus drains to both the ipsilateral and contralateral submental and submandibular nodes while deep and posterior lymphatics drain to ipsilateral level II nodes (Fig. 7.2).

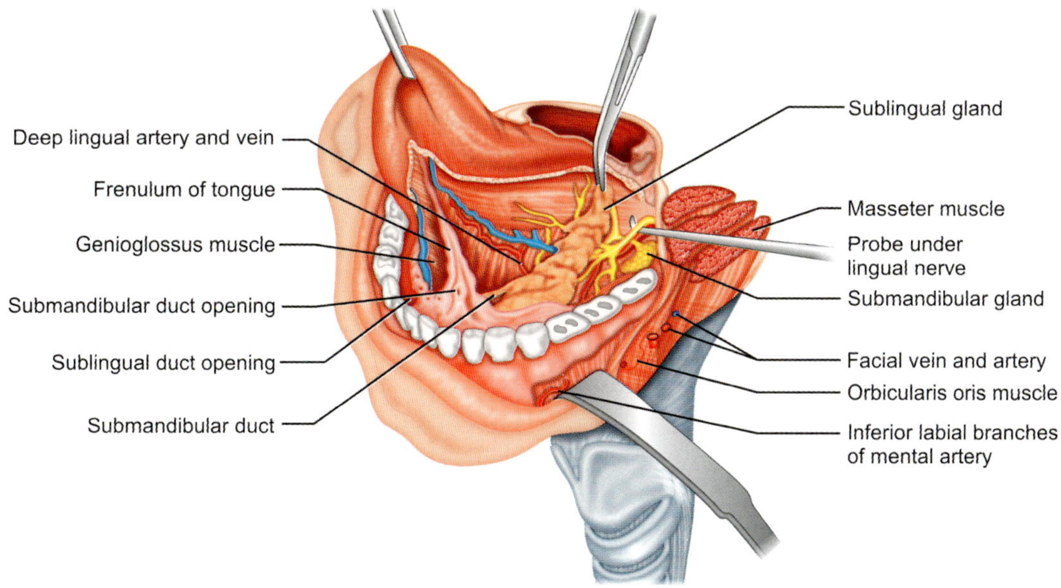

Fig. 7.1: Relevant anatomy of the floor of the mouth.

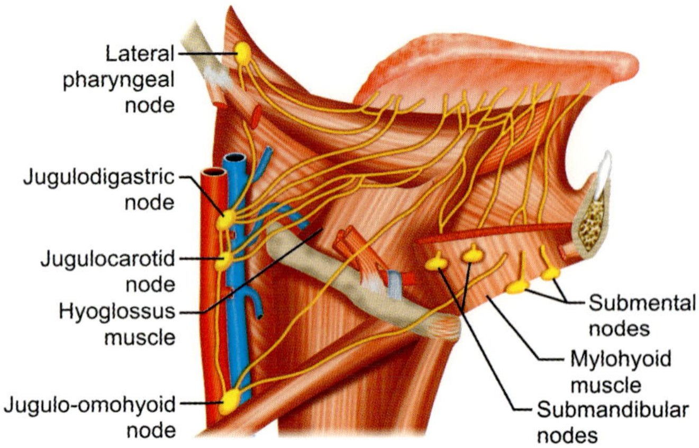

Fig. 7.2: Lymphatic drainage pattern of the floor of mouth.

SURGICAL CONSIDERATIONS

When discussing malignant neoplasms of the floor of mouth, the vast majority (>95%) are squamous cell carcinoma. Unlike other anatomic regions of the upper aerodigestive tract, malignancies of the floor of mouth are easily visible, making detection of early-stage lesions possible. Unfortunately, up to 50% of patients will present with locally advanced cancer at initial evaluation. Floor of mouth musculature, including hyoglossus, genioglossus, geniohyoid, and mylohyoid, serve as a barrier to the spread of tumor, and invasion of these muscles can lead to tongue hypomobility, fixation, dysarthria, and dysphagia.

When considering treatment strategy, the surgeon should consider two main goals of therapy—maximizing locoregional control of the tumor as well as the functional outcome with regard to speech and swallowing. Primary surgical management is the treatment of choice for floor of mouth malignancies. It affords good locoregional control, facilitates histopathologic staging, and minimizes long-term side effects of radiation therapy, including xerostomia, loss of taste, and trismus. In addition, due to the proximity of the mandibular arch to the floor of mouth, bone exposure and osteoradionecrosis of the mandible are potential devastating complications of using primary radiation therapy as curative treatment of floor of mouth malignancies.

Early-stage lesions without mandibular involvement may be resected transorally with adequate margin, and reconstruction can be achieved with primary closure, healing by secondary intention, or placement of split-thickness skin graft. Even for larger lesions not involving the mandible, anterior or lateral mandibulotomy is seldom used; instead, a pull-through technique can be used. If the tumor is closely approximated with the mandible, marginal versus segmental mandibulectomy should be considered depending on the degree of bony involvement. Advanced-staged tumors will likely require combined therapy with radical surgery followed by adjuvant radiation ± chemotherapy. Reconstructive options for advanced T-stage lesions include local or regional pedicled flap versus microvascular-free tissue reconstruction. Overall survival rates for early stages I/II are typically >80% and 40–70% for advanced stages III/IV.[1-3] The presence of nodal disease was the most significant prognostic factor of disease specific survival.[3]

SURGICAL TECHNIQUE

Transoral Excision and Split Thickness Skin Graft

This approach is best for cases that involve limited lesions of the floor of mouth that do not require marginal mandibulectomy. Careful preoperative evaluation is critical in determining the need for marginal mandibulectomy. The main indications for marginal mandibulectomy include the following: (1) the tumor is adherent to the periosteum; (2) the tumor abuts the mandible and resection of the alveolar process is necessary for adequate margin; and (3) the tumor crosses the mandible and involves the gingival buccal sulcus where resection of the alveolar process is required to obtain a third dimension on the tumor deep surface.[4]

The patient is placed in a supine position on the operating table. Perioperative antibiotics should be initiated prior to the start of the procedure. After induction of general endotracheal anesthesia, a thorough endoscopic evaluation of the upper and lower aerodigestive tract should be performed if it has not been completed already. If a split-thickness skin graft or a flap is the planned reconstructive option, a tracheostomy should be considered. Neck dissection can be performed prior to the excision of the tumor excision or delayed until after.

A Jennings mouth gag or a Doyen Jansen mouth gag is placed to provide adequate exposure. Additional mouth retractors, such as the Wieder retractor, are used to retract the buccal mucosa and the tongue. Alternatively, the tongue is retracted anteriolaterally toward the contralateral side by placing a suture in the anterior tongue in the midline. Adequate margin of at least 1 cm around the tumor is outlined using a marking pen, methylene blue, or cautery. The mucosal incision is made sharply with cutting current or a scalpel. It is best to place a marking suture at a designated orientation at this time. The soft tissue is carefully dissected, taking care to identify and ligate Wharton's duct as well as branches of the lingual artery and vein. The sublingual gland may be resected as part of the deep margin and a portion of the ventral tongue may be excised as part of the posterior-medial margin. After extirpation of the tumor, margins for frozen section analysis are selected and sent. If a close margin is identified, it is critical to excise additional tissue for permanent pathologic analysis and to examine additional margins. Finally, the wound is copiously irrigated and meticulous hemostasis is obtained.

Surgical defects from small, superficial lesions can be left open to granulate and heal by secondary intention. However, if the defect is larger and in areas essential to mobility of the tongue, coverage by split thickness skin graft can prevent the formation of fibrosis and scar contracture. Prior to harvesting a split thickness skin graft for reconstructing the floor of mouth defect, gowns, and gloves should be changed to prevent contamination of the donor site with oral secretions. A dermatome is used to harvest the split thickness skin graft in the desired dimensions. Using a pie-crusting technique, the skin graft is sutured to the floor of mouth mucosa using a 3-0 or a 4-0 chromic gut suture. Several tacking stitches are placed in the floor of mouth to assist in successful adherence of the skin graft to the underlying tissue. Finally, mesh gauze impregnated with petrolatum is used as a bolster and tacked down over the skin graft with nonabsorbable sutures. Meticulous hemostasis and immobilization are critical to optimal take and healing of the skin graft.

Transoral Excision with Marginal Mandibulectomy

If a marginal mandibulectomy is indicated based on preoperative and intraoperative evaluation, the resection should be done in an en bloc fashion with the floor of mouth specimen (Fig. 7.3). In edentulous patients, the vertical height of the mandible should be examined to assess the feasibility of marginal mandibulectomy. If the marginal mandibulectomy is included for the proper indications, it is necessary to resect only the alveolar process and not the body of the mandible. Thus, the vertical height is often adequate, even in edentulous patients, to preserve a 1 cm-thick segment of bone inferiorly.

Once optimal exposure has been obtained, the margin of the resection should be outlined on the mucosal surface of the alveolar process. The mucosal incision is made sharply down to bone, and mucoperiosteum is elevated inferiorly to facilitate exact osteotomy. Once the location of the osteotomy is identified, appropriate teeth extractions are completed. The vertical osteotomies should be made within the tooth socket or medial to it to provide adequate bone support to prevent future tooth loss and to allow eventual application of partial dentures. Vertical osteotomies are first made with a power saw and subsequently connected with a horizontal osteotomy. It is essential to ensure complete bicortical cuts through both the lingual and buccal plates prior to using an osteotome to prevent fracturing of the mandible. The free mandibular fragment is then resected with the rest of the floor of mouth specimen. Care is taken to smooth out any sharp edges or spicules at the remnant bony margin using a cutting burr. Finally, a split-thickness skin graft can be applied to provide coverage over both the cancellous and cortical bony portions of the remaining mandible. For patients who have had radiation therapy, vascularized reconstructive options should be utilized instead of the skin graft to minimize the risk of developing osteoradionecrosis.

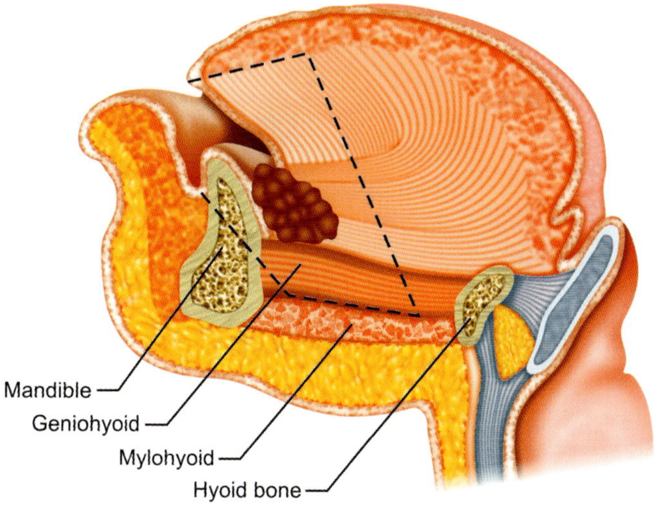

Fig. 7.3: Schematic drawing of transoral composite resection with marginal mandibulectomy.

Composite Resection with or without Segmental Mandibulectomy

For patients with advanced lesions (T3/T4) of the floor of mouth, a composite resection with or without mandibulectomy as well as ipsilateral versus bilateral neck

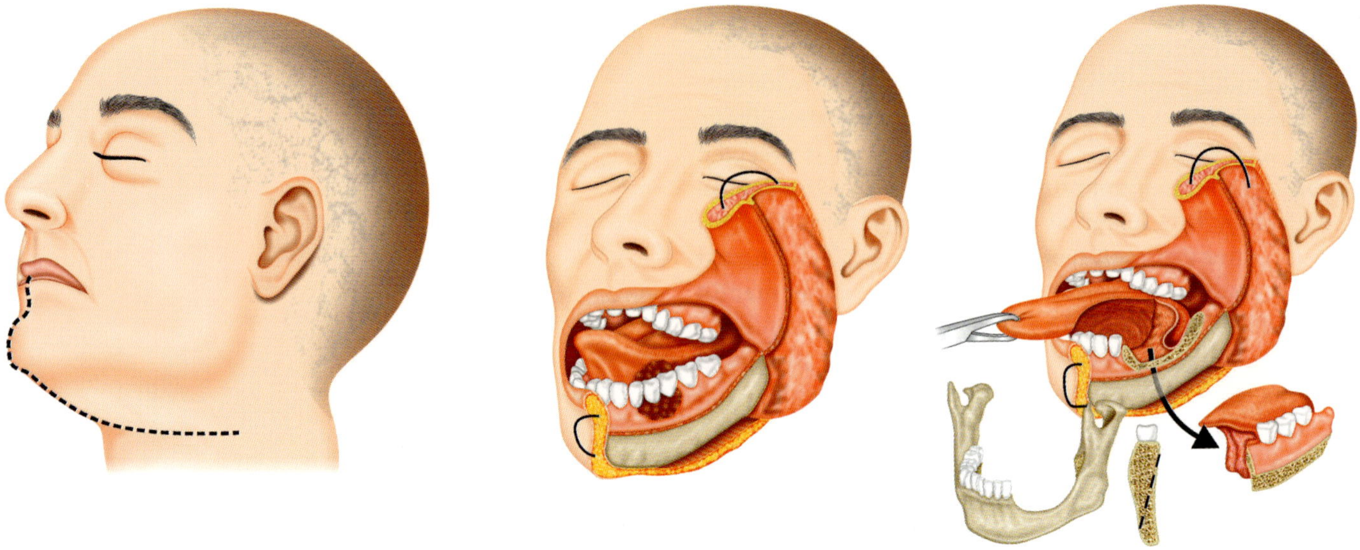

Fig. 7.4: The lip-splitting approach with marginal mandibulectomy.

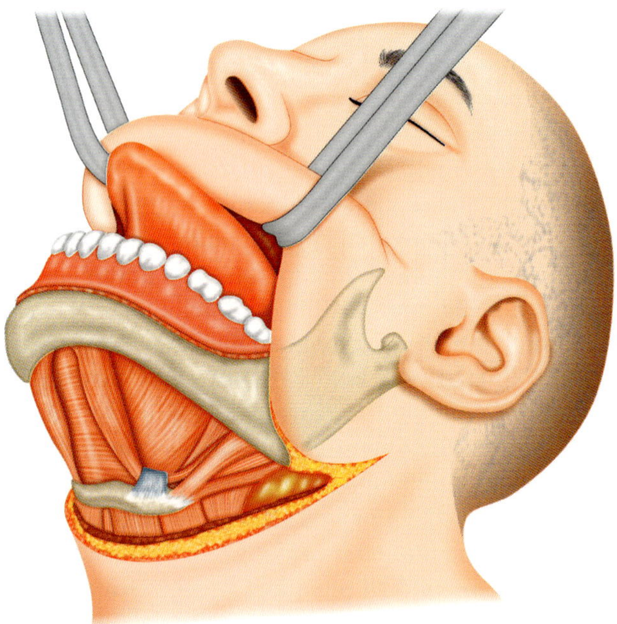

Fig. 7.5: The visor flap approach.

dissections will be required to achieve locoregional control. Transoral approach is difficult to resect large tumors with deep infiltration of the floor of mouth. Therefore, external approaches, such as a "pull-through" operation or midline mandibulotomy with a visor flap versus a lip-splitting incision, are optimal. Patients without bony invasion will require a similar approach with the addition of segmental mandibulectomy.

After a tracheostomy and an endoscopic evaluation are completed, a neck dissection is typically performed next, partly to help isolate the hypoglossal and lingual nerves as well as the branches of the external carotid artery, including the lingual and facial arteries. For anterior mandibulotomy, the ipsilateral submental cervical flap is continued as a lip-splitting incision located in the midline and around the crease of the menton (Fig. 7.4). The osteotomy site is plated prior to performing the bony cuts to achieve anatomic reduction and occlusion. Once the bone fragments are separated, floor of mouth musculature, including digastrics, mylohyoid, and geniohyoid muscles, is transected to expose the deep aspect of the floor of mouth. When making the mucosal cut along the lingual surface of the alveolus, the goal of the surgeon is to obtain adequate margin around the tumor while preserving enough cuff of mucosal tissue to facilitate later reconstruction and closure. The en bloc tumor extirpation can now be carried out in a three-dimensional fashion by approaching it from both the transcervical and transoral angles. For any involvement of the tongue, a partial or subtotal glossectomy is performed. If possible, at least one of the neurovascular bundles should be preserved without compromising the oncologic resection.

Anterior mandibulotomy can be combined with a visor flap, which is cosmetically superior to the lip-splitting incision (Fig. 7.5). While ideal for lesions involving the anterior aspect of the floor of mouth, the lip-splitting approach may provide better access to more lateral and posterior lesions. It is also important to preserve any uninvolved mental nerve, which is at an increased risk of injury with the visor flap. The visor flap is first started with a single transverse cervical incision along a natural skin crease that extends from the one mastoid tip to the other mastoid tip. The cervical subplatysmal flap is continued superiorly to the mandible. Here, marginal mandibular nerve should be preserved through direct identification or through careful elevation of the fascia overlying the submandibular gland containing the nerve branch. The periosteum is elevated off the mandible from angle to angle, again taking care around the mental nerves. Mucosal incision is made in the gingivobuccal sulcus from angle to angle and connected to the elevated periosteal incision made from the cervical approach. Finally, penrose drains are used to elevate and retract the soft tissue off the mandible to accommodate for osteotomies.

For patients with locally aggressive tumors involving the mandible, a segmental mandibulectomy should be planned. The indications for segmental mandibulectomy include the following: (1) gross invasion by the tumor; (2) tumor invasion of the inferior alveolar nerve or canal; and (3) edentulous patients in whom marginal mandibulectomy is not feasible. The initial approach is as described earlier with a lip-splitting approach or visor flap approach. After exposing the mandible and extracting teeth, vertical osteotomies are performed using a power saw. Accessing the tumor from both transoral and transcervical approaches, the floor of mouth tumor is excised with the bony segment (Fig. 7.6). Bone marrow from the remaining mandibular fragments is sent for frozen section analysis to check the margin status. Reconstruction of the mandible is best achieved with an osteocutaneous free flap reconstruction with microvascular anastomosis immediately following the tumor extirpation. However, if the patient is a poor candidate for free flap reconstruction, an alternate option would be to place a titanium plate across the bony defect and to reconstruct the floor of mouth with a pectoralis major myocutaneous flap.

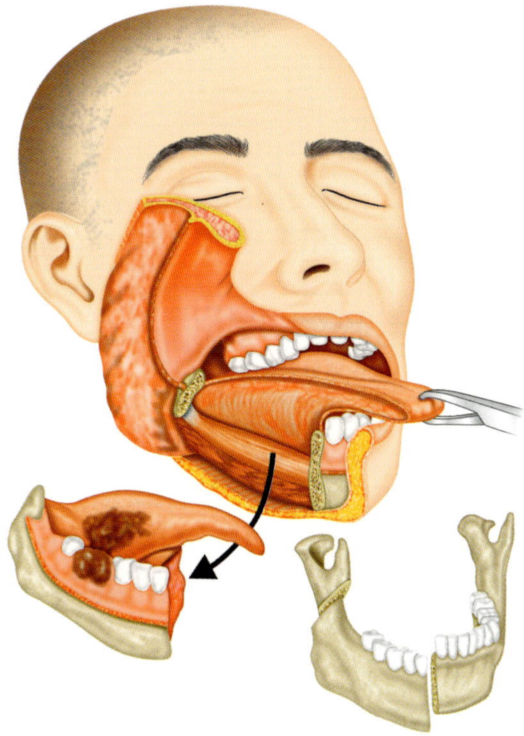

Fig. 7.6: A composite resection with segmental mandibulectomy.

Lymphatic Spread and Neck Dissection

Floor of mouth squamous cell carcinoma is characterized by a high risk of metastases to cervical lymph nodes, and uncontrolled neck disease is a common cause of treatment of failure regardless of the modality of therapy. The presence of pathologic metastatic lymph node is a significant prognostic factor and reduces survival in these patients. The incidence of occult metastases in oral squamous cell carcinoma ranges from 14% to 45%.[5-9] Therefore, elective neck dissection in patients with clinical N0 disease of the floor of mouth is recommended for certain high-risk features, which include depth of invasion, lymphatic or vascular invasion, perineural invasion, and grade/size of the primary lesion. However, studies have failed to show survival benefit of elective neck dissection compared to observation in early T1-T2N0 squamous cell carcinoma of the oral tongue and floor of mouth.[3,9-11] Thus, some advocate that N0 patients may be observed and followed closely with the neck treated for subsequent development of neck disease, especially in patients who can be followed closely with frequent examination and/or imaging.

When looking at the distribution of nodal metastases in patients with floor of mouth squamous cell carcinoma with positive neck dissection specimens, majority of patients had multiple levels involved. Most commonly involved levels were levels I and II, and levels III and IV were less involved. Only about 0–5% of patients had posterior triangle metastases (level V), usually in conjunction with disease higher in the neck.[1,12] Lesions near or crossing the midline present with an increased risk of bilateral or contralateral metastases.[13]

REFERENCES

1. Shaha AR, Spiro RH, Shah JP, et al. Squamous carcinoma of the floor of the mouth. Am J Surg. 1984; 148(4):455-9.
2. Rodgers LW Jr, Stringer SP, Mendenhall WM, et al. Management of squamous cell carcinoma of the floor of mouth. Head Neck. 1993;15(1):16-9.
3. Sessions DG, Spector GJ, Lenox J, et al. Analysis of treatment results for floor-of-mouth cancer. Laryngoscope. 2000; 110(10):1764-72.
4. Rao LP, Shukla M, Sharma V, et al. Mandibular conservation in oral cancer. Surg Oncol. 2012;21(2):109-18.
5. Yuen AP, Wei WI, Wong YM, et al. Elective neck dissection versus observation in the treatment of early tongue carcinoma. Head Neck. 1997;19(7):583-8.
6. Dias FL, Kligerman J, Matos de Sá G, et al. Elective neck dissection versus observation in stage I squamous cell carcinomas of the tongue and floor of mouth. Otolaryngol Head Neck Surg. 2001;125(1):23-9.
7. Pimenta Amaral TM, Da Silva Freire AR, Carvalho AL, et al. Predictive factors of occult metastasis and prognosis of clinical stages I and II squamous cell carcinoma of the tongue and floor of mouth. Oral Oncol. 2004;40(8):780-86.
8. D'Cruz AK, Siddachari RC, Walvekar RR, et al. Elective neck dissection for the management of the N0 neck in early cancer of the oral tongue: need for a randomized controlled trial. Head Neck. 2009;31(5):618-24.
9. Kelner N, Vartanian JG, Pinto CA, et al. Does elective neck dissection in T1/T2 carcinoma of the oral tongue and floor of mouth influence recurrence and survival rates? Br J Oral Maxillofac Surg. 2014; 52(7):590-97.
10. Fakih AR, Rao RS, Borges AM, et al. Elective versus therapeutic neck dissection in early carcinoma of the oral tongue. Am J Surg. 1989;158(4):309-13.
11. Yuen AP, Ho CM, Chow TL, et al. Prospective randomized study of selective neck dissection versus observation for N0 neck of early tongue carcinoma. Head Neck. 2009;31(6): 765-72.
12. Dias FL, Lima RA, Kligerman J, et al. Relevance of skip metastases for squamous cell carcinoma of the oral tongue and the floor of the mouth. Otolaryngol Head Neck Surg. 2006; 134(3):460-65.
13. Dias FL, Lima RA. Cancer of the floor of the mouth. Oper Tech Otolaryngol. 2005;16(1):10-17.

CHAPTER

9

Composite Resection

Jason YK Chan, Eddy WY Wong, Alexander C Vlantis

BACKGROUND AND HISTORY

Initially, the management of oral cancer followed the concept of managing breast cancer described by Halsted in which the tumor and the lymphatic drainage was removed.[1] The concept of permeative spread of malignant cells along lymphatics was well understood at that time.[2] Later, the concept of oral cancer management was expanded to include the resection of the primary tumor en bloc with the cervical lymph nodes and the intervening tissue in order to remove lymphatics through which metastases passed.[3] In this context, the intervening tissue was the mandible and this was based erroneously on the historical assumption that lymphatics from the oral cavity passed through the periosteum of the mandible to the neck so that in-transit metastases could be resected by removing the intervening mandible.[4] Marchetta et al. subsequently showed that mandibular involvement by tumor occurred only when there was direct invasion of the periosteum.[5] Further, it was policy at the time to resect the mandible purely for adequate exposure to the posterior part of the tongue, tonsil, and pharynx, the disfigurement caused by the loss of the mandible being offset by the excellent exposure and the thoroughness of the resection.[3]

A composite resection is a procedure that involves the resection of a segment the mandible in continuity with an adjacent cancer of the oral cavity or oropharynx and a neck dissection. Composite means being made up of unlike or distinct parts. A composite resection was previously known as a "COMMANDO" operation, which was an acronym for a COMbined MANDibulectomy and Neck Dissection Operation—an en bloc resection of a primary oral cavity or oropharyngeal tumor, cervical lymph nodes, and part of the mandible, a term that has been attributed to Hayes Martin.

INDICATIONS

A composite resection is indicated for advanced tumors of the oral cavity and oropharynx that abut, involve, or encase the mandible and is done in conjunction with a neck dissection as an en bloc surgical resection. In addition, extensive osteoradionecrosis of the mandible may sometimes require a composite resection and reconstruction as definitive management.

PHYSICAL EXAMINATION

The oral cavity and oropharynx must be thoroughly inspected and palpated to get an accurate impression of the extent of the local disease, and to determine which sites and structures are and are not involved by the tumor. This includes the clinical assessment of the presence of mandibular involvement or not. The challenges are twofold: firstly, to determine if the mandible is involved by tumor and if so, then secondly to determine to what extent. Involvement of the gingiva and loose dentition are suggestive of mandibular involvement. Healthy teeth are a barrier to mandibular invasion, while loose teeth or an edentulous mandible are less so, especially if the occlusal surface is involved. Palpation of the tumor, which may be painful, in relationship to the mandible may give an idea as to its mobility or fixity to the mandible, a fixed tumor being more likely to involve the mandible. Finally, paresthesia of the lower lip may suggest mandibular involvement.

IMAGING

Imaging is essential to stage the local and regional disease. Magnetic resonance imaging (MRI) is the modality of choice for soft tissue assessment. To determine mandible involvement, both computer tomography (CT) and MRI are poorly sensitive for detecting minimal bone involvement. A significant amount of bone mineral must be lost before radiographic evidence of bony invasion is apparent. CT is commonly employed as an imaging modality and can identify gross bony involvement; however, studies have suggested that findings on CT do not correlate well with histological findings.[6] The DentaScan is a software program that reformats CT images for closer inspection of buccal and lingual mandibular cortices and has been suggested to have improved accuracy in the preoperative evaluation of mandibular invasion.[7,8]

MRI is useful in detecting bone invasion, particularly if the medulla is involved by tumor. However, MRI has a high false-positive rate for this.[9] Positive emission tomography (PET) with CT may be useful in selected patients; however, the poor resolution and false-positive rate from local inflammation make its sensitivity for tumor inadequate.[10]

In addition to the determining the extent of bone resection, consideration must be given to its reconstruction as part of the preoperative workup. Attention should be given to the components of the defect needing reconstruction. For a segmental resection of the mandible, the fibula free flap is ideal for its reconstruction. When two skin paddles are needed for a through-and-through buccal defect, a scapula flap or alternatively a double-free flap, a fibular and anterolateral thigh flap, for example, could be considered. Prior to harvesting a fibula free flap, care must be taken to examine the peripheral vascular system of the leg for peripheral vascular disease (PVD) and abnormal vascular anatomy. Magnetic resonance angiography is similar to digital subtraction angiography in its accuracy in demonstrating PVD and abnormal anatomy and is non-invasive.[11] Computer tomography angiography may alternatively identify aberrant vascular anatomy and stenoses.[12] Anecdotal evidence of Monckeberg calcific stenosis on plain X-rays will eliminate the need for further investigation and indicates that microvascular reconstruction is not feasible. Other alternative flaps include the scapula free flap, particularly if two skin paddles are needed as mentioned, the osteocutaneous radial forearm free flap and the iliac crest free flap.

SURGICAL PROCEDURE

The patient is placed under general anesthesia and perioperative antibiotics are given. A tracheostomy is performed to secure the airway in the postoperative period and a fine bore nasogastric feeding tube placed and secured. If prolonged nonoral feeding is anticipated, a percutaneous endoscopic gastrostomy may be done. The patient is thoroughly re-examined under anesthesia to finalize the extent of surgery. The oral cavity is cleaned and rinsed, and the patient prepped and draped and incisions marked.

The general concept of the extent of resection: if the tumor is near to but does not abut or involve the periosteum, then the periosteum can be taken as a margin; if the tumor involves the periosteum but not the mandibular cortex, then the mandibular cortex can be taken as a margin as a marginal mandibulectomy;[1-7] and if the tumor involves the mandible cortex, or arises from the gingival ridge mucosa—allowing for invasion of bone through the vascular channels of teeth roots[13]—then the segment of mandible is resected as a segmental mandibulectomy. If the extent of the mandible involvement cannot be made preoperatively, then intraoperative periosteal stripping to assess the mandible cortex and/or frozen section examination of the periosteum has been shown to be accurate in determining mandibular invasion. This is employed to determine the type and extent of resection needed.[14]

Marginal Mandibulectomy

A clinical decision is made to determine the type of marginal mandibulectomy needed, be it an inner table mandibulectomy, an alveolar ridge or superior rim mandibulectomy, or an outer table mandibulectomy. A marginal mandibulectomy is the resection of a portion of the mandible that does not result in a segmental defect.

With mouth retractors in place, a penetrating towel clamp or a silk suture placed in the midline of the tongue roughly 1 cm posterior to the tip can be used to retract the tongue. Ideally, 1-1.5 cm of normal tissue is marked around the tongue or floor of mouth tumor with a needle tip cautery, methylene blue or a marking pen, with the resection extending to the gingivobuccal sulcus or even onto the buccal mucosa if needed.

Mucosal incisions are made with the needle tip cautery setting on "cut" and the wound deepened with the setting on "coagulation" to aid hemostasis. Over the mandible the incision is carried through the mucoperiosteum and onto the bone and a periosteal elevator used to elevate the mucoperiosteum to expose the bone and the precise place for mandibular osteotomies determined.

In a dentate patient, two teeth may need to be extracted to allow for two vertical osteotomies to be placed through

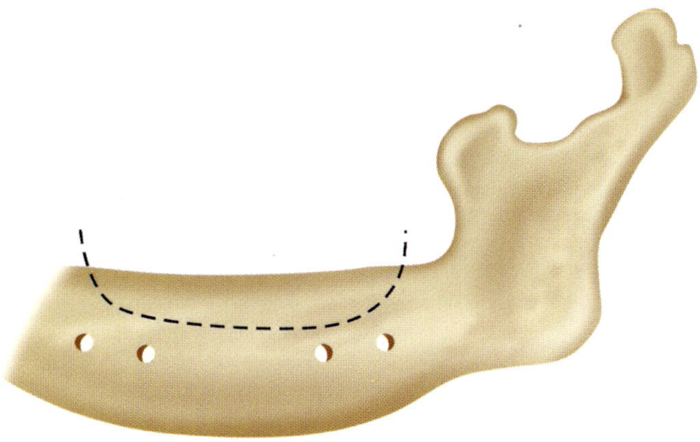

Fig. 9.1: Illustration demonstrating a mandible with the dotted line representing a curvilinear anterior marginal mandibulectomy.

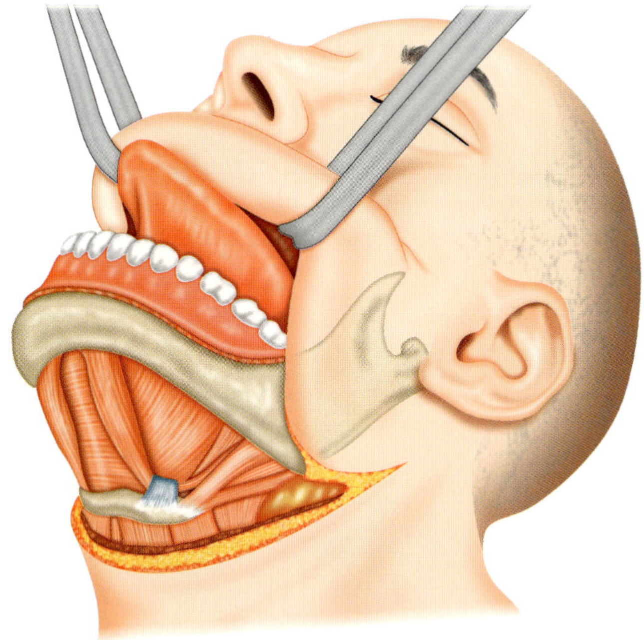

Fig. 9.2: Visor flap raised from left to right mastoid tip.

the dental sockets, thereby leaving enough bone for the adjacent teeth sockets to be preserved, preventing loosening of the teeth from a lack of bony support if the osteotomies were made too close to the tooth socket.

The osteotomies are performed with either a microsaw or focused ultrasound blade. A beveled osteotomy (Fig. 9.1) is preferentially performed as this increases the strength of the residual mandible, as opposed to right-angled osteotomies that increase the stress and strain on the remnant mandible.[15,16] Care must be taken to adequately cut through both the lingual and buccal cortex. If this is inadequate the mandible may fracture when the alveolar ridge fragment is separated from the remaining cortex. In addition, at least 11 mm of residual mandibular bone height must remain to prevent a postoperative mandibular fracture; otherwise the mandible should be reinforced with a titanium plate.

Once the bony segment is mobile, the extirpation is completed with sharp and blunt dissection deep to the tumor on the floor of mouth and tongue. The pathological specimen is then oriented appropriately with sutures. Frozen specimens are sent. Hemostasis is achieved and osteotomies are smoothed with a drill or rasp to prevent postoperative bone exposure. Reconstruction of the area will be further discussed below.

Segmental Mandibulectomy

For lateral lesions, a horizontal upper neck incision is usually made a minimum of two finger breadths below the inferior edge of the mandible in a suitable skin crease. For exposure of the mandible anteriorly, a visor flap drawn from mastoid tip to mastoid tip may be used to approach a lesion in the anterior oral cavity. When using this approach, and prior to entering the oral cavity, the intraoral mucosal incisions should be made, which facilitates the intraoral exposure and prevents the inadvertent incision into the tumor or the creation of inadequate resection margins. The intraoral gingivobuccal sulcus incision needs to cross to the contralateral gingivobuccal sulcus to provide adequate superior retraction of the flap for adequate exposure. Careful blunt dissection is used to connect the internal incisions with the external incisions and care is taken not to compromise resection margins. The primary advantage of the visor flap is the avoidance of a scar of the lip and chin. However, this does result in extensive devascularization of the mandible as the periosteum is widely stripped from the mandible, and both mental nerves are divided, resulting in unfavorable lower chin anesthesia. Lastly, there is significant disruption of lymphatic drainage of the skin flaps, resulting in more superior flap edema postoperatively than with other exposures (Fig. 9.2).

An alternative is the lower lip-splitting approach. Rather than running from mastoid tip to mastoid tip, the incision curves superiorly at the midline to extend across the submental, chin and lip area (Fig. 9.3). Intraorally this incision does not need to extend to the contralateral gingivobuccal sulcus and has the advantage of preserving the contralateral mental nerve and

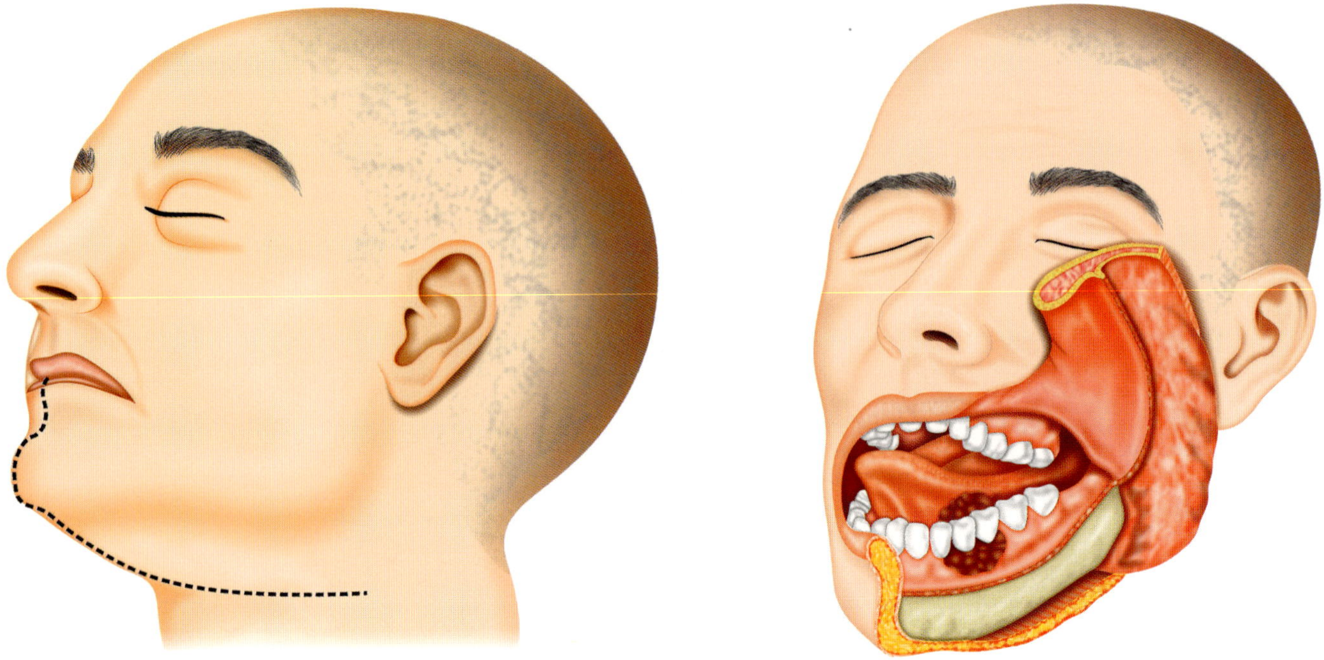

Fig. 9.3: Lip-split approach to the composite resection.

periosteum while providing wide exposure, which is preferred by most surgeons.

When raising either flap, care is taken to preserve the marginal mandibular nerve and, if possible, the facial artery, which is particularly useful as a donor artery in microvascular reconstruction. For lesions of the oral cavity, most surgeons prefer to remove perifacial lymph nodes and directly identify and preserve the marginal mandibular nerve to prevent its injury. It may not be feasible to preserve the marginal mandibular nerve in all situations; for example, if tumor is found to involve tissue lateral to the buccal cortex of the mandible, both the marginal mandibular nerve and facial artery may need to be sacrificed to achieve an adequate oncological resection.

Once adequate exposure of the mandible and tumor has been achieved and with the buccal cortex of the mandible exposed, both anterior osteotomy and posterior osteotomy sites can be marked with at least a 2-cm margin of resection on either side of the tumor. This then allows for the placement of a prefabricated reconstruction plate for postablative reconstruction. If the lateral extent of the tumor or the presence of a primary mandibular tumor results in the reconstruction plate not being accurately placed, an external fixating device can be used to maintain the correct occlusion. Figures 9.4A and B demonstrate a completed lip-split approach composite resection and a prefabricated reconstruction bar placement, respectively.

The osteotomies are then performed. Teeth that will have their roots exposed adjacent to the osteotomy sites are removed. The anterior osteotomy is made first and then the posterior osteotomy. This provides a free mandible segment, permitting easier oncologic resection of the tumor. The location of the posterior cut depends on the tumor. If the ramus is not involved then the osteotomy can be placed below the sigmoid notch; if involved, then the resection needs to be above the sigmoid notch and include the coronoid process with part of the temporalis tendon. Disarticulation of the temporomandibular joint is avoided if possible, and the native condyle preserved and used in the reconstruction. Care must be taken when performing osteotomies of the ramus not to injure the internal maxillary artery by placing a malleable retractor medial to the osteotomy site. The inferior alveolar artery will also be encountered when cutting through the ramus, but injury to it can be minimized by performing the osteotomy close to the sigmoid notch.

With both osteotomies completed the tumor will be readily visible; however, the temptation to retract the segment of mandible too forcefully must be resisted to avoid inadvertent tearing of the specimen. Mucosal incisions can now be made around the tumor in the oral

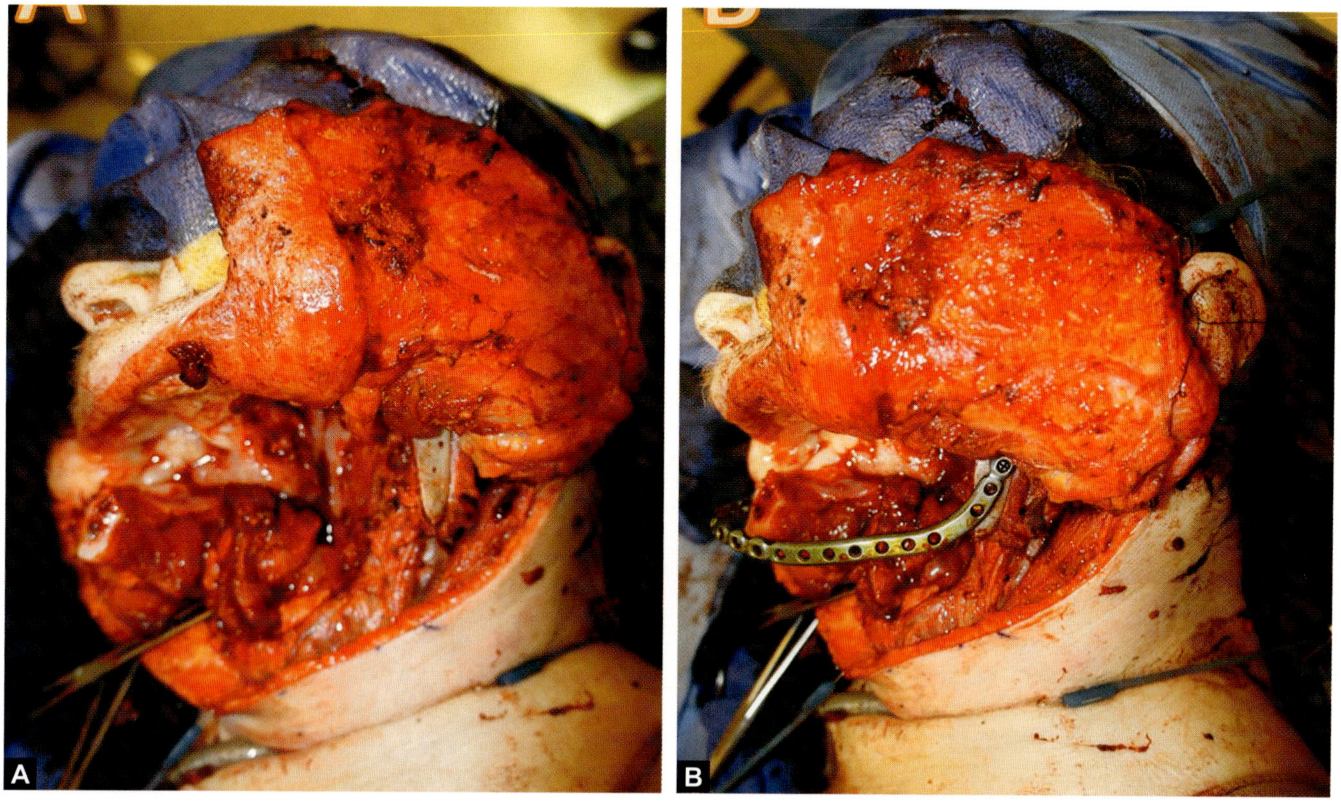

Figs. 9.4A and B: (A) Lip-split approach with composite resection tumor removed. (B) Prebent reconstructive bar placement prior to free flap reconstruction.

cavity. This may involve the soft palate superiorly; the pterygoid musculature, in particular the medial pterygoid muscle; and the branches of the mandibular division of the trigeminal nerve. Care must be taken within this region to protect the carotid artery posteriorly since it is likely that bleeding from the pterygoid venous plexus will obscure the field, and hemostasis should be adequately achieved before further resection in this region continues. Branches of the internal maxillary artery will also be encountered and will need ligation. Figure 9.5 shows a completed composite resection, and Figure 9.6 shows the resected specimen. Figure 9.7 is a schematic representation of a composite resection without neck dissection.

Once the resection has been completed, frozen margins are sent, appropriate orientation of the specimen is performed, the wound is irrigated and hemostasis ensured, and reconstruction of the defect is commenced.

RECONSTRUCTION OF THE DEFECT

Reconstruction of the defect has been important for functional and aesthetic rehabilitation. There is also a need to close the intraoral wound to cover exposed bone to prevent osteomyelitis and to prevent the oral cavity from contaminating the neck wound, as a wound infection will delay adjuvant therapy if needed. Following ablative resection and confirmation that the surgical margins are clear on frozen section, the wound is washed, and gloves and instruments are changed, reconstruction can then begin.

Primary Closure

When soft tissue loss is minimal and the defect small, it can be closed primarily, which is relatively simple and is a traditional technique. However, with healing there may be scarring resulting in tethering of the tongue, which may significantly affect speech and swallowing and therefore primary closure is rarely used in both marginal and segmental mandibulectomy resections.

Split Thickness Skin Graft

Split thickness skin grafts (STSGs) can be used for defects involving a marginal mandibulectomy. The exposed cancellous bone provides an adequate vascular supply for the

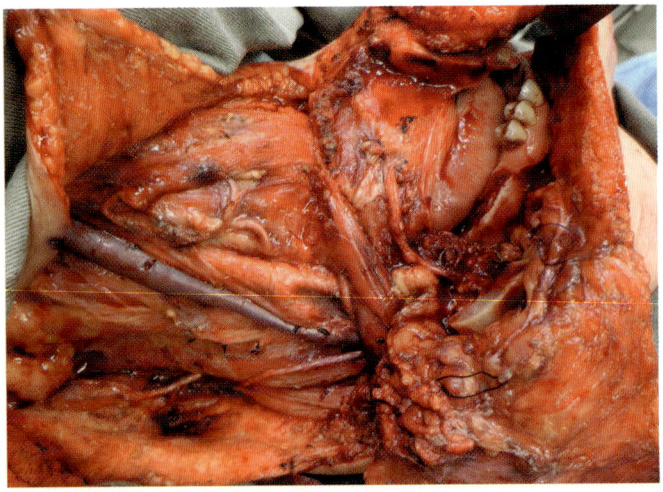

Fig. 9.5: Picture of a surgical defect after composite en-bloc resection of a 3 cm × 3 cm left retromolar trigone/buccal carcinoma, segmental mandibulectomy with preservation of the arch and upper ramus of the left mandible, and an extended modified radical neck dissection (the anterior belly of digastric was also resected).

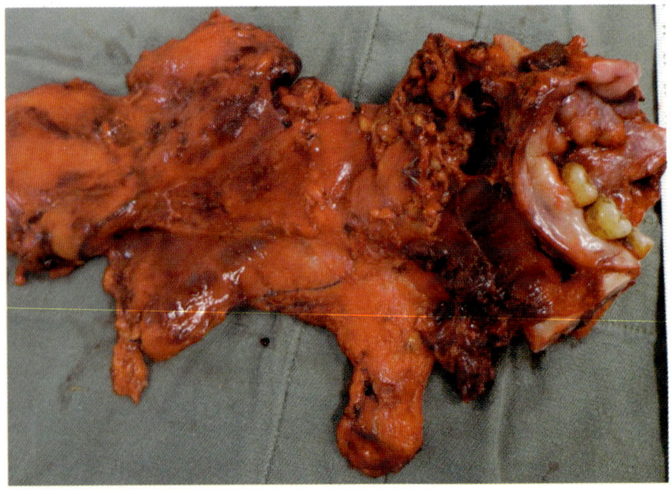

Fig. 9.6: This photograph shows the surgical specimen of a composite en-bloc resection of a 3 cm × 3 cm left retromolar trigone/buccal carcinoma, segmental mandibulectomy, and modified radical neck dissection.

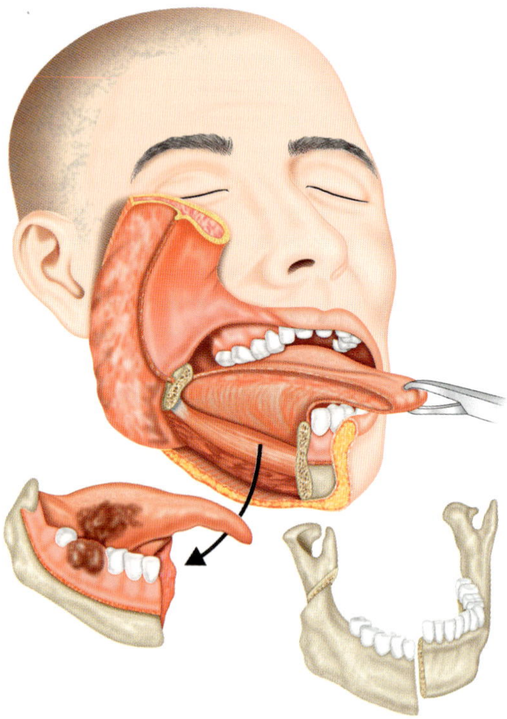

Fig. 9.7: Schematic representation of a composite resection through a lip-splitting approach without the attached neck dissection.

skin graft. A thickness of 4.3 mm. is typically used and the graft is sutured to the surrounding mucosa with absorbable sutures and pie crusting done, whereby small incisions are made in the graft. The graft is then bolstered with Xeroform (antiseptic impregnated) gauze sutured down with silk ties that allow contouring of the skin graft to the defect and also creates a watertight closure. However, care must be taken if the tissue has been previously irradiated or irradiation is anticipated as wound complications are more likely.[17,18]

Local Flaps

In a previously irradiated or an anticipated irradiated field, vascularized tissue would preferentially be used to close the defect. Local pedicled flaps that can be considered for this purpose include inferiorly based nasolabial flaps, island platysma flaps with STSG,[19] infrahyoid fasciocutaneous flaps,[20] facial artery musculomucosal flaps,[21] and mylohyoid advancement flaps.[22] However, these are not widely used.

Regional Myocutaneous or Myofascial Flaps

The most widely used pedicled flap is the pectoralis major flap that is based on the thoracoacromial artery; this flap may include chest wall skin for a myocutaneous flap or muscle only for a myofascial flap. The goal of the flap is to provide vascularized tissue for bulk, improved cosmetic appearance, coverage of the carotid artery and coverage of reconstruction plates. Consequently this flap is very useful in composite resections needing a segmental mandibulectomy and in patients not suitable for a free flap reconstruction.

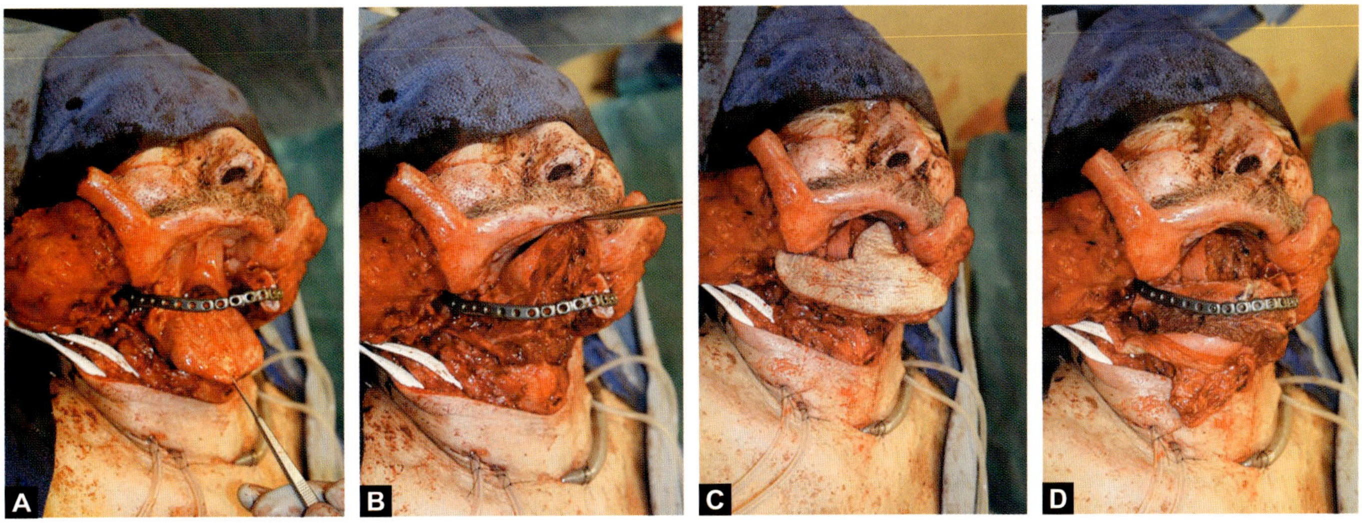

Figs. 9.8A to D: (A) Reconstructive bar in place following reconstruction with the remnant tongue retracted inferiorly. (B) Tongue retracted superiorly demonstrating resection on inferior aspect of togue onto. (C) Skin paddle of fibula free flap with anterior projecting skin paddle to prevent tethering of the tongue. (D) Fibula free flap bone attached to reconstructive bar with monocortical screws and skin paddle folded inferiorly prior to inset.

Microvascular Free Flap Reconstruction

Free flap reconstruction plays an important part in both marginal and segmental mandibulectomy defects. In marginal mandibulectomy defects that have been previously irradiated, the radial forearm free flap may be selected to provide pliable vascularized tissue to the cover the soft tissue and bony defect and to prevent tongue tethering. For segmental mandibular defects, the fibula free flap is typically used. It provides good bone stock for implants and allows osteotomies to be performed that accurately contour the flap to the mandibular defect, while also providing adequate soft tissue coverage as can be seen in Figures 9.8A to D. Three-dimensional planning is now available, and with the use of prebent plates and cutting guides, it further improves the reconstruction result.[23] Alternative flaps that may be considered include the anterolateral thigh flap (which has become a workhorse of the head and neck reconstructive surgeon as it allows for two teams to be operating simultaneously), the rectus abdominis myocutaneous flap, and the scapula free flap.

Postoperative Management

The patient is monitored closely postoperatively for 24–48 hours. Careful management of the drains is important. Regular chest physiotherapy and suctioning of the trachea is necessary, regardless of sputum production. Bolsters for STSGs are kept in place for 5 days and then removed. Free microvascular flaps require regular monitoring, hourly for the first 24 hours, with Doppler ultrasound and skin paddle monitoring to detect flap congestion, which is an indication to re-explore the wound and check on the vascular anastomoses, which may have to be redone in order to save the flap. Perioperative antibiotics are continued for 24 hours.

The drains can start to be removed after 48 hours as long as the output is <30 mL/24 h, leaving one drain adjacent to the closure until a gastric diet is commenced.

Feeding is via a nasogastric or percutaneous endoscopic gastrostomy tube. Mouth care is avoided for the first 72 hours. A clear liquid diet can be introduced on day 5 if the drains show no sign of a leak. Bolsters are removed from the skin grafts and the patient is advanced to a full-liquid diet. Decannulation can begin 72 hours after surgery, first changing to an uncuffed tube and followed by capping or spigotting of the tracheostomy once bolsters are removed and the patient tolerates capping or spigotting with appropriate monitoring of oxygen saturation.

COMPLICATIONS

Marginal Mandibulectomy

A mandibular fracture is the major complication that occurs with a marginal mandibulectomy. Care must be taken during the resection to perform a curved osteotomy, that an adequate remnant and mandibular height is left, and that forceful prying of mandibular fragments is avoided. If there is any concern, then the mandible should be reinforced with a titanium plate to prevent a future mandibular fracture.

Segmental Mandibulectomy

An orocutaneous fistula is one major complication of a composite resection involving a segmental mandibulectomy. Most cases can be managed with local wound care and continued nonoral feeding via a feeding tube. However, more severe cases may require further surgery and vascularized tissue such as a pectoralis major flap placed to ensure wound closure or to reduce wound size.

Complications such as malocclusion, nonunion, or malunion may occur if care is not taken when insetting the fibula free flap, when it is important to ensure that occlusion is maintained and that there is adequate bony contact. Longer-term care involves the placement of dental implants, which must be done with minimal stripping of the periosteum, especially after adjuvant therapy, as bone necrosis may occur from overaggressive stripping.

REFERENCES

1. Slaughter DP, Roeser EH, Smejkal WF. Excision of the mandible for neoplastic diseases; indications and techniques. Surgery. 1949;26(3):507-22.
2. McGregor AD. A classic paper revisited—Polya and von Navratil (1902). Head Neck Surg. 1987;9(6):325-8.
3. Ward GE, Robben JO. A composite operation for radical neck dissection and removal of cancer of the mouth. Cancer. 1951;4(1):98-109.
4. Jay O, Boyle EWS. Oral cavity cancer. In: Jatin P, Patel S (eds.). Cancer of the Head and Neck. Shelton, CT: PMPH; 2001. p. 112.
5. Marchetta FC, Sako K, Murphy JB. The periosteum of the mandible and intraoral carcinoma. Am J Surg. 1971;122(6): 711-13.
6. Gu DH, Yoon DY, Park CH, et al. CT, MR, (18)F-FDG PET/CT, and their combined use for the assessment of mandibular invasion by squamous cell carcinomas of the oral cavity. Acta Radiol. 2010;51(10):1111-19.
7. Brockenbrough JM, Petruzzelli GJ, Lomasney L. DentaScan as an accurate method of predicting mandibular invasion in patients with squamous cell carcinoma of the oral cavity. Arch Otolaryngol Head Neck Surg. 2003;129(1):113-17.
8. Talmi YP, Bar-Ziv J, Yahalom R, et al. DentaCT for evaluating mandibular and maxillary invasion in cancer of the oral cavity. Ann Otol Rhinol Laryngol. 1996;105(6):431-7.
9. Vidiri A, Guerrisi A, Pellini R, et al. Multi-detector row computed tomography (MDCT) and magnetic resonance imaging (MRI) in the evaluation of the mandibular invasion by squamous cell carcinomas (SCC) of the oral cavity. Correlation with pathological data. J Exp Clin Cancer Res. 2010;29:73.
10. Babin E, Desmonts C, Hamon M, et al. PET/CT for assessing mandibular invasion by intraoral squamous cell carcinomas. Clin Otolaryngol.2008;33(1):47-51.
11. Klein S, Van Lienden KP, Van't Veer M, et al. Evaluation of the lower limb vasculature before free fibula flap transfer. A prospective blinded comparison between magnetic resonance angiography and digital subtraction angiography. Microsurgery. 2013;33(7):539-44.
12. Ribuffo D, Atzeni M, Saba L, et al. Clinical study of peroneal artery perforators with computed tomographic angiography: implications for fibular flap harvest. Surgical and radiologic anatomy: SRA. 2010;32(4):329-34.
13. McGregor IA, MacDonald DG. Spread of squamous cell carcinoma to the nonirradiated edentulous mandible—a preliminary report. Head Neck Surg. 1987;9(3):157-61.
14. Brown J. Mechanisms of cancer invasion of the mandible. Curr Opin Otolaryngol Head Neck Surg. 2003;11(2):96-102.
15. Melugin MB, Oyen OJ, Indresano AT. The effect of rim mandibulectomy configuration and residual segment size on postoperative fracture risk: an in vitro study. J Oral Maxillofac Surg. 2001;59(4):409-13; discussion 413-4.
16. Ertem SY, Uckan S, Ozden UA. The comparison of angular and curvilinear marginal mandibulectomy on force distribution with three dimensional finite element analysis. J Craniomaxillofac Surg. 2013;41(3):e54-58.
17. Deleyiannis FW, Dunklebarger J, Lee E, et al. Reconstruction of the marginal mandibulectomy defect: an update. Am J Otolaryngol. 2007;28(6):363-6.
18. Alvi A, Myers EN. Skin graft reconstruction of the composite resection defect. Head Neck. 1996;18(6):538-43; discussion 543-4.
19. Pogrel MA. Anterior floor of mouth resection with marginal mandibulectomy. Atlas Oral Maxillofac Surg Clin North Am. 1997;5(2):37-54.
20. Deganello A, Manciocco V, Dolivet G, et al. Infrahyoid fascio-myocutaneous flap as an alternative to free radial forearm flap in head and neck reconstruction. Head Neck. 2007;29(3):285-91.
21. Ayad T, Kolb F, De Mones E, et al. Reconstruction of floor of mouth defects by the facial artery musculo-mucosal flap following cancer ablation. Head Neck. 2008;30(4):437-45.
22. Sawhney R, Young L, Ducic Y. Mylohyoid advancement flap for closure of composite oral cavity defects. Laryngoscope. 2011;121(11):2313-16.
23. Stirling CE, Yuhasz M, Shah A, et al. Simulated surgery and cutting guides enhance spatial positioning in free fibular mandibular reconstruction. Microsurgery. 2015;35(1): 29-33.

CHAPTER

10

Mandibulotomy

Ryan Orosco, Steven S Chang

INTRODUCTION

The mandibular "swing" via vertical osteotomy and lip split was first proposed by Roux in 1836 for access to the oral cavity and oropharynx.[1] Variations were later described by Sedillot,[2] vonLangenbeck,[3] Billroth,[4] and Trotter.[5] Hayes Martin popularized the median labiomandibulotomy as a variation on the theme.[6]

Today, surgical access to the oral cavity and pharynx can be achieved through a variety of techniques including lingual release, lateral or transhyoid pharyngotomy, and mandibulotomy, as well as endoscopic and robotic techniques. Lingual release and other transoral techniques avoid osteotomy and may be advantageous in select cases of patients with an atrophic mandible or to avoid facial incisions as with a lip split. Pharyngotomy approaches offer direct access to the oropharynx and larynx, but come with the risk of pharyngocutaneous fistula and the added morbidity associated with disruption of pharyngeal musculature. Endoscopic approaches compromise the manual dexterity afforded by open surgery, and may be inadequate when dealing with large tumors or when considerable retraction is required. Although the role of robotic surgery is likely to continue to expand, mandibulotomy will remain an important surgical technique whenever increased exposure is required to access and effectively excise tumors of the oral cavity, oropharynx, parapharyngeal space, and more rarely the nasopharynx and skull base.

In cases that necessitate mandibulotomy, improved intraoperative exposure comes with additional risk of postoperative complications related to the wound, dentition, osteotomy site, bony integrity, and added dissection through the floor of the mouth. Importantly, mandibulotomy can have comparable esthetic and functional outcomes when compared to transoral approaches.[7]

INDICATIONS AND PATIENT SELECTION

Relevant Anatomy

After the trigeminal nerve divides into its three major segments, the inferior alveolar nerve branches off of the mandibular nerve (CN V3). It travels medial to the mandibular ramus and enters the mandibular foramen before running in a canal through the body of the mandible. The nerve exits at the mental foramen where it supplies sensory innervation to the lower lip, gingiva, and chin (Figs. 10.1A and B). In dentate patients, the foramen is halfway between the upper and lower borders of the body of the mandible, and between the two premolars.

Mandibulotomy can be lateral to the inferior alveolar foramen (lateral approach) or medial to the mental foramina (medial approach). Lateral mandibulotomy is rarely used today due to the risk of nonunion and osteoradionecrosis (ORN), which arise from division of the inferior alveolar artery[8] and periosteal vessels.[9] Additionally, lateral osteotomies divide the inferior alveolar nerve, causing bothersome paresthesia of the ipsilateral chin, jaw, and gingiva. Medial osteotomies are generally preferred, and they should always be made with respect to the mental foramen.

Patient Evaluation

The history, physical, and radiographic assessment is aimed at choosing the optimal surgical approach to provide the best chance for success. Decisions regarding the selection of transoral, transmandibular, or transcervical approaches depend on the tumor location, unique patient factors and surgeon experience. Understanding the

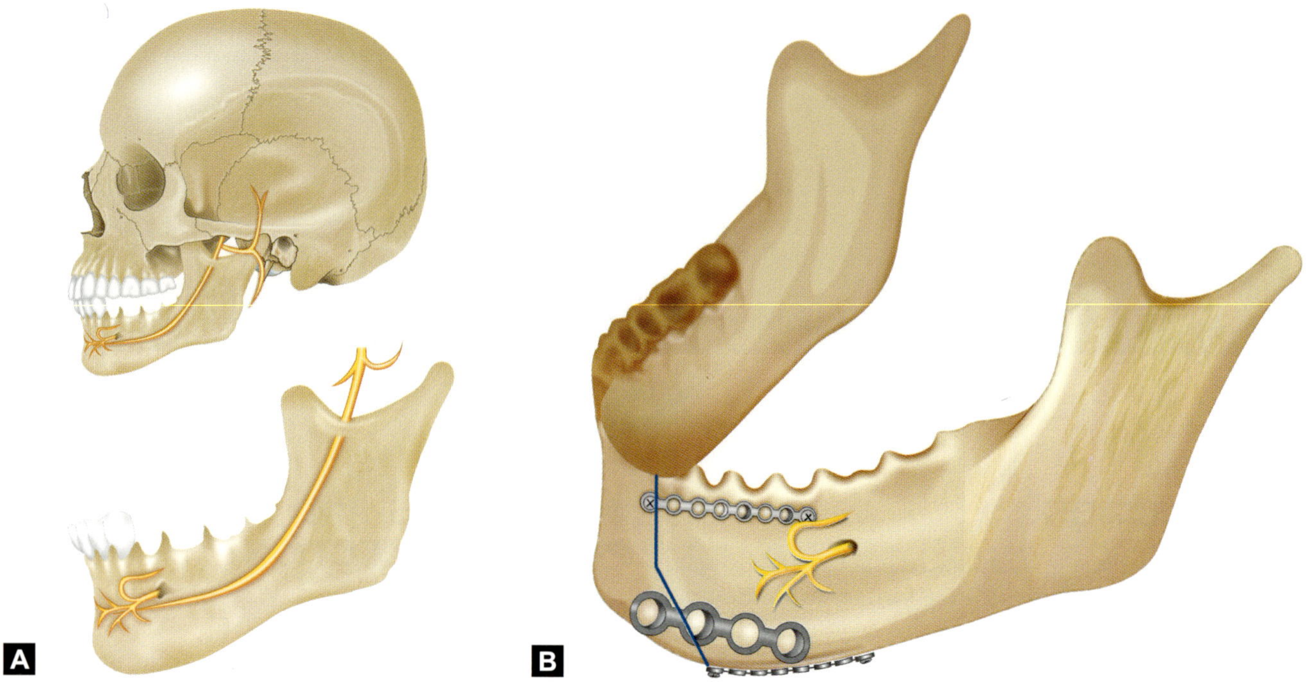

Figs. 10.1A and B: (A) The inferior alveolar nerve branches from the mandibular nerve (CN V3) and runs medial to the mandibular ramus. It enters the mandibular foramen on the medial cortex and runs through the mandibular body before exiting at the mental foramen where it supplies sensory innervation to the lower lip, gingiva, and chin. (B) Medial osteotomy geometry. Reconstruction plates are placed away from the infraorbital nerve.

strengths and limitations of all of the surgical options will help guide the selection for operative approach.

Anterior tumors are well-suited for mandibulotomy, but for tumors that extend posteriorly and inferiorly into the pharynx, exposure requires more dissection and exposure becomes compromised. In some cases, transcervical exposure may be combined with mandibulotomy in order to access the parapharyngeal space.[10] Neck adiposity may limit or impinge on exposure through transcervical pharyngotomy routes. Trismus can prevent transoral resections and even mandibulotomy. If osteotomy is undesirable, a lingual release approach can be employed to provide access to tumors in many of the same subsites of the oral cavity and pharynx.[11]

If mandibulotomy is chosen as the optimal approach, any history of mandibular trauma and prior hardware fixation is carefully noted. The patient's dentition and occlusion are documented, and particular attention is paid to anterior mandibular teeth. Missing or nonviable incisors are ideal for the placement of medial osteotomies. Mandibulotomy should be avoided in patients with an atrophic mandible or prior radiation therapy due to the increased risk of nonunion, ORN, or fracture. The presence of CN V3 paresthesia, tumor fixed to the mandible or adjacent to tooth roots or loose teeth may indicate osseous invasion and mandibulotomy should be supplanted by mandibulectomy.

Radiographic imaging is used to better define the tumor location, extension, and relationship with surrounding structures. Combining imaging findings with information gathered from the history and physical examination will help solidify the choice of a particular exposure method.

MANDIBULOTOMY SURGICAL TECHNIQUE

Tracheotomy affords optimal transoral exposure and is commonly employed in order to ensure a safe airway in the acute postoperative period. If tracheotomy is not necessary, nasotracheal intubation simplifies oral cavity instrumentation and improves visualization. The tumor extent is again judged once the patient is under general anesthesia to verify that mandibulectomy is not indicated.

The common skin incision is a lip-split technique. The proposed incision is carefully planned, with particular attention to the vermillion border and the aesthetic subunit of the chin. Various incision designs have been described

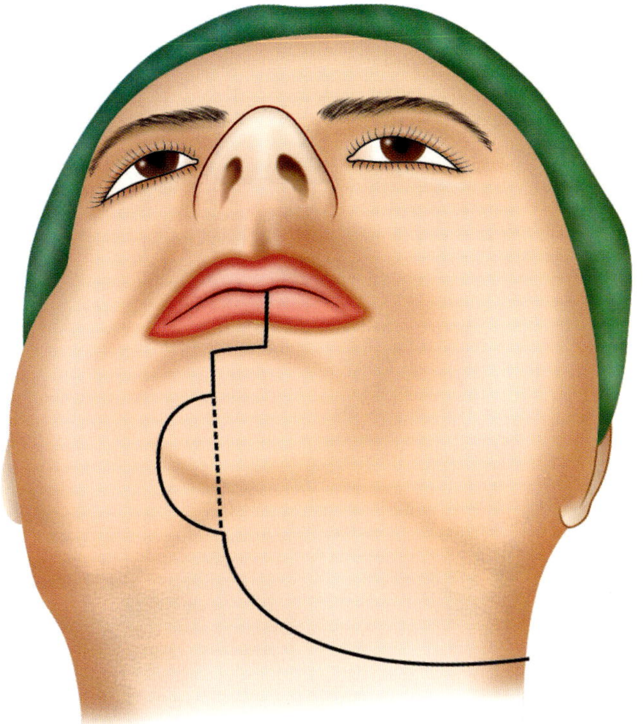

Fig. 10.2: If a neck dissection is performed in conjunction with the primary site resection, the lip incision is extended into the mental crease in a geometric or curvilinear path to meet the neck incision.

including linear or Z-type, and chin button geometries. If a neck dissection is performed in conjunction with the primary site resection, the lip incision is extended into the mental crease in a geometric or curvilinear path to meet the neck incision (Fig. 10.2).

The skin incisions are carried through the lip and down to the mandible. The periosteum is exposed on either side of the planned osteotomy. Attention is paid to preserving the inferior alveolar nerves.

A visor flap is an alternative to the lip-split approach, but is oftentimes less desirable for several reasons. It requires bilateral facial flaps that are extended over the lateral mandibular cortex, placing the marginal mandibular branch of the facial nerve at risk for injury. Elevation of the "visor" also necessitates bilateral division of the inferior alveolar nerves. Following vertical osteotomy, transoral exposure may be hindered if the flap restricts lateral swing of the mandibular segments.

Current reconstructive practices favor plate fixation of the mandibular segments with monocortical (miniplates) and bicortical plates. Modern bicortical rigid fixation techniques obviate concerns about multiplanar forces affecting the mandible during speech, mastication, and deglutition. The historical solution to these concerns was angular or stair-step osteotomies to aid in force distribution and to promote rigid fixation. The reconstruction plates are contoured to span the planned mandibulotomy. The plates are predrilled with care to ensure that bicortical screws are placed below the level of the tooth roots. The plates are removed and set aside until needed for reconstruction.

There are several variations of the medial mandibulotomy. A median mandibulotomy is performed between the central incisors, and the paramedian approach splits the lateral incisor and canine.[12] Modified straight midline mandibulotomy has demonstrated excellent results, and is preferred by some.[13]

The central incisors are at increased risk of injury during median osteotomies.[14] Alternatively, some advocate for the paramedian approach because the distance[14] and angle[8] between the lateral incisor and canine are significantly larger than that between the central incisors. Another advantage of paramedian approaches is that the skin incision and osteotomy do not directly overlap, providing full-thickness tissue coverage over the healing bone (Figs. 10.3A and B).

The majority of patients who have medial mandibulotomy do not require tooth extraction to obtain space for osteotomy.[15] Care is taken to preserve viable dentition, particularly the canine, which is useful as an abutment if a dental prosthesis is needed. When dental extraction is required for access, or to remove carious teeth, it is performed prior to osteotomy.

The osteotomy is performed using a powered reciprocating sagittal saw (or gigli saw). After completion of the osteotomy, swinging the mandibular segments laterally provides the desired exposure. This requires division of oral musculature that includes the genioglossus, geniohyoid, and mylohyoid muscles if a medial approach is used.[16] Though rarely used, lateral mandibulotomy offers the advantage of leaving the genioglossus and geniohyoid muscles intact.[17] The glossogingival sulcus is opened along the floor of the mouth, with preservation of a cuff of mucosa along the alveolar side that facilitates suturing during closure (Fig. 10.4). The incision can be extended into a pharyngotomy if additional exposure of tongue base or pharyngeal tumors is required.

If exposure with a traditional mandibulotomy and pharyngotomy is judged to be inadequate preoperatively, a midline labiomandibuloglossotomy may be required (Figs. 10.5A and B). This technique is generally reserved for midline oropharynx and base of tongue tumors not

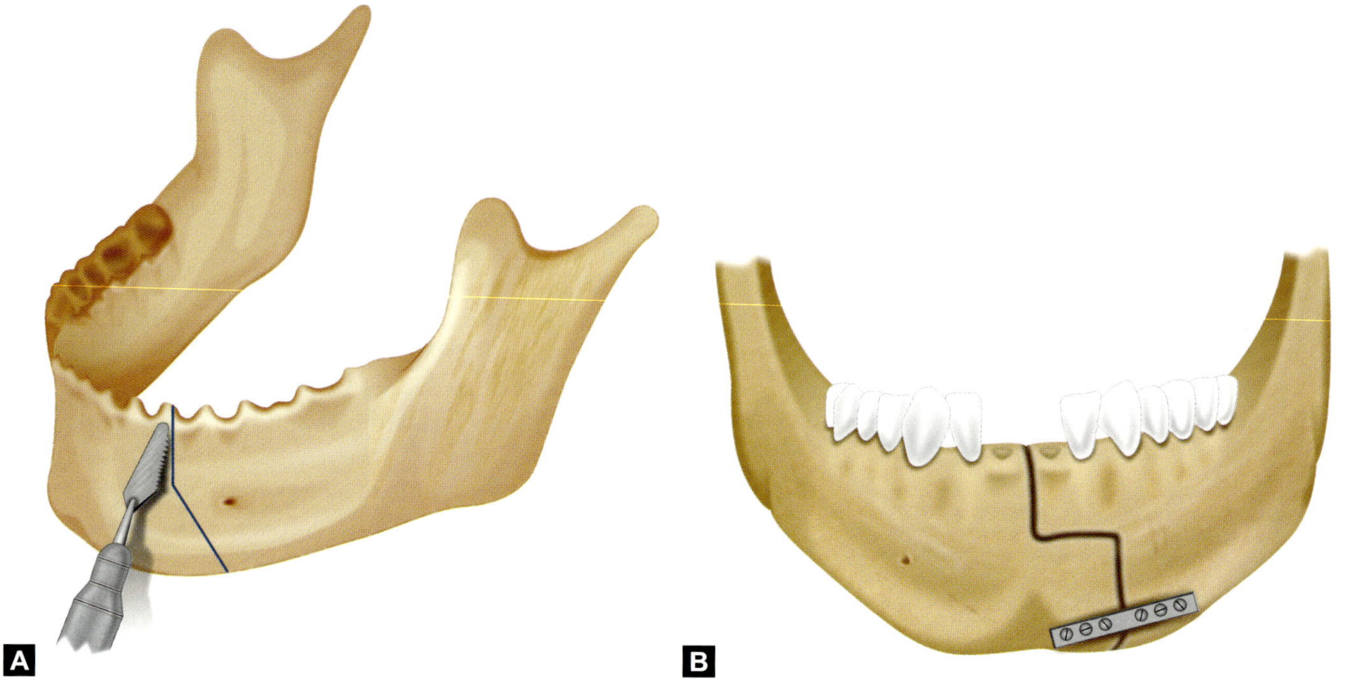

Figs. 10.3A and B: Medial osteotomies are performed with respect to the infra-orbital nerve and can have obtuse angle (A) or stairstep (B) geometry.

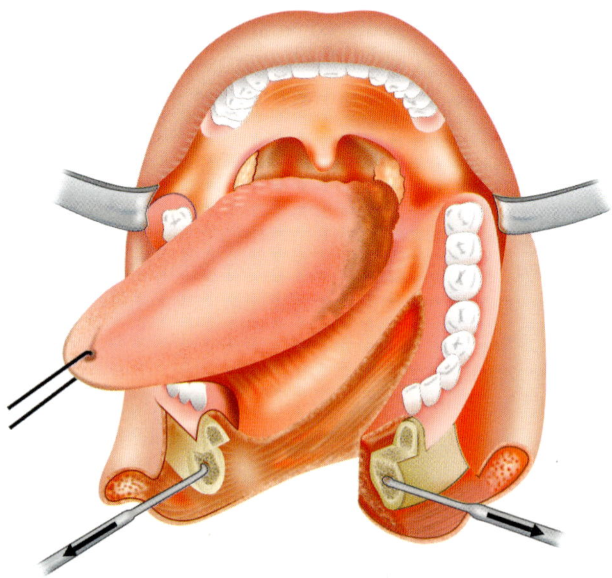

Fig. 10.4: The glossogingival sulcus is opened along the floor of mouth, with preservation of a cuff of mucosa along the alveolar side that facilitates suturing during closure.

accessible via transoral or transhyoid approaches. It can also provide access to large nasopharyngeal and clival tumors when combined with a palatal split. Initial skin and osseous steps are the same as described above. However, instead of incising the mucosa along the lateral floor of mouth, the anterior floor of mouth is divided in the midline between the submandibular papillae. The geniohyoid and genioglossus muscles are divided in the midline, and the tongue is split back to the vallecula precisely along the mid-sagittal plane.

Once the desired exposure is achieved, the tumor is resected and margins are assessed by intraoperative frozen section analysis.

RECONSTRUCTION

Depending on the site and extent of the defect, reconstruction is achieved by various methods. Smaller defects can often be treated with primary closure, skin graft, tissue matrix, or other biologic materials, or local tongue flap. Larger defects may require an axial flap such as the pectoralis major or supraclavicular artery island, or free tissue transfer such as the radial forearm fasciocutaneous free flap. Functional considerations are important in choosing the reconstructive technique, but establishing a physical barrier between the oral and neck compartments is paramount. The inlay suturing of graft of flap tissue is facilitated by the cuff of mobile mucosa that was previously created during the exposure dissection.

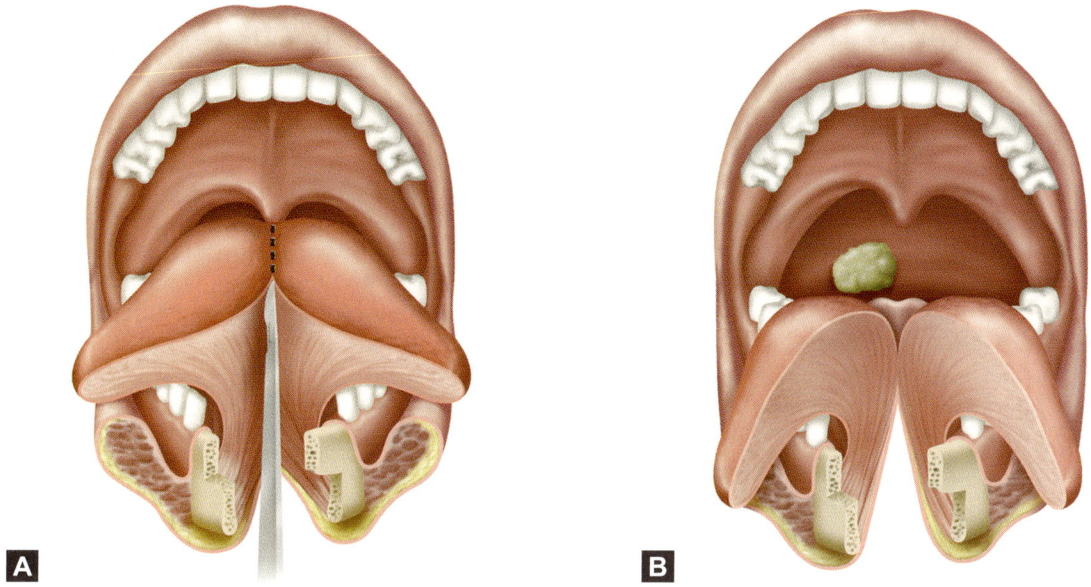

Figs. 10.5A and B: If exposure with a traditional mandibulotomy and pharyngotomy is judged to be inadequate preoperatively, a midline labiomandibuloglossotomy may be required.

Following reconstruction, any remaining open oral mucosa is closed in a watertight manner and the mandibular segments are fixed using the predrilled holes and contoured plate(s). The skin incisions are closed and care is taken to align the vermillion border if a lip incision was created. A nasogastric feeding tube is placed if the patient does not already have a gastrostomy tube.

POSTOPERATIVE CARE AND COMPLICATIONS

Postoperative management is focused on maintaining a secure airway, appropriate nutrition, oral and wound care, as well as encouraging recovery of function and quality of life. Alimentation protocols vary by surgeon and depend on the extent of dissection and reconstruction method. Oral hygiene should be practiced diligently with rinses (hydrogen peroxide, saline, or chlorhexidine) until the mucosal incisions are healed.

Common complications following mandibulotomy include injury to the inferior alveolar nerve, wound infection, fistula formation, bony nonunion, ORN, plate complications, malocclusion, and dental complications. Complication rates from large mandibulotomy series have been reported to range from 10% to 22%.[15,18-20] Rate of nonunion and ORN have been reported in the single digits.[15] Rigid fixation of the mandibular segments has been found to decrease complications.[15] Preoperative radiation increases the risk for nonunion and ORN.[15,21] Adjuvant chemoradiation likely increases this risk as well.

REFERENCES

1. Butlin HT. Diseases of the Tongue. London: Cassell; 1885.
2. Sedillot A. Paper presented to Academie des Sciences. Gaz d'Hop. 1844;17:83.
3. Esmarch Fv, Kowalzig E, Grau LH, et al. Surgical Technique: A Text-book on Operative Surgery. New York: The Macmillan company; London: Macmillan & Co, Ltd; 1901.
4. Folz BJ, Silver CE, Rinaldo A, et al. An outline of the history of head and neck oncology. Oral Oncol. 2008;44:2-9.
5. Trotter W. Operations for malignant diseases of the pharynx. Br J Surg. 1929;16:485-95.
6. Martin H, Tollefsen HR, Gerold FP. Median labiomandibular glossotomy. Trotter's median (anterior) translingual pharyngotomy. Am J Surg. 1961;102:753-9.
7. Dziegielewski PT, O'Connell DA, Rieger J, et al. The lip-splitting mandibulotomy: aesthetic and functional outcomes. Oral Oncol. 2010;46:612-17.
8. Pan WL, Hao SP, Lin YS, et al. The anatomical basis for mandibulotomy: midline versus paramidline. Laryngoscope. 2003; 113:377-80.
9. Bradley JC. Age changes in the vascular supply of the mandible. Br Dent J. 1972;132:142-4.
10. Chang SS, Goldenberg D, Koch WM. Transcervical approach to benign parapharyngeal space tumors. Ann Otol Rhinol Laryngol. 2012;121:620-24.

11. Stringer SP, Jordan JR, Mendenhall WM, et al. Mandibular lingual releasing approach. Otolaryngol Head Neck Surg. 1992;107:395-8.
12. McGregor IA, MacDonald DG. Mandibular osteotomy in the surgical approach to the oral cavity. Head Neck Surg. 1983;5:457-62.
13. Amin MR, Deschler DG, Hayden RE. Straight midline mandibulotomy revisited. Laryngoscope. 1999;109:1402-5.
14. Shinghal T, Bissada E, Chan HB, et al. Medial mandibulotomies: is there sufficient space in the midline to allow a mandibulotomy without compromising the dentition? J Otolaryngol Head Neck Surg. 2013;42:32.
15. Nam W, Kim HJ, Choi EC, et al. Contributing factors to mandibulotomy complications: a retrospective study. Oral Surg Oral Med Oral Pathol Oral Radiol Endod. 2006;101:e65-70.
16. Spiro RH, Gerold FP, Shah JP, et al. Mandibulotomy approach to oropharyngeal tumors. Am J Surg. 1985;150:466-9.
17. Krespi YP, Sisson GA. Transmandibular exposure of the skull base. Am J Surg. 1984;148:534-8.
18. Dubner S, Spiro RH. Median mandibulotomy: a critical assessment. Head Neck. 1991;13:389-93.
19. Dziegielewski PT, Mlynarek AM, Dimitry J, et al. The mandibulotomy: friend or foe? Safety outcomes and literature review. Laryngoscope. 2009;119:2369-75.
20. El-Zohairy MA. Straight midline mandibulotomy: technique and results of treatment. J Egypt Natl Canc Inst. 2007; 19: 292-8.
21. McCann KJ, Irish JC, Gullane PJ, et al. Complications associated with rigid fixation of mandibulotomies. J Otolaryngol. 1994;23:210-15.

CHAPTER

11 Segmental and Marginal Mandibulectomy

Ryan Orosco, Steven S Chang

INTRODUCTION

Segmental mandibular resection was historically a routine approach to malignancies of the mouth.[1,2] This practice was driven by the improved exposure and advantages related to defect closure, as well as the belief that squamous cell carcinoma invaded bone via lymphatics. We now know that tumors gain access to periosteum and cortex via direct invasion,[3-5] and mandibular resection is no longer utilized solely for exposure. Our knowledge of tumor growth patterns has matured and our modern surgical techniques have opened the door for mandibular conservation with marginal mandibulectomy, which necessitates appropriate patient selection and surgical planning.

SEGMENTAL VERSUS MARGINAL MANDIBULECTOMY

Adhering to oncologic principles, completeness of surgical resection is germane to preventing local recurrence and achieving favorable outcomes in head and neck cancer.[6-8] For oral cavity and oropharynx malignancies that do not abut or involve the mandible, soft tissue resection is sufficient. When a cancer is frankly invading the mandible, or even in close approximation, mandibulectomy is indicated in order to obtain circumferential surgical margins that are not otherwise possible with soft tissue resection alone. The selection of either segmental or marginal mandibulectomy depends on the surgeon's assessment of tumor infiltration of periosteum and bone. Underestimation of bone invasion can lead to incomplete resection and unfavorable outcomes.

Segmental resection disrupts mandibular continuity by removing the portion of the involved mandibular arch. If mandibular bony involvement is identified clinically or radiographically, a segmental resection should be performed with wide clearance of osseous and soft tissue margins.

Mandibular conservation with marginal mandibulectomy removes a rim of bone with adjacent periosteum and preserves mandibular continuity while still providing a bony surgical margin. Marginal mandibulectomy is reserved for tumors that abut and involve the periosteum, but do not invade the cortex. First described by Crile in 1923,[9] rim resection did not gain widespread acceptance for decades. Werning and colleagues reported good outcomes in 222 patients with oral cavity squamous cell carcinomas that were treated without segmental mandibulectomy.[10] They concluded that mandibular conservation surgery is oncologically safe for patients with involvement of the periosteum. Multiple other groups have reported good oncologic and functional outcomes in patients who undergo marginal resection.[11-15] In properly selected cases, marginal (rim) resection of the mandible is well established as an oncologically safe procedure with a favorable cosmetic and functional profile. Today, both segmental and marginal mandibulectomies serve well-defined roles in the surgical management of advanced head and neck cancer.

INDICATIONS AND PATIENT SELECTION

Relevant Anatomy

By design, mandibulectomy techniques alter the osseous mandibular framework, so its form and function should be understood. When performing segmental mandibulectomy with reconstruction, the preoperative dental occlusion should be noted, as care will be given to the preservation of remaining occlusive dentition following tumor extirpation. In addition to disrupting occlusion, mandibulectomy affects the inferior alveolar nerve, mandibular arch strength, and osseous blood supply.

The inferior alveolar nerve branches from the third division of the trigeminal nerve and courses deep to the mandibular angle, entering at the mandibular foramen. It passes through the mandibular body and exits at the mental foramen adjacent to the first and second premolars. This nerve may be grossly or microscopically involved with tumor spread. Segmental resection will likely involve transection of at least one nerve, and the nerve can sometimes be spared with marginal resection in patients with adequate mandibular height.

Mandibular height is defined as the vertical distance from the lower border of the mandible to the alveolar crest. Edentulous patients with hypoplastic mandibles may have increased susceptibility to bony invasion and are poor candidates for marginal resection. Segmental resection is preferred, even when there is minimal loss of vertical height in an edentulous mandible. When performing marginal mandibulectomy in a dentate patient, at least 1 cm of mandibular height should be preserved in order to preserve arch integrity.

An understanding of the mandibular blood supply is important when performing mandibulectomy because devascularized bone predisposes to complications. The arterial supply to the mandible changes with aging and is thought to be predominantly via subperiosteal vessels as opposed to the inferior alveolar artery.[16] The buccal, lingual, and facial arteries contribute to this periosteal blood supply,[17] and the anterior mandible is fed via mental vessels carried in adjacent muscles.[18]

Patient Evaluation

When approaching oral cavity malignancies, preoperative evaluation of mandibular involvement is crucial because bone margins cannot be evaluated with intraoperative frozen sections. Frozen section analysis of the marrow is possible, but is not routinely used. The importance of obtaining wide osseous margins cannot be overemphasized because bony invasion is generally not responsive to radiation or chemotherapy and can only be treated with surgery. If the mandible is thought to be involved, a segmental resection should be performed with wide clearance of gross margins.

The first step toward evaluating mandibular involvement is a thorough history that inquires about chin or lip paresthesia and loose teeth, which could indicate nerve or osseous involvement.

Next, a complete head and neck examination is performed, including an assessment of cranial nerves with particular attention to trigeminal, facial, and hypoglossal function. Additionally, bimanual palpation of the oral cavity will help assess the degree of tumor fixation and relationship between the alveolus, dentition, tongue, and adjacent soft tissue. Tumors that are not mobile, and by palpation feel to be fixed, are likely to have invaded the periosteum or mandibular cortex. Tumors adjacent to dentition should trigger a high suspicion for mandibular invasion because extension can occur along the tooth root and into the marrow.

Physical examination may be limited by patient discomfort and trismus, which is indicative of tumor spread to the masseteric space or pterygoid muscles. Clinical suspicion of mandibular involvement is influenced by multiple factors, not the least of which is tumor size. Larger tumors are more likely to invade adjacent structures. Fixation to underlying bone and inferior alveolar nerve paresthesia are also indicative of bony invasion. After a thorough clinical examination, additional information is provided by radiographic studies.

Previously irradiated mandibles are more susceptible to multifocal tumor infiltration with unpredictable patterns of invasion,[19] and segmental rather than marginal mandibulectomy is advised. Segmental resection is also employed in cases of primary bone tumors, osteoradionecrosis, and in other select nononcologic cases.

Imaging

Clinical evaluation, in the office and the operating room, remains a highly reliable method of determining the extent of tumor infiltration,[20,21] but does not obviate the utility of radiographic imaging.[22] Radiographic studies can provide supplemental information in evaluating for mandibular osseous invasion, but the images do not provide enough diagnostic accuracy to be relied upon exclusively.

A variety of methods have been employed to investigate mandibular invasion, including plain and panoramic X-rays, computed tomography (CT), magnetic resonance imaging,[7] single positron emission computed tomography (SPECT), and bone scans.[20,21,23-25] CT scans are commonly used for staging of the primary site and regional nodes, but has been shown to have low sensitivity for detecting bony involvement.[20] Bone scans and MRI can be helpful in evaluating the marrow and in patients with significant tooth artifact on CT.

Evaluate images to detect bone invasion by cortical erosion, medullary space enhancement, or widening of or extension into the mental or mandibular foramen.

SURGICAL TECHNIQUE

Tracheotomy is not universally performed with mandibulectomy procedures, but should be considered in cases of large resection or extensive reconstruction that may compromise the airway postoperatively. Tracheotomy serves to protect the airway during the acute postoperative period, and is usually intended to be temporary. If a surgical airway is not required, nasotracheal intubation is helpful because it optimizes exposure to allow for optimal tumor resection.

Once the patient is under anesthesia, a thorough manual and visual examination is performed that may confirm preoperative findings and at times can identify mandibular invasion that was not previously evident.

Neck dissection can be performed prior to, or after, mandibular resection. Advantages of starting with the neck are that the major vessels can be dissected and controlled, and the surgical field is not yet contaminated from the oral cavity. Alternatively, starting with tumor extirpation can accelerate the start of surgical margin evaluation and allows additional time to assess the defect and begin reconstruction steps while the neck dissection proceeds.

Particularly if the floor of the mouth is not violated by the tumor, the neck dissection specimen can be removed separately. However, if the tumor is in direct extension or continuity with neck nodes, an en bloc resection is preferred to prevent tumor spillage.

Segmental Mandibulectomy

Wide exposure of the lateral mandibular cortex is required in order to perform the osteotomies necessary for segmental resection. A lip-splitting approach and the visor flap are the two options to gain this exposure. Both require transection of the inferior alveolar nerve, but each has unique advantages and disadvantages.

To perform a visor flap, the neck incision is carried across the midline and subplatysmal flaps are extended superiorly and lateral to the mandible (Figs. 11.1A and B). A Hayes Martin maneuver is performed to preserve the marginal mandibular nerve by retracting the facial vein superiorly and sweeping the fascial contents overlying the submandibular gland. The inferior alveolar nerve(s) is divided, and the outer mandibular cortex is exposed. The advantage of this approach is avoiding a chin and lip scar, but tumor exposure may still be limited by the chin soft tissue and oral aperture.

The lip-split approach trades a facial incision for direct exposure of the lateral and posterior mandible (Fig. 11.2). Additionally, in the case of lateral tumors, an ipsilateral neck incision can be extended up to the lip, therefore avoiding the need for bilateral neck incisions.

Once the tumor is exposed, the extirpation begins with soft tissue cuts around the tumor. Next, the uninvolved mandible is exposed along the lateral and lingual cortices. At least 1 cm is planned for bony and soft tissue margins. The remaining mucoperiosteum is back-elevated to facilitate later reconstruction. Dentition that interferes with the proposed osteotomies should be removed. Carious and nonviable dentition should also be removed, with attention to complete extraction of root fragments.

Plating is required if mandibular continuity is to be maintained postoperatively. If the contour of the lateral cortex is preserved, it is exposed, and a reconstruction plate is contoured. Alternatively, customized or prebent plates are available from several manufacturers. The reconstruction plate is predrilled with bicortical screw holes that are placed below the level of any remaining tooth roots, and set aside until frozen section surgical margins are cleared.

Osteotomies can be created using a sagittal saw, oscillating saw, or reciprocating saw. The mandibulectomy geometry is dictated by the tumor location (Figs. 11.3 and 11.4). The cuts are made in the center of the tooth socket to avoid damage to adjacent viable dentition, if present. It is preferable to make the lateral cut prior to making the medial cuts to stabilize the bone. Soft tissue medial to the mandible should be protected with malleable retractors. Large posterior tumors may require partial soft palate resection and transection of pterygoid musculature. In such cases, the superior osteotomy can be through the sigmoid notch or below the coronoid. The condyle may need to be disarticulated and removed during the resection. For retromolar trigone tumors and other cases where the ramus is involved, brisk bleeding from the internal maxillary artery should be anticipated.

Care should be taken to orient the resection specimen. Whenever possible it is preferable to take the margins

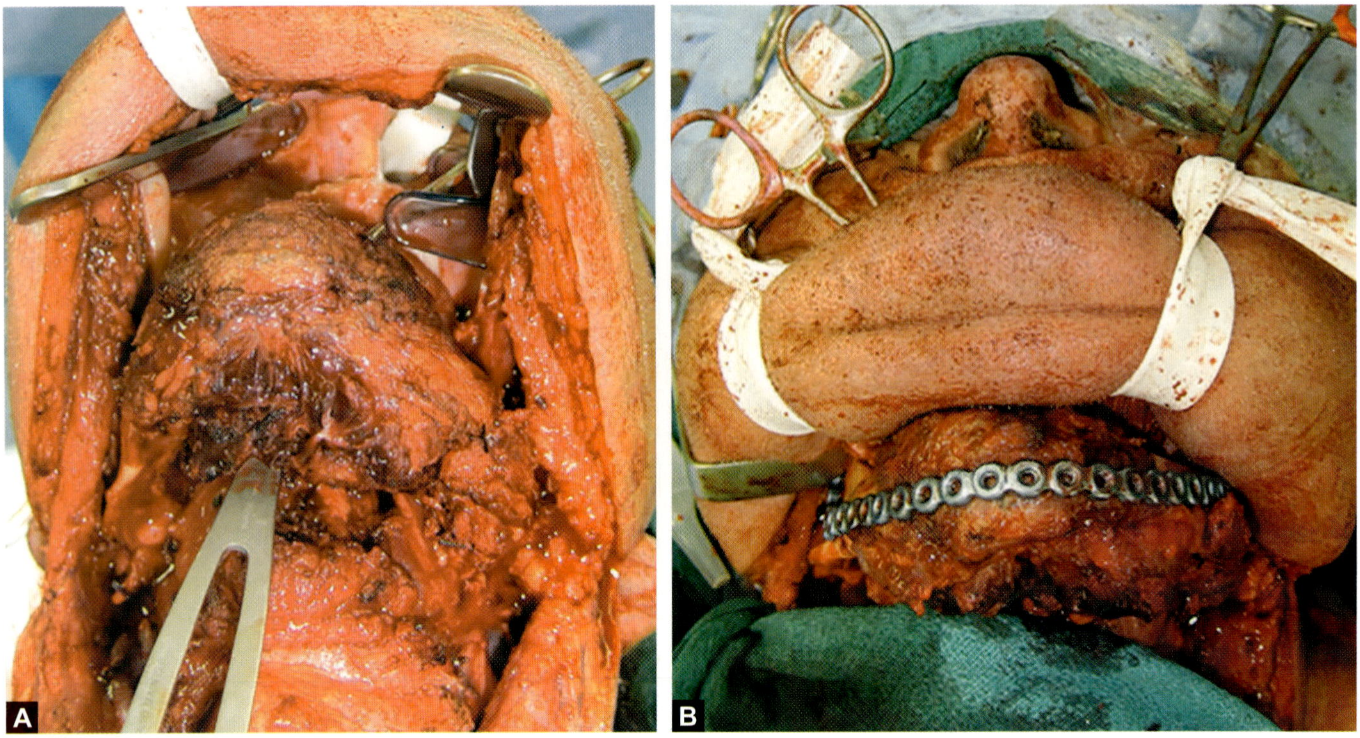

Figs. 11.1A and B: Visor flap. The visor flap is retracted superiorly to expose the lateral cortex of the mandible (A). With the visor flap retracted superiorly, a reconstruction plate is bent to follow the contour of the mandible. This step is not possible if the tumor alters the lateral mandibular contour (B).

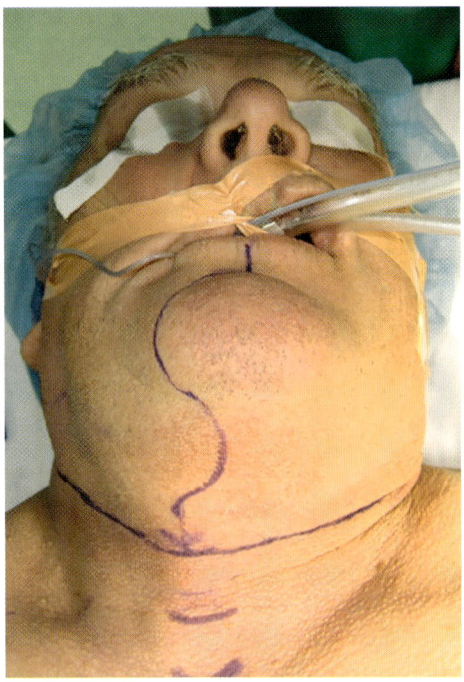

Fig. 11.2: Lip-split incision. The bilateral neck incision is joined by a vertical lip-split incision. Note the preservation of the chin aesthetic subunit. The submental incision is nonlinear in anticipation of scar contracture.

off the specimen rather than the patient. This allows for better hemostasis and it encourages wide margins of resection. Additional margins can be taken from the inferior alveolar nerve and marrow. Specimens are clearly labeled and sent for frozen section analysis because positive intraoperative histopathology necessitates a wider margin of resection.

Marginal Mandibulectomy

Marginal mandibulectomy is generally possible via direct transoral exposure, and can be improved with visor flap or lip-splitting approaches described above. Once the desired exposure has been obtained, the gingiva is incised down to bone. The mandibular cortex is exposed along the proposed mandibulectomy lines, and the remaining periosteum distal and proximal to the tumor is not elevated. The goal should be at least a 1-cm margin when planning the osteotomies. Nonviable dentition and teeth that interfere with osteotomy lines are removed (Figs. 11.3A to F). If overt mandibular involvement is suspected at any time during the procedure, the surgeon should be prepared to convert to segmental resection.

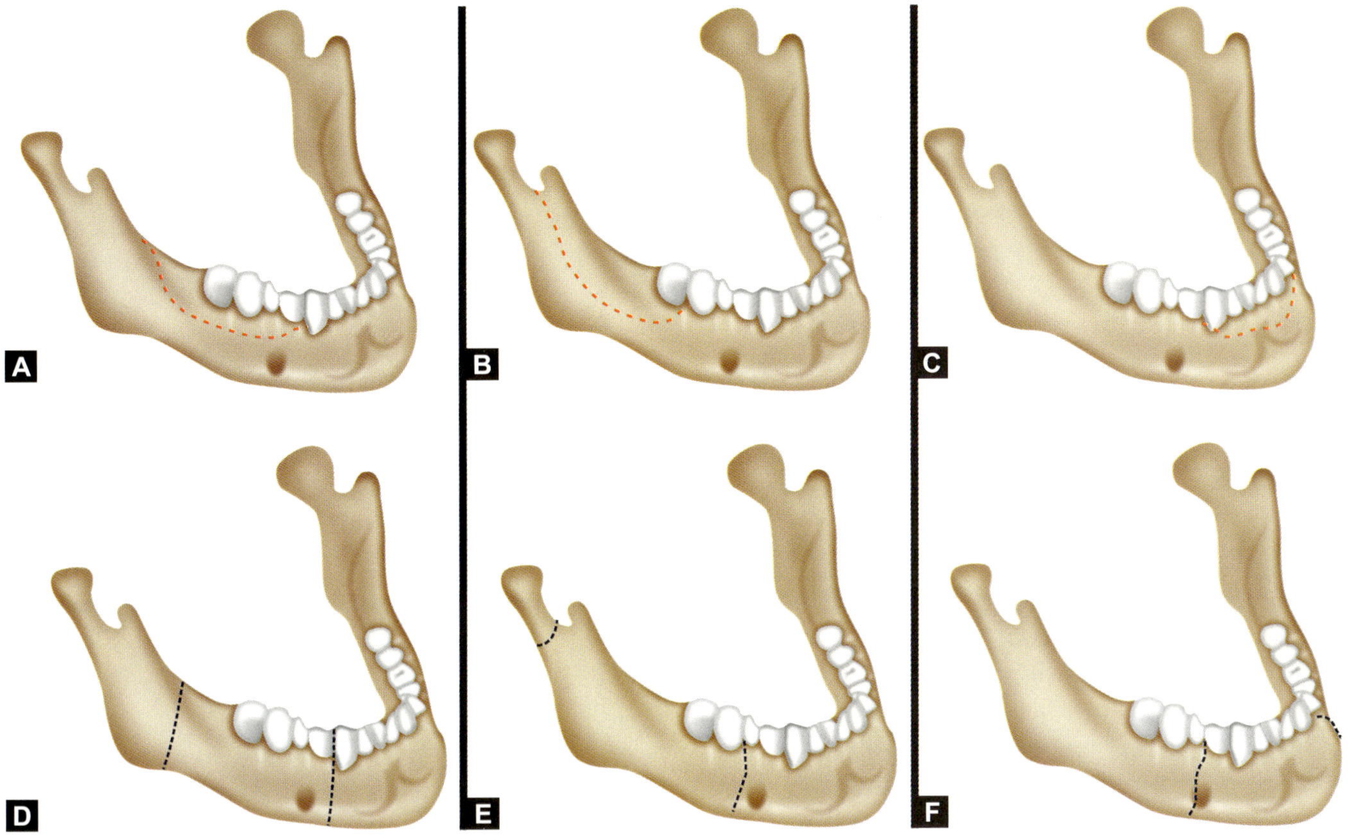

Figs. 11.3A to F: Marginal mandibulectomy geometries and segmental mandibulectomies for corresponding tumor locations. Proposed osteotomy lines are shown: red, marginal osteotomies; orange, segmental osteotomies. Note that any dentition in the proposed osteotomy path is removed and care taken to avoid damaging adjacent teeth by performing osteotomies in the center of the resultant tooth socket. (A) Lateral marginal mandibulectomy. (B) Posterior mandibulectomy for retromolar trigone tumors. The rim resection can be designed to preserve the coronoid. If the posterior cut is through the sigmoid notch, the temporalis muscle is divided above its bony attachment. (C) Anterior marginal mandibulectomy for lip, alveolar, or floor of mouth lesions encroaching on the mandible, but without bony involvement. (D) Lateral segmental mandibulectomy. (E) More extensive segmental mandibulectomy involving the ramus and body. (F) Anterior segmental mandibulectomy.

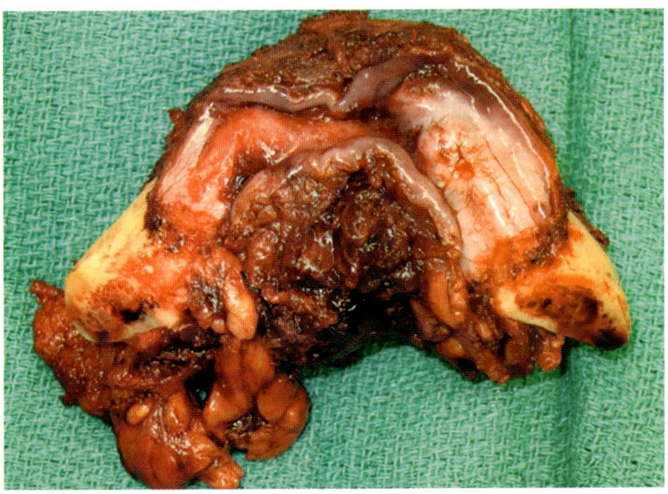

Fig. 11.4: Anterior mandible composite resection specimen. Note the cuff of soft tissue and bone removed around the tumor specimen. The goal of resection should be for at least 1 cm of margin clearance.

As with segmental mandibulectomy, the soft tissue cuts are performed first so that the tumor can be removed in continuity with the bony segment.

For tumors of the alveolar ridge, a horizontal osteotomy is created using a sagittal saw, oscillating saw, or osteotomes. The distal edges are tapered to avoid leaving square corners that serve as sites of weakness. A cutting and diamond burr may also be used to remove the involved bone but it is not preferred because it does not allow for pathologic evaluation of the bone—soft tissue interface. Floor of mouth and other tumors that primarily involve the lingual cortex are approached similarly with a vertical rim mandibulectomy. In addition to anterior and lateral tumors, posterior marginal mandibulectomy has been used successfully for tumors of the retromolar trigone.[26,27] An example of an inferior marginal mandibulectomy for an osteoma is shown in Figures 11.5A to C. Complete

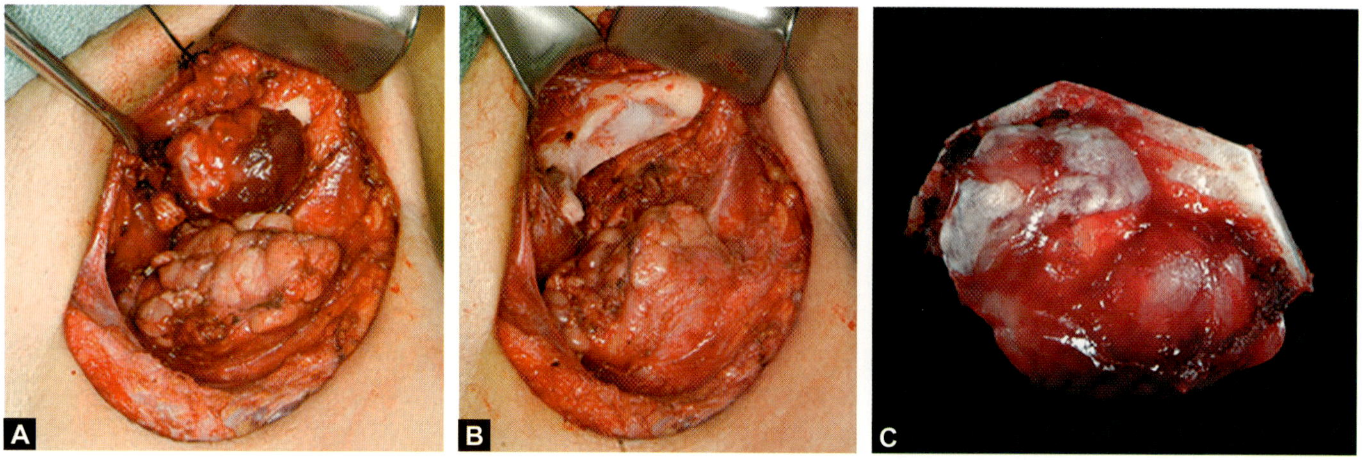

Figs. 11.5A to C: (A) Osteoma of the right mandibular angle. (B) Post-resection marginal mandibulectomy defect along the mandibular angle. (C) Surgical specimen with osteotomies well seen.

osteotomies should be ensured because prying or manipulating an incompletely mobilized bony specimen can lead to inadvertent fracture of the native mandible. Bone wax may be helpful with achieving hemostasis.

The pathology review of frozen specimens of the surgical resection margins is the same process described above for segmental mandibulectomy.

RECONSTRUCTION

The resulting defect following mandibulectomy poses unique functional and cosmetic issues related to occlusion, mandibular contour, mastication, deglutition, and airway. Reconstructive techniques depend on the size and location of the soft tissue and osseous defect as well as the patient's presurgical dental status, functional state, prognosis, donor site availability, and associated comorbidities. Urken and colleagues developed a classification scheme that is helpful when approaching mandibular defects.[28]

Freely swinging mandibular segments should be avoided whenever possible, but may be unavoidable in cases of advanced tumors in patients with increased surgical risk. Autogenous bone grafting is the preferred technique in modern mandibular reconstruction,[29] and has demonstrated excellent long-term cosmetic and functional outcomes.[30] Reconstruction of anterior mandibular defects is preferred because of the significant cosmetic deformity and possibility of airway compromise from tongue prolapse (Fig. 11.6). Free flap reconstruction of lateral defects is less imperative, but preferred when feasible.

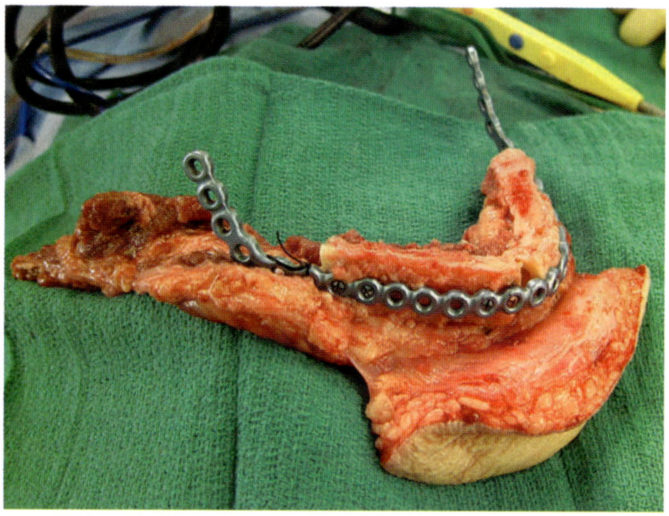

Fig. 11.6: Fibula free flap and reconstruction bar. The fibula is plated prior to securing the plate back into the predrilled holes in the mandible.

The fibular osteocutaneous free flap is the workhorse for mandibular reconstruction, and other options include iliac crest, scapular, and radial forearm. Endosseous implants may be possible in many cases and further improve functional outcomes. Short mandibular defects in nonirradiated, healthy wound beds have also been reconstructed using nonvascularized bone grafts and distraction osteogenesis.[31,32]

Small soft tissue defects can be left open to heal by secondary intention, or can be covered using skin grafts, local flaps (tongue, buccal), regional flaps (submental or supraclavicular artery island), or myocutaneous free tissue transfer. Regardless of the reconstruction technique, it is critical to ensure a barrier of vascularized tissue between the oral cavity and the neck.

POSTOPERATIVE CARE

Patients with advanced oral cavity tumors requiring mandibulectomy are best served in the postoperative period through a collaborative, multidisciplinary approach. Decisions regarding every realm of postoperative care largely depend on surgeon preference and will vary according to the extent of mandibular resection and reconstructive technique. Patients who undergo segmental mandibulectomy and free flap reconstruction will require more in-depth postoperative care than those who receive marginal resection and skin graft.

Perioperative antibiotics are generally continued for 24 hours. Nutrition is provided by gastrostomy or nasogastric feeding tube for patients who undergo segmental resection, whereas early resumption of oral intake may be possible in patients receiving marginal mandibulectomy. Oral hygiene regimens may entail saline, peroxide, or chlorhexidine rinses. Surgeons should consider obtaining a speech pathology evaluation to address speech and deglutition. Once the patient is able to perform safe and effective swallow function, an oral diet can be initiated and advanced. When applicable, routine tracheostomy care is provided, and patients are progressed along weaning, voice-rehabilitation, and capping protocols.

REFERENCES

1. Slaughter DP, Roeser EH, Smejkal WF. Excision of the mandible for neoplastic diseases; indications and techniques. Surgery. 1949;26:507-22.
2. Ward GE, Robben JO. A composite operation for radical neck dissection and removal of cancer of the mouth. Cancer. 1951; 4:98-109.
3. Carter RL, Tsao SW, Burman JF, et al. Patterns and mechanisms of bone invasion by squamous carcinomas of the head and neck. Am J Surg. 1983;146:451-5.
4. Brown JS, Browne RM. Factors influencing the patterns of invasion of the mandible by oral squamous cell carcinoma. Int J Oral Maxillofac Surg. 1995;24:417-26.
5. Brown JS, Lowe D, Kalavrezos N, et al. Patterns of invasion and routes of tumor entry into the mandible by oral squamous cell carcinoma. Head Neck. 2002;24:370-83.
6. Zieske LA, Johnson JT, Myers EN, et al. Squamous cell carcinoma with positive margins. Surgery and postoperative irradiation. Arch Otolaryngol Head Neck Surg. 1986;112: 863-6.
7. Chen TY, Emrich LJ, Driscoll DL. The clinical significance of pathological findings in surgically resected margins of the primary tumor in head and neck carcinoma. Int J Radiat Oncol Biol Phys. 1987;13:833-7.
8. Loree TR, Strong EW. Significance of positive margins in oral cavity squamous carcinoma. Am J Surg. 1990;160: 410-14.
9. Crile GW. Carcinoma of the jaws, tongue, cheek, and lips. Surg Gynecol Obstet. 1923;36:159-62.
10. Werning JW, Byers RM, Novas MA, et al. Preoperative assessment for and outcomes of mandibular conservation surgery. Head Neck. 2001;23:1024-30.
11. Barttelbort SW, Bahn SL, Ariyan SA. Rim mandibulectomy for cancer of the oral cavity. Am J Surg. 1987;154:423-28.
12. Munoz Guerra MF, Naval Gias L, Campo FR, et al. Marginal and segmental mandibulectomy in patients with oral cancer: a statistical analysis of 106 cases. J Oral Maxillofac Surg. 2003;61:1289-96.
13. Guerra MF, Campo FJ, Gias LN,et al. Rim versus sagittal mandibulectomy for the treatment of squamous cell carcinoma: two types of mandibular preservation. Head Neck. 2003;25:982-9.
14. Shaha AR. Marginal mandibulectomy for carcinoma of the floor of the mouth. J Surg Oncol. 1992;49:116-19.
15. Wald RM, Jr, Calcaterra TC. Lower alveolar carcino ma. Segmental v marginal resection. Arch Otolaryngol. 1983;109:578-82.
16. Bradley JC. Age changes in the vascular supply of the mandible. Br Dent J. 1972;132:142-4.
17. Bradley JC. The clinical significance of age changes in the vascular supply to the mandible. Int J Oral Surg. 1981;10: 71-6.
18. Hamparian AM. Blood supply of the human fetal mandible. Am J Anat. 1973;136:67-5.
19. McGregor AD, MacDonald DG. Routes of entry of squamous cell carcinoma to the mandible. Head Neck Surg. 1988;10:294-301.
20. van den Brekel MW, Runne RW, Smeele LE, et al. Assessment of tumour invasion into the mandible: the value of different imaging techniques. Eur Radiol. 1998;8:1552-7.
21. Shaha AR. Preoperative evaluation of the mandible in patients with carcinoma of the floor of mouth. Head Neck. 1991;13:398-402.
22. Rao LP, Shukla M, Sharma V, et al. Mandibular conservation in oral cancer. Surg Oncol. 2012;21:109-18.
23. Bolzoni A, Cappiello J, Piazza C, et al. Diagnostic accuracy of magnetic resonance imaging in the assessment of mandibular involvement in oral-oropharyngeal squamous cell carcinoma: a prospective study. Arch Otolaryngol Head Neck Surg. 2004;130:837-43.
24. Imola MJ, Gapany M, Grund F, et al. Technetium 99m single positron emission computed tomography scanning for assessing mandible invasion in oral cavity cancer. Laryngoscope. 2001;111:373-81.

25. Soderholm AL, Lindqvist C, Hietanen J, et al. Bone scanning for evaluating mandibular bone extension of oral squamous cell carcinoma. J Oral Maxillofac Surg. 1990;48:252-7.
26. Petruzzelli GJ, Knight FK, Vandevender D, et al. Posterior marginal mandibulectomy in the management of cancer of the oral cavity and oropharynx. Otolaryngol Head Neck Surg. 2003;129:713-19.
27. Ayad T, Guertin L, Soulieres D, et al. Controversies in the management of retromolar trigone carcinoma. Head Neck. 2009;31:398-405.
28. Urken ML, Weinberg H, Vickery C, et al. Oromandibular reconstruction using microvascular composite free flaps. Report of 71 cases and a new classification scheme for bony, soft-tissue, and neurologic defects. Arch Otolaryngol Head Neck Surg. 1991;117:733-44.
29. Mehta RP, Deschler DG. Mandibular reconstruction in 2004: an analysis of different techniques. Curr Opin Otolaryngol Head Neck Surg. 2004;12:288-93.
30. Hidalgo DA, Pusic AL. Free-flap mandibular reconstruction: a 10-year follow-up study. Plast Reconstr Surg. 2002; 110:438-49; discussion 450-451.
31. Kuriakose MA, Shnayder Y, DeLacure MD. Reconstruction of segmental mandibular defects by distraction osteogenesis for mandibular reconstruction. Head Neck. 2003;25: 816-24.
32. Gonzalez-Garcia R, Rodriguez-Campo FJ, Naval-Gias L, et al. The effect of radiation in distraction osteogenesis for reconstruction of mandibular segmental defects. Br J Oral Maxillofac Surg. 2007;45:314-16.

Section 3

Surgery of the Larynx and Hypopharynx

Section Editor: *David Goldenberg*

Chapters

CHAPTER

12 Surgery for Larynx Cancer

Richard Goldman, Joseph Curry, Adam Luginbuhl, David Cognetti

INTRODUCTION

When the open surgical management of laryngeal tumors was first introduced with the use of laryngofissure in the late 19th century, patients were fortunate to survive their surgery, let alone their cancer. Lack of anesthesia, antibiotics, and proper airway control led to unacceptably high operative mortality. This, coupled with a limited understanding of oncologic principles, made cure almost nonexistent.[1] Fortunately, over the past 100 years, the surgical and nonsurgical approaches to the larynx have evolved, with current cure rates for early-stage lesions exceeding 85%.

When cure becomes the expectation, there is a greater emphasis on functional outcomes. In modern practice even select late-stage lesions can be successfully managed with preservation of the larynx. The appropriate treatment selection based on both tumor and patient characteristics is critical to the successful management of laryngeal cancer. A thorough knowledge of laryngeal anatomy and its impact on the route of spread and metastatic potential of each individual tumor is imperative. Equally important is the understanding of the functional role of the larynx and the impact that any functional change would have on comorbid disease and quality of life.

Smoking is the major cause of laryngeal cancer, with squamous cell carcinoma accounting for 95% of laryngeal malignancies. Beginning in the early 20th century, the smoking rate in the United States sharply increased, peaking at over 40% of the adult population in 1963, which led to a rise in the rate of laryngeal cancer as well. Due to increased awareness and public measures to curb tobacco use since the first Surgeon General's report on the hazards of tobacco use in 1964, the smoking rate in the United States has declined to under 20%. Fortunately, this has led to a downward trend in laryngeal cancer rates in recent decades. Tobacco abstinence is the key to laryngeal cancer prevention, and it is paramount to the success of any treatment approach for laryngeal cancer.

ANATOMY

The larynx is positioned in the neck as the doorway to the airway. It separates the pharynx from the trachea. For staging and treatment purposes it is anatomically divided into the supraglottis, the glottis, and the subglotttis (Figs. 12.1A and B).

The supraglottis extends from the tip of the epiglottis to the inferior edge of the false vocal folds at the laryngeal ventricle. It includes the epiglottis, the aryepiglottic folds, the false vocal folds, and the arytenoid cartilages. Approximately 40% of laryngeal cancers in the United States arise

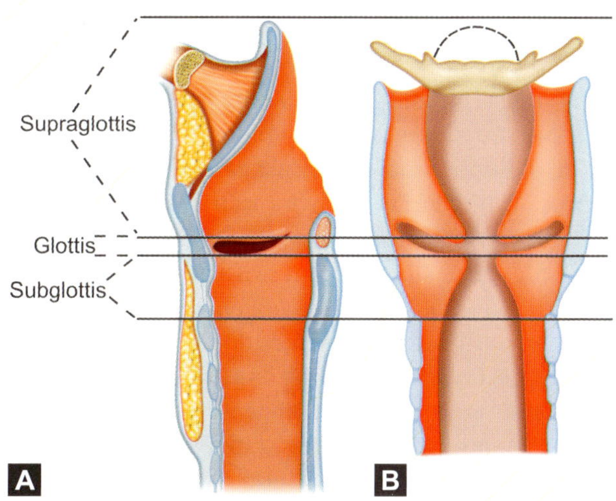

Figs. 12.1A and B: Laryngeal anatomy. The larynx is divided into three sites as depicted in (A) sagittal and (B) coronal views.

from the supraglottis. Supraglottic cancers are often diagnosed at a late stage because early-stage tumors produce relatively vague symptoms without significant impact on voice, breathing, or swallowing. Supraglottic cancers have a high propensity for nodal metastases due to the rich lymphatic drainage of this portion of the larynx. Nodal metastases can be occult and can occur on both sides of the neck even in unilateral primary tumors. Therefore, bilateral necks must be addressed in the treatment of supraglottic carcinomas.

The glottis refers to the true vocal folds. It extends from the inferior extent of the supraglottis at the laryngeal ventricle to 5 mm below the free edge of the true vocal folds. Glottic carcinoma accounts for approximately 60% of laryngeal cancers in the United States. These tumors tend to be diagnosed at an early stage due to the early impact on voice. There is a paucity of lymphatic drainage at the glottic level. Due to this, nodal metastases are rare for early-stage glottic tumors. The combination of these factors results in higher cure rates for glottic cancers in comparison to supraglottic cancers.

The subglottis extends for the inferior edge of the glottis to the inferior edge of the cricoid cartilage. Primary tumors in this location are rare and account for < 1% of laryngeal cancers in the United States. Tumors at this level are particularly challenging to manage with both endoscopic and open surgical approaches.

FUNCTION

As demonstrated by the moniker "voicebox," the production of sound is frequently perceived as the main function of the larynx, particularly by patients who require treatment for laryngeal cancer. However, from the surgeon's perspective, voice may be the least important of the laryngeal functions. The larynx must also be able to provide an adequate glottic opening to allow for respiration. In addition, the larynx must be able to protect the airway from aspiration to allow for safe deglutition. These complex functional demands require adequate sensation and dynamic glottic opening and closure.

Any treatment of laryngeal cancer, both surgical and nonsurgical, must account for functional considerations. Anatomic preservation without intact function is not an acceptable goal in organ-preserving strategies. The landmark VA laryngeal cancer trial and its follow-up RTOG 91-11 trial led to great enthusiasm for the use of definitive chemoradiation as an organ-preserving approach for the treatment of laryngeal cancer.[2,3] Since the early 1990s the rate of chemoradiotherapy has significantly increased, whereas the rate of surgery has decreased. Over the same time period, epidemiological data indicate that laryngeal cancer is the only malignancy for which survival rates have decreased.[4] In addition, more than two decades after the landmark chemoradiotherapy trials, there is evidence that the late toxicity of chemoradiotherapy is substantial.[5] Given these concerns, there may be an increased role of primary surgical management in the future.

OPEN PARTIAL LARYNGECTOMY

The management of laryngeal cancer requires a comprehensive understanding of all available treatment modalities, both surgical and nonsurgical. The American Society of Clinical Oncology has published clinical practice guidelines for the use of organ preservation strategies in the treatment of laryngeal cancer (Table 12.1). Endoscopic and open surgical management continue to play an important role in both early- and late-stage disease. While voice outcomes of radiation therapy (RT) and surgery for early-stage cancers have not been adequately compared, superior local control rates have been demonstrated with surgical management in numerous case series.[6] It should be emphasized that to achieve adequate functional outcomes, a single treatment modality should be pursued for early-stage tumors. For late-stage tumors, open partial laryngectomies can be selectively used. Here, we review the most commonly described open techniques, with an emphasis on the most commonly applied.

Vertical Partial Laryngectomy

Advances in endoscopic laser surgery have limited the role of open vertical partial laryngectomy (VPL) to highly selected cases. Best results in terms of local control and functional outcome are achieved with mobile midcord lesions. Local failure rates increase to 14–20% for anterior commissure involvement or T2 lesions.[7] As such, the best candidates can often be managed with endoscopic surgery. A role still exists for VPL for cases in which endoscopic exposure is inadequate. In addition, some authors would argue that VPL can provide the opportunity to reconstruct what would be large defects with endoscopic surgery. The hope is that glottic reconstruction would improve the sphincteric and vocal function in these cases. A variety of different vertical partial approaches and reconstructions have been described. Here, we provide an overview of the most commonly described methods.

Table 12.1: Clinical practice guidelines for laryngeal preservation strategies.[6]

Cancer type	*Recommended treatment*	*Other treatment options*
T1 glottic	Endoscopic resection or RT	Open OPS
T2 glottic, favorable*	Open OPS or RT	Endoscopic Resection
T2 glottic, unfavorable*	Open OPS or CRT (for select N+ patients)	RT or Endoscopic resection
T1-2, supraglottic favorable†	Open OPS or RT	Endoscopic resection
T2 supraglottic, unfavorable†	Open OPS or CRT (for select N+ patients)	RT or Endoscopic resection
T3-4 glottic or supraglottic‡	CRT, Open OPS (for highly selected patients)	RT

(RT: Radiation therapy; OPS: Organ preservation surgery; CRT: Concurrent chemoradiotherapy).

*Favorable T2 glottic: Superficial tumor on radiographic imaging with normal vocal cord mobility.Unfavorable T2 glottic: deeply invasive tumor on radiographic imaging, with impaired cord mobility.

†Favorable supraglottic: T1 or T2 with superficial invasion on imaging and preserved cord mobility and/or tumor of the aryepiglottic fold with minimal involvement of medial pyriform sinus. Unfavorable supraglottic tumors are more locally advanced and more deeply invasive.

‡Total laryngectomy will frequently be the appropriate treatment for advanced laryngeal cancer in lieu of organ preservation.

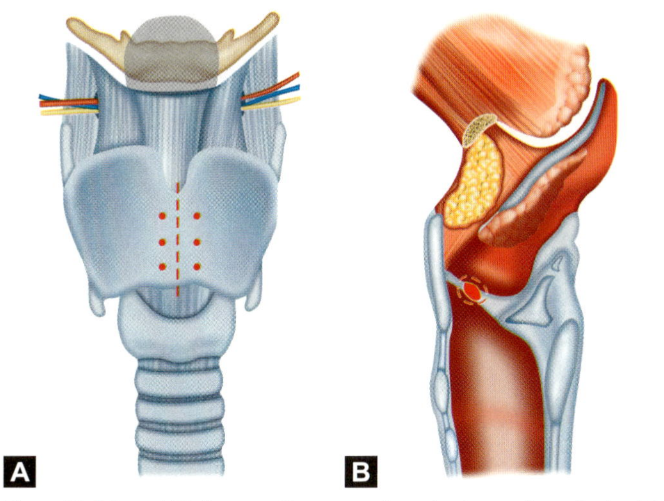

Figs. 12.2A and B: Laryngofissure and cordectomy. A vertical midline thyrotomy provides open tumor exposure. Before opening paired drill holes can be made to aid in reconstruction (A). The procedure is most appropriate for mobile mid cord lesions as demonstrated in sagittal view (B).

Laryngofissure with Cordectomy

Conceptually, this technique is the most straightforward. A vertical midline thyrotomy is performed with the drill, scalpel, or saw. The anterior commissure is opened and exposure achieved for cordectomy (Figs. 12.2A and B). With larger resections, small subglottic and supraglottic mucosal advancement flaps can allow for primary closure. The laryngofissure is closed with 2-0 Vicryl sutures, which can be passed through paired drill holes on the anterior lamina.

Vertical Hemilaryngectomy with Imbrication Laryngoplasty

This method described by Weinstein and Laccourreye involves a midline thyrotomy along with the resection of a horizontal strut of the midthyroid lamina.[7] Following resection, the defect is closed with mucosal flaps followed by imbrication of the upper and lower segments of the thyroid lamina. The overlapping cartilages thereby provide bulk for the reconstructed glottis (Figs.12.3A and B).

Frontolateral and Extended Approaches

These techniques involve the resection of additional thyroid cartilage, including the anterior commissure, with a variety of possible reconstructions utilizing the epiglottis (epiglottic laryngoplasty) or strap muscles and perichondrium. The frontolateral approach involves a paramedian vertical thyrotomy on the less involved side. A variety of different cartilaginous resections can then be performed, including the anterior thyroid cartilage and portions on the more involved side (Figs. 12.4A to D). Given the variety of resections and reconstructions possible, the functional outcome with these extended procedures is uncertain. Supracricoid partial laryngectomy is likely to provide a more reliable and reproducible result.

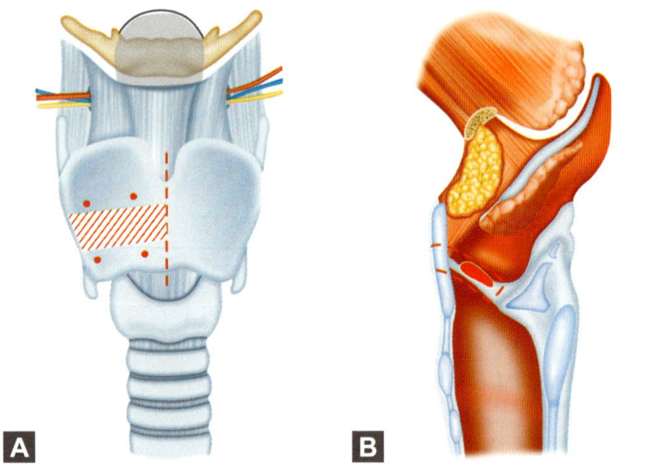

Figs. 12.3A and B: Vertical partial laryngectomy with imbrication laryngoplasty. A vertical midline thyrotomy is made and a horizontal strut of the thyroid lamina is resected (A) along with the tumor seen in sagittal view (B).

Open Supraglottic Partial Laryngectomy

The open supraglottic partial laryngectomy (SGPL) removes the larynx above the level of the true vocal folds (Figs. 12.5A and B). It may be indicated for T1 and T2 lesions of the supraglottis and select T3 lesions with limited preepiglottic space invasion and mobile vocal cords. This procedure includes the resection of the entire preepiglottic space along with a portion of the thyroid cartilage superior to the anterior commissure. After laryngeal exposure, the thyroid cartilage incision is made approximating the level of the glottis. A variety of different cartilaginous incisions have been employed. A pharyngotomy is then made into the vallecula. The epiglottis is retracted anteriorly and endolaryngeal cuts are made anterior to the arytenoids. Cuts are extended inferiorly to the level of the lateral extent of the ventricle, that is, to the glottis. Cuts are then extended in a horizontal plane at the inferior border of the supraglottis and connected with the cartilaginous incision. The specimen can then be removed and frozen sections obtained. A thyrohyoid impaction must then be performed (Figs. 12.6A and B).

With the advent and demonstrated viability of endoscopic transoral SGPL, we feel that there is a limited role for open SGPL, which is mostly confined to cases in which adequate endoscopic exposure cannot be achieved. For more advanced stage disease, a variety of extended open

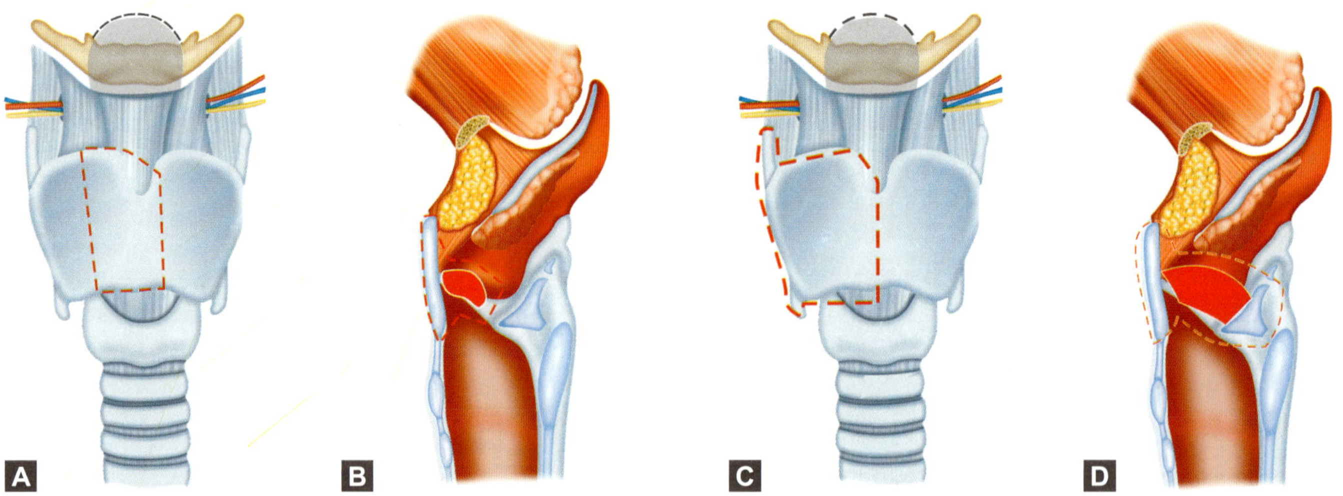

Figs. 12.4A to D: Frontolateral and extended vertical partial laryngectomy. A paramedian thyrotomy is made in the frontolateral approach and variable amounts of the ipsilateral thyroid cartilage can be resected, including the anterior commissure (A and B). A more extensive resection including the arytenoid is possible (C and D).

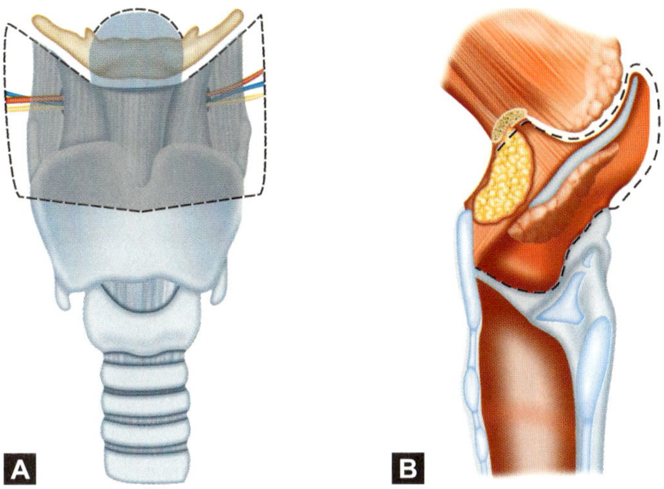

Figs. 12.5A and B: Open supraglottic partial laryngectomy (SGPL). The extent of resection in open SGPL is indicated in frontal (A) and sagittal (B) views. This procedure is classified as a Type 1 open partial laryngectomy by the European Laryngological Society.[8]

SGPL techniques have been described, which can address tumors extending to the arytenoid, to one vocal cord, to the hypopharynx or to the tongue base and hyoid. In cases where such extended approaches would be required, patients may be better served by organ preservation chemoradiation protocols or total laryngectomy with partial pharyngectomy.

Supracricoid Partial Laryngectomy with Cricohyoidoepiglottopexy or Cricohyoidopexy (SCPL with CHEP or CHP)

Indications and Patient Selection

The SCPL removes the entire thyroid cartilage, both vocal cords, most of the paraglottic space and a variable amount of the supraglottis (Figs. 12.7 and 12.8). It is indicated for the surgical management of early-stage and select advanced-stage glottic cancers but is infrequently the first-line treatment choice and would rarely be recommended for superficial focal lesions. For more extensive and invasive early-stage lesions, it provides superior local control with the tradeoff of potentially worse vocal outcome when compared with RT. It may be preferable to endoscopic resection when there is inadequate endoscopic exposure or when it is anticipated to provide improved local control and/or functional outcome. This situation may be likely in lesions with significant involvement of both vocal cords, deep extension at the anterior commissure, as well as deeply invasive unilateral lesions. For select late-stage lesions, it provides the possibility of a curative resection with laryngeal preservation and reliable voice and swallowing outcomes.

Special Considerations

With both true vocal folds removed, the production of voice and the protection against aspiration rely upon the dynamic opposition of the arytenoid against the residual epiglottis or base of tongue. The preservation of the cricoarytenoid joint and its innervation is, therefore, critical, and the functional importance of the crico-arytenoid unit is a key concept in conservation laryngeal surgery. Although resection of one arytenoid is feasible, preservation of both arytenoids permits optimal functional outcome. Involvement of both arytenoids is a strict contraindication to SCPL.

All patients will have at least temporary aspiration after SCPL. Patient motivation and close follow-up with an experienced speech therapist are critical to swallowing rehabilitation. Patient comorbidities and performance status must be carefully evaluated prior to the procedure. Poor pulmonary status is a contraindication to SCPL. This assessment can be based on pulmonary function tests, although many surgeons accept the ability to climb two flights of steps without dyspnea as adequate evaluation of respiratory status. Patient motivation is also an important factor as significant speech and swallowing rehabilitation is required. At our institution, all patients meet with the speech therapist prior to surgery. This provides the patients with a better understanding of postoperative expectations and an opportunity to practice swallowing exercises and techniques. We favor placement of a percutaneous endoscopic gastrostomy tube in all patients undergoing SCPL. This practice avoids a foreign body in the pharynx and allows a more gradual transition to PO intake, although use of a temporary nasogastric tube is another common practice.

Frozen section analysis of margins is imperative for SCPL. This is especially true in the salvage setting where there is a greater chance of unrecognized submucosal extent. All patients must be counseled and consented for the possibility of total laryngectomy based on intra-operative findings.

Contraindications

The SCPL may be contraindicated due to tumor extent or individual patient characteristics. Extension to the cricoid cartilage or to both arytenoids would not permit complete

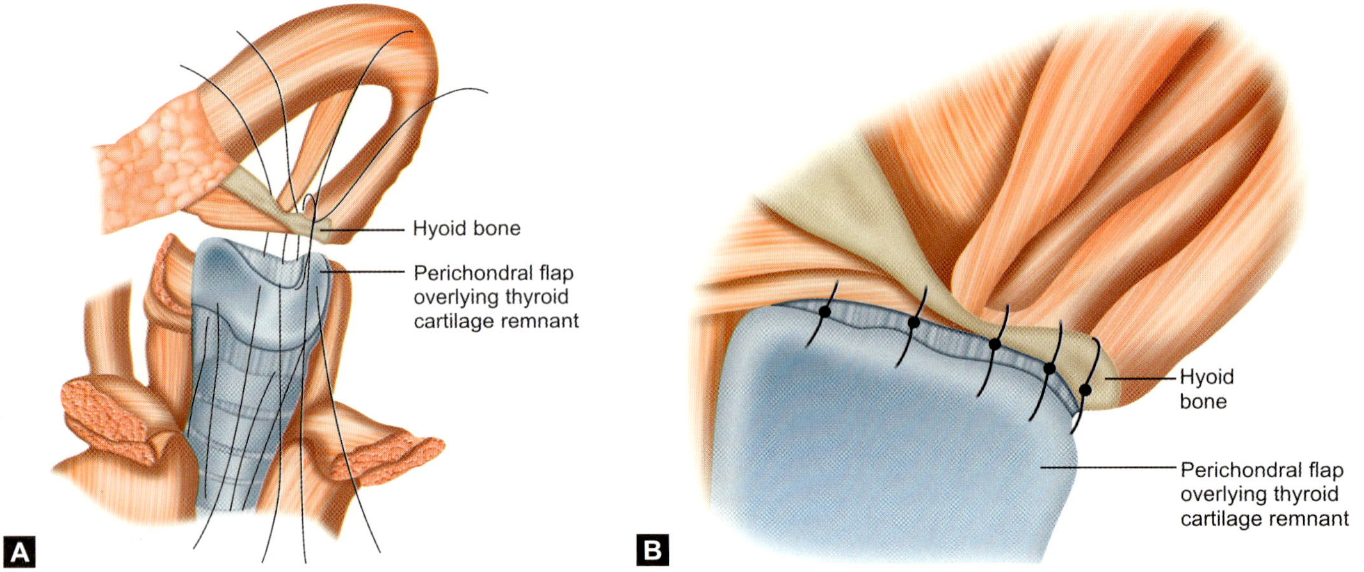

Figs. 12.6A and B: Thyrohyoid impaction. After open supraglottic partial laryngectomy the remaining cartilage must be approximated to the hyoid and tongue base.

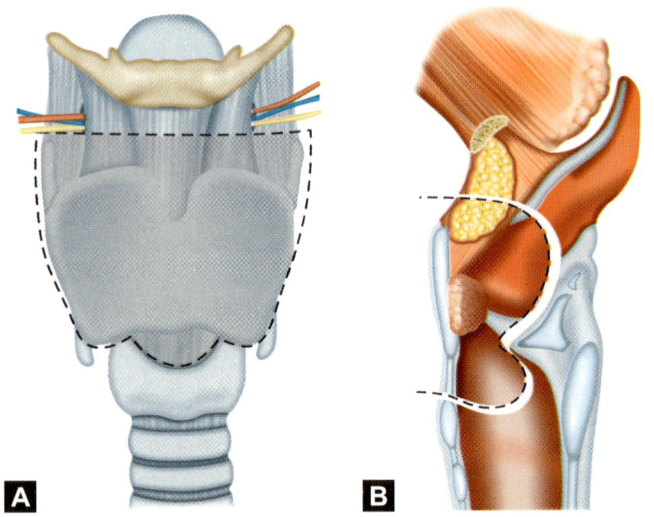

Figs. 12.7A and B: Supracricoid partial laryngectomy with cricohyoidoepiglottopexy. The extent of resection is demonstrated in frontal (A) and sagittal (B) views. This procedure is classified as a type IIa open partial horizontal laryngectomy.[8]

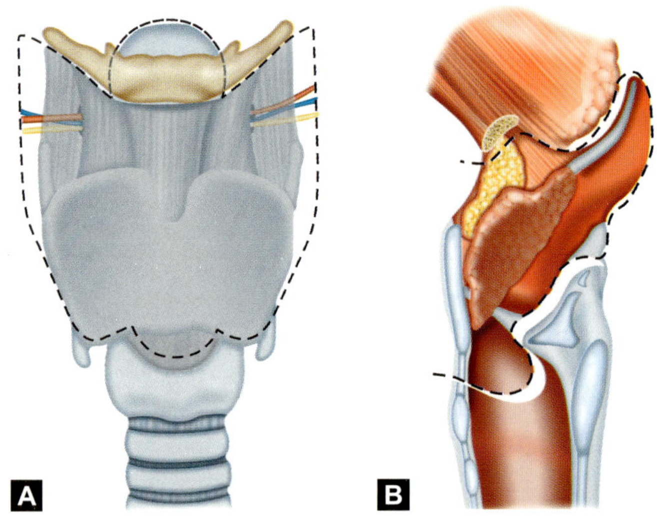

Figs. 12.8A and B: Supracricoid partial laryngectomy with cricohyoidopexy. The extent of resection is demonstrated in frontal (A) and sagittal (B) views. This procedure is classified as a type IIb open partial horizontal laryngectomy.[8]

resection of tumor with SCPL. Significant edema from prior radiation frequently limits the use of SCPL in the salvage setting. The key patient characteristic that precludes SCPL is poor baseline pulmonary status, which would not allow patients to tolerate the expected postoperative aspiration. In addition, advanced age and dementia are relative contraindications due to the intensive swallowing rehabilitation required postoperatively. Contraindications are listed in Table 12.2.

Operative Technique

1. Preoperative endoscopy is performed in all cases to confirm tumor characteristics and operative plan. Special attention should be given to the sites of laryngeal entry, specifically mucosal involvement of the subglottis and epiglottis.
2. A thyroidectomy-type or apron incision is designed with its nadir approximately 2 cm above the sternal

Table 12.2: Contraindications to supracricoid partial laryngectomy.

Inadequate pulmonary reserve	Extensive preepiglottic space or hyoid invasion
Major comorbidity	Cricoarytenoid joint invasion
Thyroid cartilage invasion*	Extension below upper border of cricoid†
Extralaryngeal extension*	Mucosal involvement of both arytenoids
Cricoid cartilage invasion	Posterior commissure or interarytenoid involvement

*Except focal invasion/extension amenable to resection with a margin of uninvolved tissue.
†Extended technique involving partial resection of anterior cricoid may be selectively used.

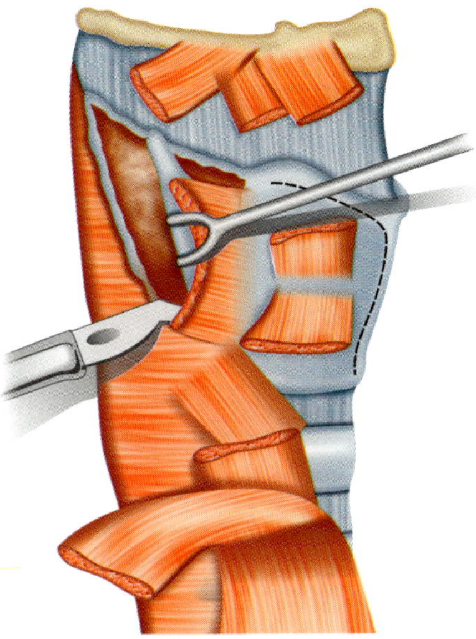

Fig. 12.9: Constrictor release and pyriform sinus elevation. After the anterior trachea is released from the mediastinum and the strap muscles are divided, the larynx is rotated and the constrictors are divided along the posterolateral thyroid cartilage.

notch. It can be extended more laterally and superiorly to facilitate lateral neck dissections.

3. Subplatysmal flaps are elevated to the level of the clavicles and 1–2 cm above the hyoid.
4. The strap muscles are separated along the midline raphe. Fibrofatty tissues including any delphian nodes along the anterior central compartment are resected.
5. The thyroid isthmus is divided and the lobes mobilized laterally maintaining their attachment at Berry's ligament. Paratracheal dissection can be performed at this time. Preservation of the recurrent laryngeal nerves (RLNs) is critical. In cases where paratracheal dissection is not performed, identification of the RLNs is not necessary for preservation.
6. Blunt dissection along the anterior trachea is performed in the mediastinum. This is best performed with finger dissection approximately to the level of the carina. Tracheal mobilization facilitates impaction during the reconstructive portion of the procedure.
7. The sternohyoid muscles are divided along the superior border of the thyroid cartilage and the sternothyroid and thyrohyoid muscles are released at their attachments to the thyroid cartilage. Any necessary vessels are ligated but care is taken to avoid injury to the superior laryngeal nerve.
8. The larynx is rotated and the inferior constrictor muscles are released along the lateral border of the thyroid cartilage down to the level of the cricoid. The pyriform sinus mucosa is mobilized away from the inner cortex of the thyroid cartilage. This can be accomplished with a Freer elevator or a cottonoid (Fig. 12.9).
9. With great care, the cricothyroid joint is disarticulated with a Cottle or Freer elevator along the thyroid cartilage in an anterior to posterior fashion to avoid injury to the RLN running just posterior to the joint. Remaining ligamentous and constrictor muscle attachments are carefully divided sharply. The above two steps are performed bilaterally (Fig. 12.10).
10. A cricothyrotomy is then made wide enough to accommodate an endotracheal tube closely following the upper cricoid cartilage. The transoral tube is withdrawn and an endotracheal tube is passed through the cricothyrotomy.
11. The appropriate approach to the endolarynx is selected according to the tumor extent. In a CHP, the hyoepiglottic ligament is cut and the vallecula is entered such that the epiglottis and preepiglottic space may be included in the resection. In CHEP, a cut is made through the preepiglottic space and the epiglottis in an axial plane at the level of the thyroid notch.

12. The petiole (in CHEP) or the tip of the epiglottis (in CHP) is then retracted anteriorly and cuts are extended starting on the less involved side first through the aryepiglottic fold and then down through the supraglottis just anterior to the arytenoids. The true vocal cord is then transected anterior to the vocal process (Fig. 12.11). Inferiorly, the cut then follows the upper border of the cricoid cartilage dividing the cricothyroid muscle and connecting with the previously made cricothyrotomy.

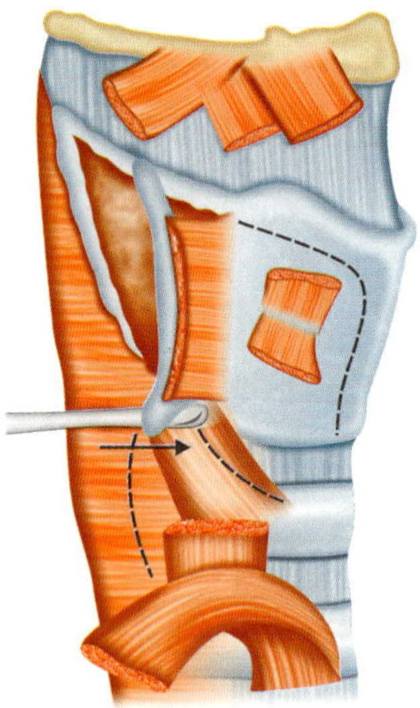

Fig. 12.10: Cricoarytenoid joint separation. The joint is carefully separated in a posterior to anterior direction along the thyroid facet.

13. The thyroid cartilage is then grasped and fractured along the midline to better visualize the endolarynx and tumor on the more involved side. This allows an "open book" view of the endolarynx.
14. Cuts are then made on the more involved side in a similar fashion. Alternatively, resection may include the arytenoid if necessary. Frozen section margins are then taken circumferentially from the defect.
15. The cut mucosa may be advanced over the arytenoid to reduce cartilage exposure or to add bulk to replace the resected arytenoid with 3 or 4-0 absorbable suture. The anterior aspect of the arytenoid is then sutured to the anterior cricoid cartilage with a 2-0 or 3-0 absorbable suture reapproximating the tension of the true vocal cord. The arytenoid does not close that distance, thus leaving the naked suture crossing the laryngeal lumen as an air knot (Figs. 12.12A and B).
16. Three impaction sutures are then placed and tagged with hemostats. Using a 1-0 Vicryl on a large needle, the suture is passed inferiorly around the cricoid cartilage in the midline to the laryngeal lumen. In CHEP, it is then passed through the full thickness of the epiglottis and then regrasped and passed over the hyoid bone (Figs. 12.13A and B). In CHP, the suture is passed through the mucosa of the tongue base and over the hyoid bone with a generous bite of the tongue base. Two additional sutures are placed 1 cm lateral to the midline and tagged. The hypoglossal nerves must

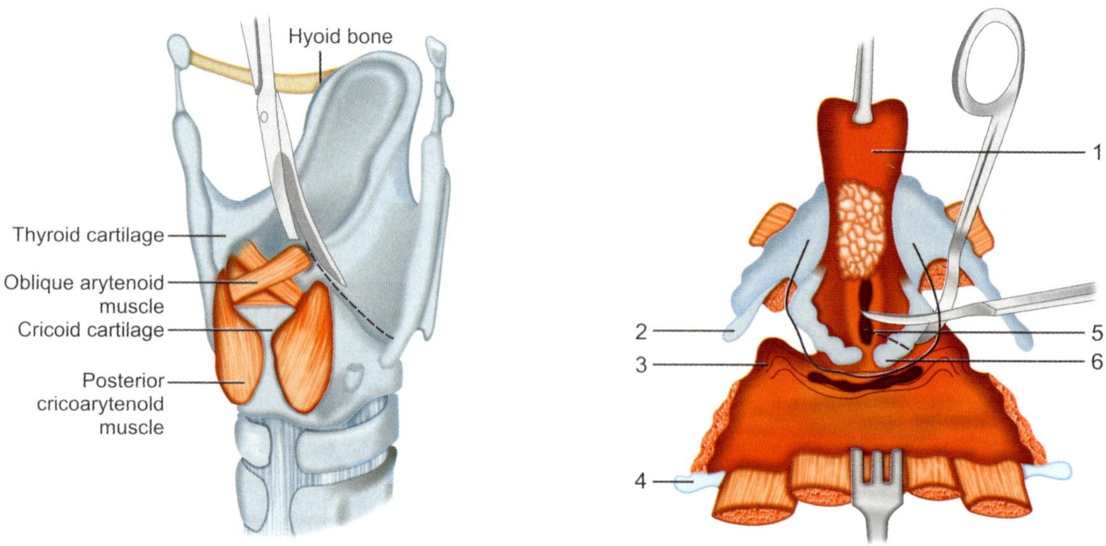

Fig. 12.11: Tumor resection with exposure through the laryngotomy or pharyngotomy and anterior retraction; the tumor can be directly visualized and incisions through the supraglottis and glottis of the less involved side are made.
1. Epiglottis; 2. Thyroid cartilage; 3. Pyriform sinus; 4. Hyoid bone; 5. Prearytenoid incision; 6. Arytenoid cartilage.

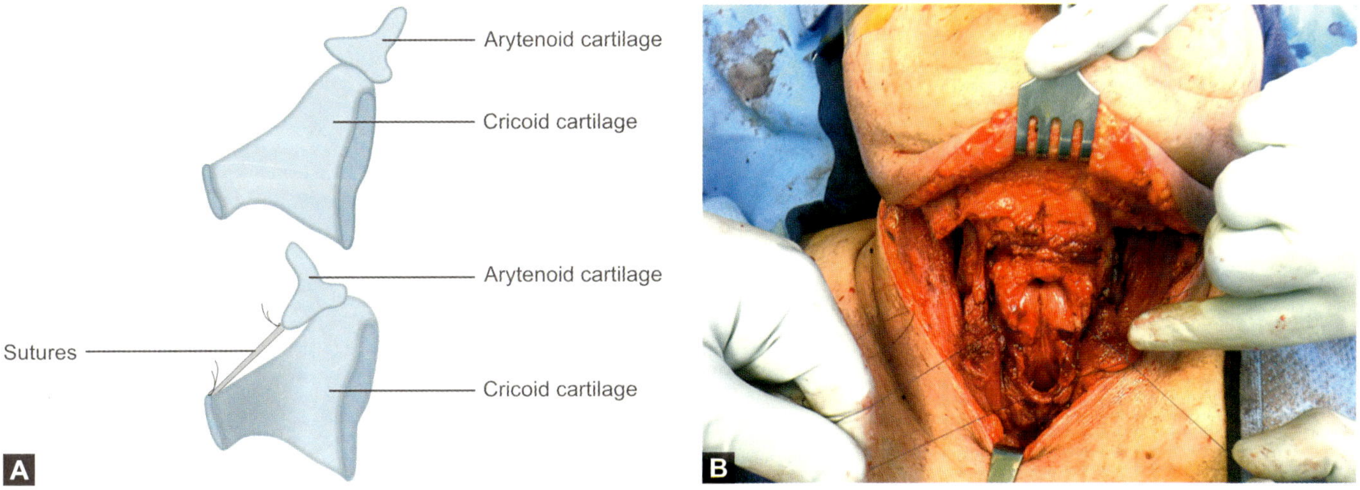

Figs. 12.12A and B: Arytenoid sutures. A suture replaces the tension of the vocal cord to maintain the arytenoid in more anatomic position as demonstrated in the diagram (A) and photograph (B).

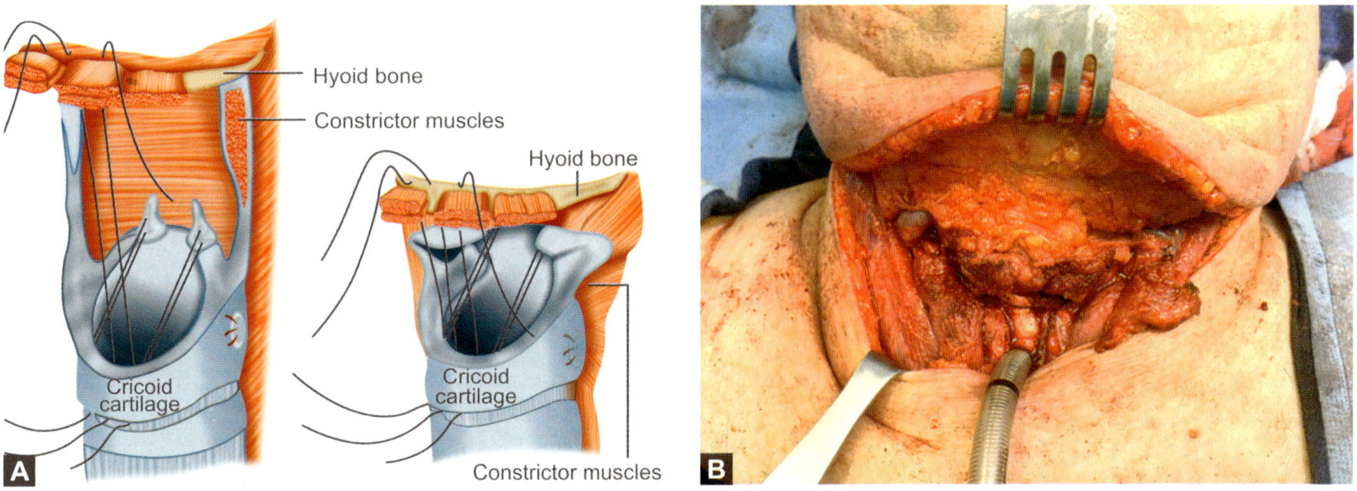

Figs. 12.13A and B: Impaction sutures. Three heavy impaction sutures pass around the cricoid and hyoid for reconstruction as demonstrated in the cricohyoidoepiglottopexy diagram (A) and photograph (B).

be avoided. Some authors describe passing these sutures submucosally around the cricoid, but doing so is likely to result in further mucosal disruption in the subglottis and risks damage to the cricoid cartilage. With the use of absorbable suture, submucosal suturing is unnecessary and decreases risk of future extrusion and chondritis.

17. The sutures are then pulled tightly to approximate the impaction so that the tracheostomy site can be appropriately selected. This is typically lower on the trachea itself than a standard tracheostomy but corresponds to a more typical position in the anterior neck due to tracheal mobilization. The tracheotomy is then made and the endotracheal tube relocated.
18. With the aid of assistants the impaction sutures are simultaneously tightened and then tied sequentially maintaining the impaction. During this process, the anterior border or the cricoid and hyoid must be aligned vertically (Fig. 12.14).
19. The constrictors can then be reapproximated to suspend the pyriform sinuses in a more anatomic position. This can be accomplished by passing sutures the fascia of the constrictors in mattress fashion. The suture can then be tied anteriorly across the front of

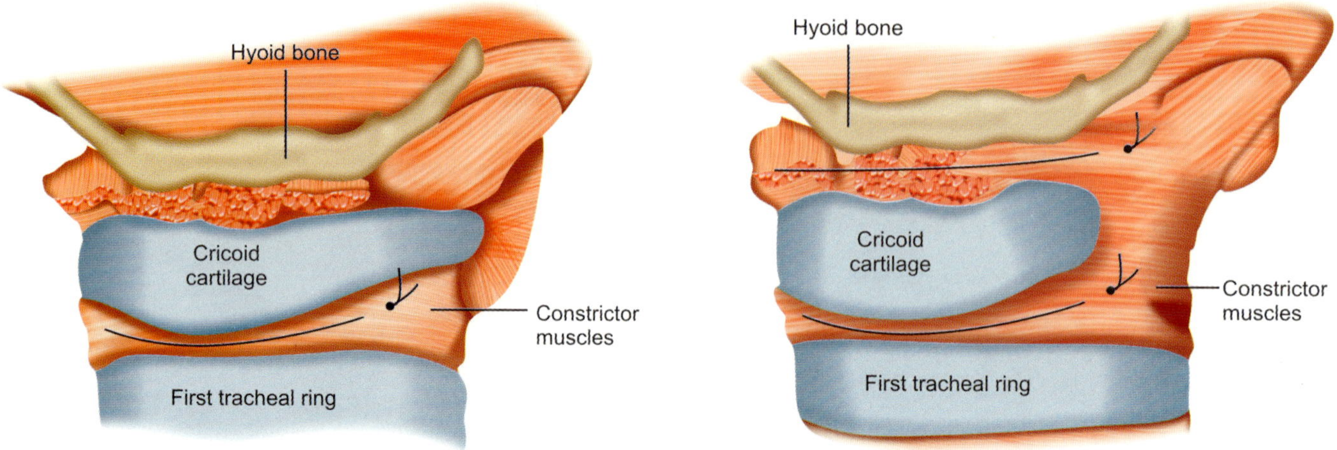

Fig. 12.14: Impaction and constrictor suspension. The impaction sutures are tightened and tied. The mobile cut edges of the constrictors are tied across the midline to each other to suspend the pyriform sinuses in more anatomic position.

the impaction. This maneuver has been shown to reduce the risk of aspiration (Laccourreye). The divided strap muscles are then reapproximated in another layer to provide additional tissue coverage over the impaction.

20. Drains are placed laterally and the neck is closed in layers with the tracheostomy positioned centrally. We prefer to replace the endotracheal tube with a cuffed tracheostomy tube with the cuff inflated postoperatively.

Operative Considerations

In select cancers, the procedure can be modified to include resection of a single arytenoid or the upper portion of the cricoid ring anteriorly. It is important to note that these extensions are for the management of mucosal spread to these locations. Gross involvement of the cricoarytenoid joint or the cricoid cartilage is a contraindication to SCPL due to oncologic compromise. Select T4 lesions with focal thyroid cartilage involvement can be addressed with SCPL in experienced hands. Care must be taken to maintain an adequate margin with the overlying strap muscles. Extensive thyroid cartilage destruction is a contraindication to SCPL.

Postoperative Management

We prefer the use of a cuffed tracheostomy tube in the immediate postoperative period. The cuff can be deflated on the first postoperative day to avoid prolonged pooling of secretions along the impaction. We proceed with tracheostomy tube change on the fifth postoperative day and then begin Passy-Muir valve (PMV) use or capping trials if possible. A standard decannulation algorithm can then be followed. Most patients can be decannulated by the second postoperative week. Aspiration is expected and use of a PMV or cap will increase compensatory mechanisms until decannulation. Patients receive perioperative antibiotics and are maintained on proton pump inhibitors throughout their recovery. Once patients are using a PMV or cap and are managing their own secretions, they may begin sips of water. An oral diet can then be advanced as tolerated to thickened liquids and soft foods. Patients should work closely with speech pathologists to develop compensatory strategies for successful swallowing rehabilitation. A mild degree of aspiration is tolerated in the early postoperative period as the diet is advanced. More severe aspiration and silent aspiration raise the concern for damage to the superior laryngeal nerves, which will limit progression to an oral diet. The amount of time before patients return to an oral diet is variable and has been reported to be 9–50 days.[9] This variation is a result of preoperative factors such as prior radiation and comorbid illness, as well as certain operative factors. Resection of the entire epiglottis, resection of one arytenoid, and damage to the superior laryngeal nerve may be expected to prolong tube feeding. Damage to the RLN is catastrophic and must be avoided.

Complications

Reported complications include wound infection, perichondritis, aspiration pneumonia, laryngeal stenosis, laryngocele, and ruptured pexy.[9,10] Postoperative laryngocele is likely the result of retained mucosa within the ventricle so care should be taken to ensure that all is removed during resection. Ruptured pexy should be suspected in the event of severe aspiration and tracheostomy dependence. A palpable gap may be present between the hyoid and cricoid cartilage. This event is rare, reported in only 0.8% of cases.[9] Interestingly, fistula is not a reported complication. Laryngeal stenosis is also rare, occurring in <5% of cases and may occur as a delayed complication.[10]

TOTAL LARYNGECTOMY

Indications and Patient Selection

Total laryngectomy is indicated for the management of advanced laryngeal cancer when partial laryngectomy techniques are not feasible and when definitive chemoradiation is not expected to control the tumor or is not expected to result in satisfactory functional outcome. Total laryngectomy is an excellent treatment option for many patients and has predictable oncologic and functional outcomes.

Chemoradiotherapy must be selectively offered. It should not be offered as a means to avoid total laryngectomy when tumor or patient characteristics do not allow. In general, T4 tumors should undergo laryngectomy. In addition, if a patient's comorbidities or performance status makes completion of chemoradiation unlikely, then it is best avoided. Significant pretreatment laryngeal dysfunction will seldom improve with nonoperative treatment and must be considered in the treatment selection process. Patient refusal of laryngectomy should not be viewed as an indication for chemoradiation as it often reflects insufficient patient counseling.

Due to the increased use of chemoradiation, total laryngectomy is frequently performed in the salvage setting. When performed as salvage, there is an increased rate of complications, especially pharyngocutaneous fistula, and additional reconstructive measures may be required. Due to the recurrent nature of the tumor, local control and cure are lower in the salvage setting. Initial treatment planning must consider these factors to minimize the need for salvage laryngectomy.

Operative Technique

- Direct laryngoscopy is always performed to evaluate tumor extent and plan for pharyngeal and tracheal entry, as well as to anticipate the potential need for flap reconstruction of the pharynx or tongue base.
- A variety of skin incisions may be considered. Most commonly an apron incision extending to approximately 2 cm above the sternal notch is used. If a preoperative tracheostomy is present, it is incorporated into the incision such that an ellipse of skin and the tracheostomy tract are incorporated into the incision and resection.
- Alternatively, we tend to use a higher incision within an existing neck crease and then create the stoma in a separate circular incision 2 cm inferior to the upper border of the lower skin flap (Figs. 12.15A and B). This eliminates the trifurcation at the stoma, which is

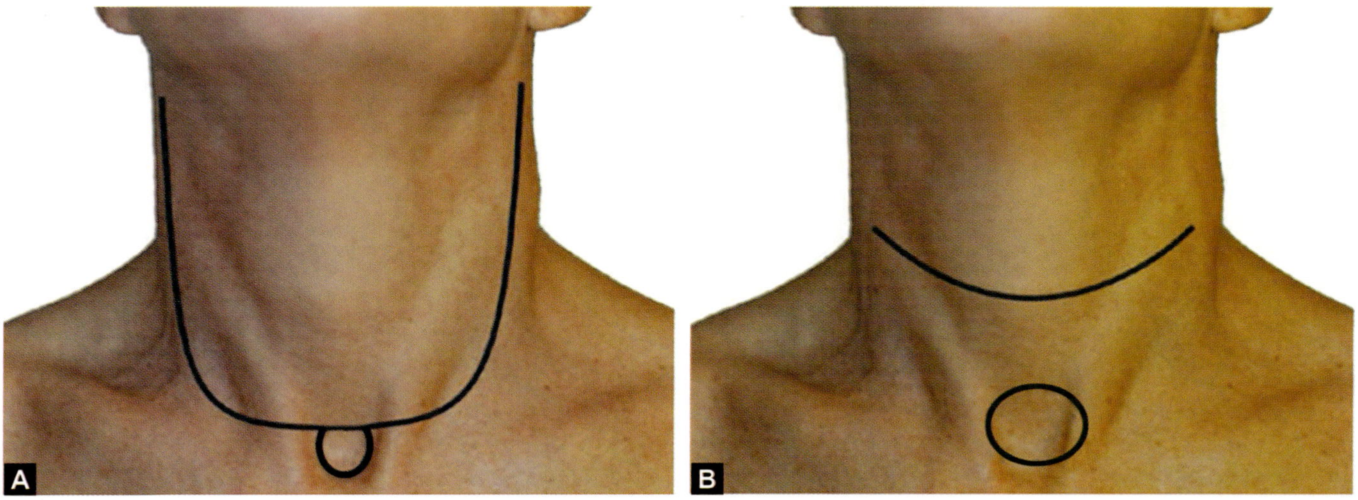

Figs. 12.15A and B: Total laryngectomy incisions. An apron incision can be used and the stoma positioned at its inferior aspect (A). Alternatively a higher incision can be used with a separate stoma incision (B).

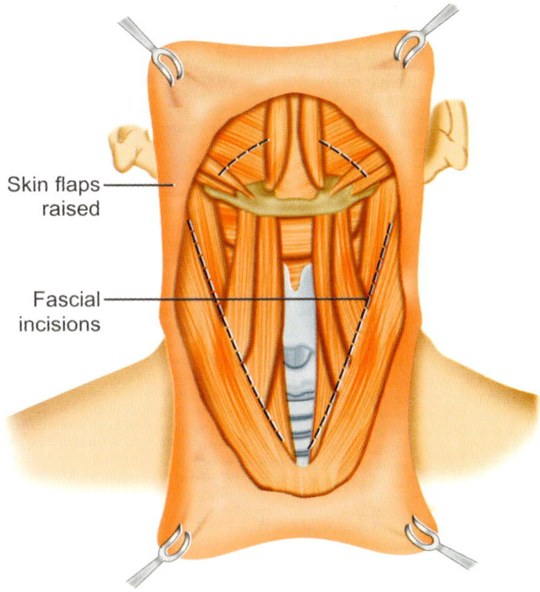

Fig. 12.16: Skin flaps and fascial incisions. After elevation of subplatysmal flaps, the superficial layer of the deep cervical fascia is incised to expose the deeper neck structures.

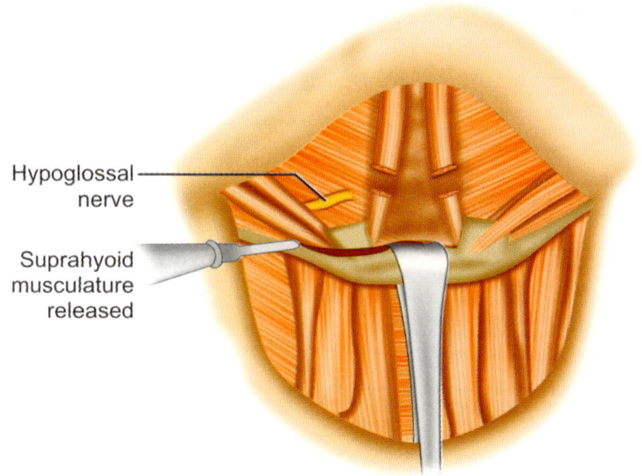

Fig. 12.17: Suprahyoid muscle release. Closely following the upper border of the hyoid, the muscles are released and the lateral hyoid bone is skeletonized.

a frequent site of wound breakdown. We have found that this technique allows for the creation of a large and stable stoma and in the event of postoperative fistula, drainage tends to manifest in the neck incision rather than at the trifurcation of the stoma where it leads to aspiration and is closer to the carotid artery. The midneck incision extended horizontally along a natural crease typically allows exposure for the laryngectomy as well as neck dissections without the need for vertical limb extensions.

- Subplatysmal flaps are elevated to the level of the clavicles and to 2 cm above the hyoid. When lateral neck dissections are to be performed, we usually proceed with one or both at this point. Some surgeons advocate completing the laryngectomy prior to both neck dissections to prevent pharyngeal edema from interfering with reconstruction.
- As in a neck dissection, the posterior belly of the digastric is widely exposed bilaterally. This can be accomplished by dividing the fascia superficial to the fibrous loop attachment to the hyoid and following it posteriorly (Fig. 12.16). Alternatively, the fascia inferior to the submandibular gland can be incised and the muscle belly is encountered deep to the gland. Care must be taken to avoid injury to the marginal mandibular branch of the facial nerve, although its routine identification is unnecessary. In the event of a planned microvascular reconstruction, the facial vein or common facial trunk should be skeletonized and preserved.
- If not already done during neck dissections, the superficial layer of the deep cervical fascia is incised along the anterior border of the sternocleidomastoid muscle (SCM) bilaterally (Fig. 12.16). The sternal heads of the SCMs are then separated at their attachments medially. The purpose of this maneuver is to allow for a flat contour and a wide stoma, but we prefer to perform it early to improve exposure during the neck dissection and dissection of the midline neck structures.
- A plane is then developed medial to the carotid artery down to the prevertebral fascia. We prefer to perform this procedure bluntly and maintain as much fascial covering of the carotid as possible to provide protection in the event of fistula. The superior thyroid artery, laryngeal vessels, and superior laryngeal nerve will bridge this plane superiorly and are preserved at this point. Inferiorly, the omohyoid muscle is divided.
- The suprahyoid muscles (mylohyoid, geniohyoid, hyoglossus, stylohyoid, and digastric sling) are then released from the hyoid with electrocautery by closely following the upper border of the bone (Fig. 12.17). Laterally, this requires rotation of the bone out of the deeper neck to access the greater horn, which is then skeletonized. Injury to the hypoglossal nerve can be avoided by incising precisely on the bone. Alternatively, it can be dissected and exposed to

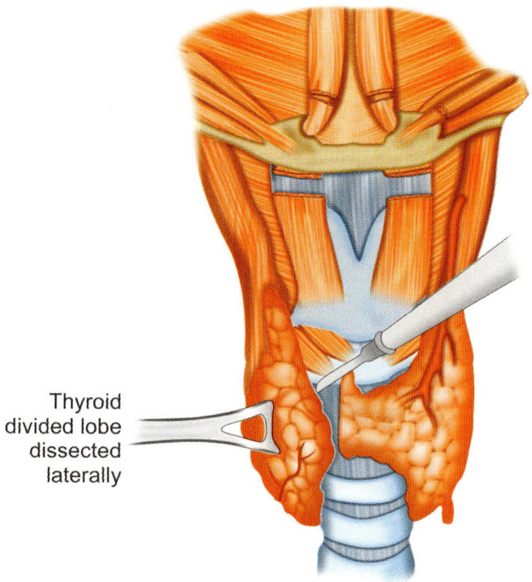

Fig. 12.18: Thyroid division. The isthmus is divided and the lobe to be preserved is retracted laterally and separated from the airway. The lobe included in resection is separated from its fascial and vascular attachments.

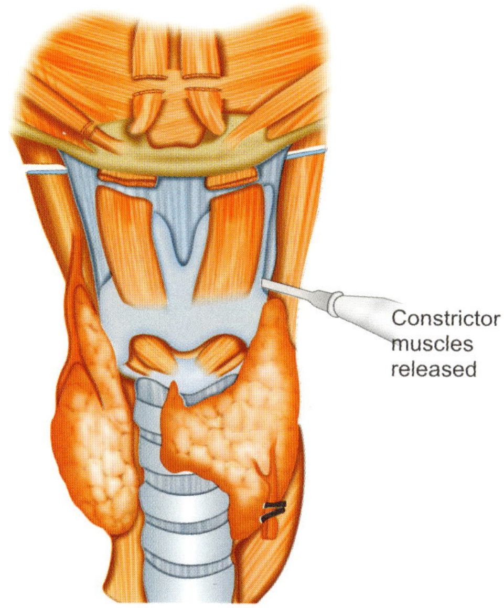

Fig. 12.19: Constrictor release. The larynx is rotated to create tension and the constrictors are divided along the posterolateral thyroid cartilage.

ensure identification and preservation. Dissection ceases when the plane deep to the muscle fibers is encountered.

- The strap muscles are divided inferiorly at the manubrium and anterior jugular veins are ligated. The midline raphe may be opened inferiorly to facilitate this dissection and subsequent thyroid dissection.
- Based on tumor extent, the decision is made to perform ipsilateral, subtotal or total thyroidectomy. With ipsilateral thyroidectomy, the isthmus is divided and the contralateral lobe is retracted laterally (Fig. 12.18). It is separated from the trachea such that it can be fully mobilized and reflected laterally with the parathyroid glands and the superior vascular pedicle preserved. Alternatively, the lobe itself can be divided and mobilized to similarly preserve its posterolateral portion. On the ipsilateral lobe or on both lobes in the case of total thyroidectomy, a capsular dissection is performed posterolaterally to identify and preserve the parathyroid glands. It may be helpful to tag them with a clip for identification during paratracheal dissection. Frozen section sampling and reimplantation of parathyroid glands may be necessary.
- The larynx is then rotated to create tension over the constrictors and then with the aid of palpation, the constrictors are divided along the posterolateral border of the thyroid cartilage from the greater cornu down to the cricoid cartilage. Electrocautery is used to divide these muscles and the perichondrium along the posterior border of the cartilage (Fig. 12.19). The ligamentous attachments to the cornu are separated superiorly, and then the perichondrium and pyriform sinus mucosa can be elevated from the inner cortex of the thyroid lamina with a cottonoid or Freer elevator (Fig. 12.20). This step is not performed when tumor is present beyond the endolarynx on that side.
- During or after the separation of the constrictors, the superior laryngeal vessels can be identified. They are divided and ligated medially. In this manner the superior thyroid pedicle and branches to the constrictors and pharyngeal mucosa can be preserved. The superior laryngeal nerve is next encountered and divided (Fig. 12.21).
- At this point a tracheotomy can be made between the first few rings or below the existing tracheotomy. If a paratracheal dissection is performed, it should be done prior to tracheotomy. Indications for paratracheal dissection are reviewed in Table 12.3. The existing endotracheal tube is withdrawn and the airway is entered. The cut can follow a ring horizontally or be beveled superiorly through one ring. When a separate stoma is planned, the tracheotomy typically follows a single ring and is not beveled. If it appears necessary, the trachea can be secured to the lower skin flap with a suture to prevent mediastinal retraction while the laryngectomy is completed.

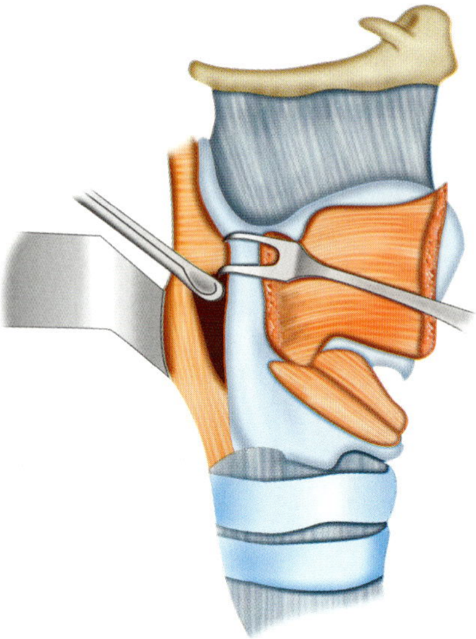

Fig. 12.20: Pyriform sinus elevation. The superior cornu is skeletonized and the pyriform sinus is elevated away from the inner cortex.

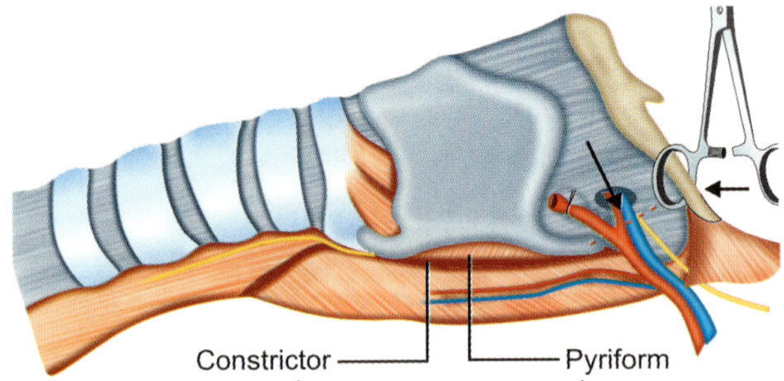

Fig. 12.21: The skeletonized larynx. The superior laryngeal vessels and superior laryngeal nerve are divided. The pedicle to the remaining thyroid lobe may be preserved.

Table 12.3: Indications for paratracheal dissection
Subglottic extension
Hypopharyngeal extension or primary
Advanced T stage
Clinically positive paratracheal nodes

- For endolaryngeal tumors the trachea can then be elevated from the esophagus and hypopharynx until the postcricoid musculature is visible on its deep surface (Figs. 12.22A and B). If not already done, the RLNs are transected. If there is hypopharyngeal extension, then the larynx should not be elevated in this manner and the remainder of the resection should be performed from the top down.
- The pharynx is then entered, usually in the vallecula. A Yankauer suction or Deaver retractor can be placed into the vallecula transorally to provide tension on the mucosa and then electrocautery is used to make entry. The tip of the epiglottis can frequently be identified transmucosally and the mucosa is divided superior to it (Fig. 12.23). It is then grasped with an Allis clamp and retracted anteriorly, facilitating direct visualization of the tumor through the pharyngotomy (Fig. 12.24).
- Maintaining visualization of the tumor, mucosal cuts are then made following the lateral aspect of the aryepiglottic folds to preserve uninvolved pharyngeal mucosa. The deeper tissues are then divided taking care to preserve the pyriform mucosa but include the paraglottic space. These cuts are done first on the less involved side and may require more extensive mucosal resection depending on the tumor extent. The cuts are then connected along the postcricoid mucosa. The larynx is then fully mobilized and can be removed from the field. Mucosal margins are taken and sent for frozen section analysis.
- If the esophageal introitus is felt to be tight, as is often the case in the salvage setting, a myotomy may be performed. A finger is placed within the esophagus and the muscle fibers are transected with a scalpel.
- The stomaplasty is performed. When a separate incision is used for the stoma, the incision is placed at least 2 cm inferior to the edge of the lower skin flap thus creating a bipedicled skin flap to serve as a bridge of skin above the stoma. A circle of skin 2 cm in diameter is then excised. In severely fibrotic tissues such a flap will be much less robust and should be avoided. The trachea is then sutured to the skin edges with "vertical half-mattress" sutures. In this technique the needle is passed through the skin from superficial to deep, then from outside to inside the trachea beneath the superior most ring, and then back up through the skin closer to the edge. These are performed around the cartilaginous trachea oriented radially. The sutures through the membranous trachea may be simple interrupted or mattress sutures. We use 3-0 Vicryl sutures but 2-0 Prolene sutures are frequently used as well.
- In the more traditional stomaplasty, interrupted sutures are used to secure the cartilaginous portion of the trachea to the lower skin flap, thus pulling the

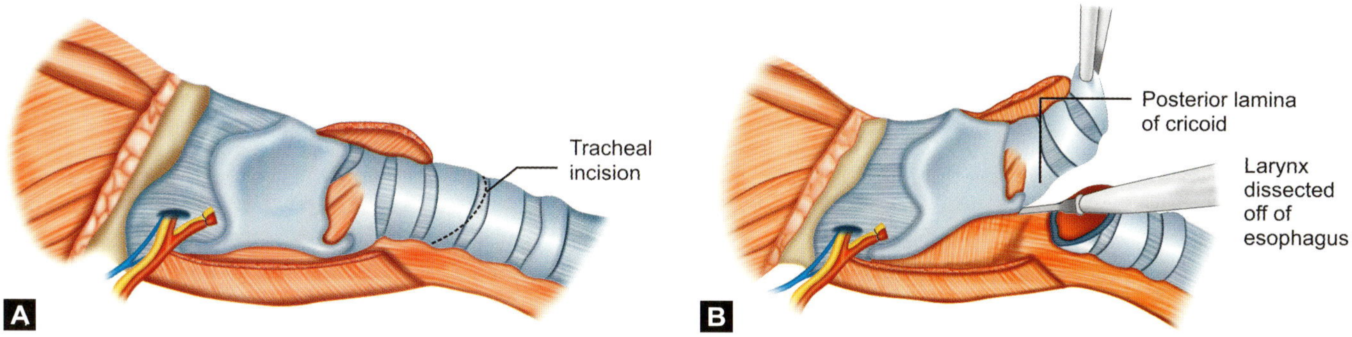

Figs. 12.22A and B: Tracheotomy and laryngeal elevation. A tracheotomy is made following a tracheal ring for a separate stoma. In a more traditional stoma, it can be beveled up through one ring (A). The membranous trachea can then be incised or bluntly dissected away from the esophagus and then divided. Dissection continues superiorly to mobilize the larynx (B). In a bottom-up approach for tongue base involvement the pharynx may be entered here.

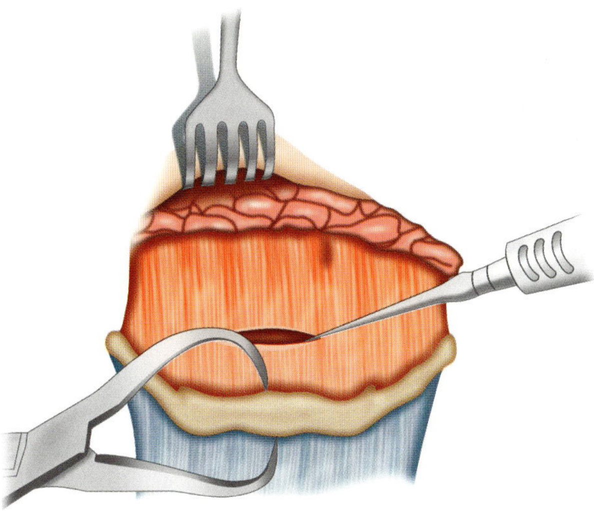

Fig. 12.23: Pharyngotomy. The pharynx is entered above the hyoid and epiglottis.

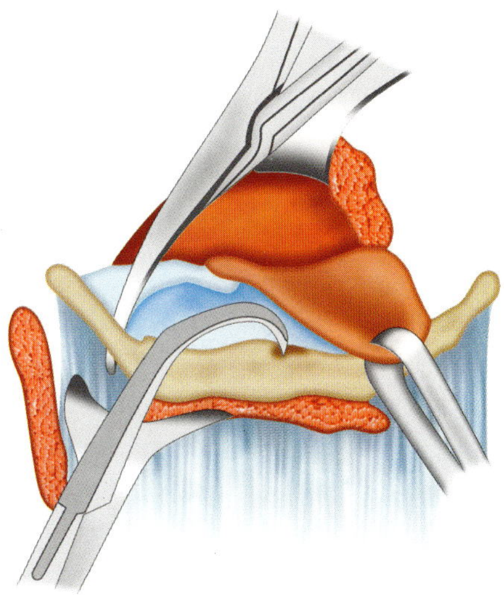

Fig. 12.24: Pharyngeal incisions. The epiglottis is retracted anteriorly to directly visualize pharyngeal incisions.

tracheal wall laterally and ensuring a widely patent stoma. The "half mattress" technique can also be used here as it helps maintain skin coverage of the cut tracheal edge. The upper skin flap is closed to the membranous trachea. Care should be taken to ensure adequate closure at the trifurcation.

- After stomaplasty and before pharyngeal reconstruction, a primary tracheoesophageal puncture (TEP) can be performed. Primary TEP at the time of laryngectomy is not recommended in irradiated patients and we prefer to delay this procedure in all cases.
- The pharyngeal defect is then primarily repaired when possible. A minimum width of approximately 3 cm of pharyngeal mucosa is required to perform primary closure with an adequate diameter of the neopharynx.

Prior to closure a nasogastric feeding tube is placed if the patient does not have a gastrostomy. A variety of closure techniques have been described without any one technique demonstrating superiority. When possible we prefer to close the pharynx in a straight vertical line, starting inferiorly with a running Connell suture using a 3-0 Vicryl. Alternatively, interrupted sutures may be used in an inverting mattress fashion. If there is excessive tension superiorly, then a T-shaped closure is performed with the free ends of the suture meeting medially to be tied (Figs. 12.25A to C). When performing the running suture, it is important to ensure that mucosal edges are appropriately inverted with each advancement and that tension is maintained by an assistant throughout the entire

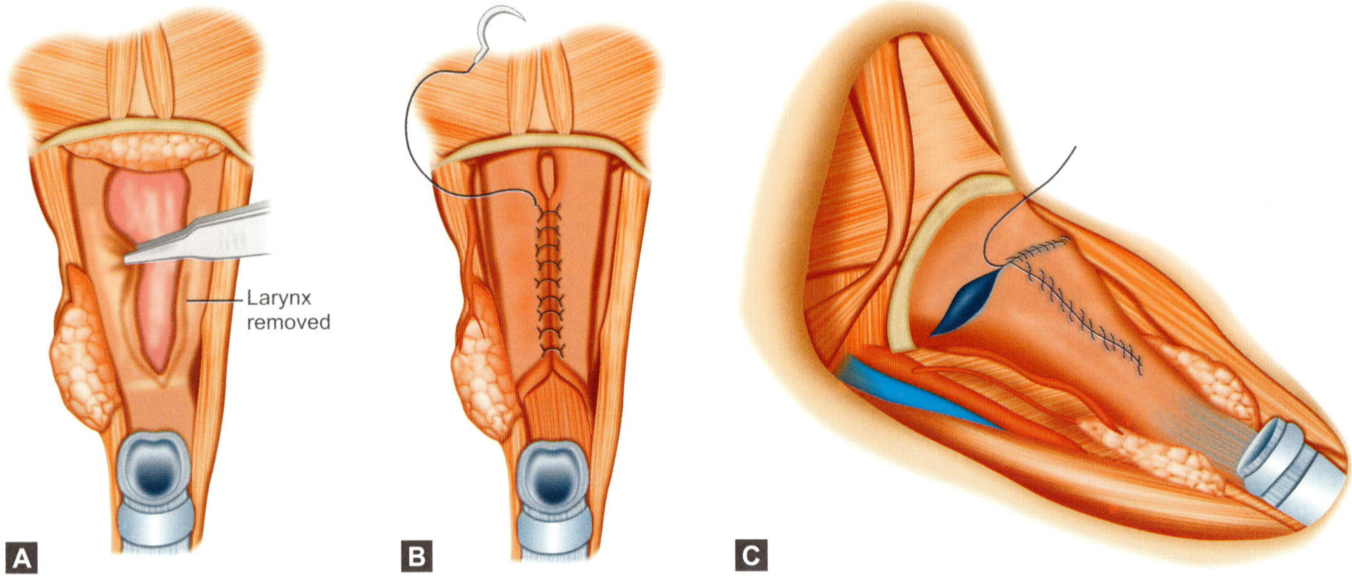

Figs. 12.25A to C: Pharyngeal reconstruction. The remaining pharyngeal mucosa is assessed (A) and if adequate a primary closure is performed. Most commonly a vertical straight line closure (B) is used but a T-shape closure (C) may be used if tension is excessive.

closure to prevent loose areas. Straight line horizontal closures can occasionally be utilized.

- After the first layer of closure, the neopharynx is tested. A catheter is advanced transorally or transnasally and palpated in the neopharynx. With a finger applying pressure to seal the esophagus, the neopharynx is filled with saline or diluted peroxide until it is visibly distended. Any areas of leaking are reinforced or the closure is revised. When a water-tight closure has been achieved, then a second reinforcing layer can be performed. This layer pulls adjacent tissue over the first layer with a series of submucosal inverting mattress sutures. The remaining thyroid lobe may also be used to reinforce a part of the closure. Care should be taken not to tighten the constrictors around the neopharynx, which may result in delayed stenosis.
- The neck is copiously irrigated and checked for bleeding or chyle leakage. Drains are placed laterally away from the pharyngeal closure line and the neck is closed in layers. We routinely perform bronchoscopy to clear any aspirated blood, which may have entered the airway during surgery. If the patient requires ventilation, then a cuffed tracheostomy tube can be placed. Otherwise, no appliance is required in the stoma but a laryngectomy or tracheostomy tube can be placed. We prefer to use a soft silicone laryngectomy tube, which decreases the need for frequent debridement of obstructing crusts in the early postoperative period and allows for early use of a heat moisture exchange device.

Operative Considerations

For tumors confined to the endolarynx, a primary closure of the neopharynx can usually be achieved as described above. When inadequate pharyngeal mucosa (<3 cm width) remains after tumor resection, reconstruction with an interposed regional or free flap is required. Even when primary closure can be achieved, flap reconstruction may be of value in the salvage setting. Myofascial pectoralis major flaps used in an onlay fashion to reinforce the primary closure have been shown to significantly lower the fistula rate and free tissue transfer used as an interposition or onlay flap may also lower the fistula rate or at least reduce the severity and duration of the fistula.[11]

The above stepwise procedures are not intended to impose a rigid framework for operative technique. Instead the goal is to provide an understanding of the key maneuvers involved in laryngectomy. The exact approach and order of maneuvers will frequently need to be altered and customized to individual tumor characteristics, specifically as they relate to extralaryngeal origin or extension. "Top-down" approaches can address hypopharyngeal tumors and "bottom-up" approaches can address extension to the base of the tongue. A thorough knowledge of anatomy and an individualized approach is critical to sound oncologic technique.

Postoperative Management

If not done preoperatively, thyroid hormone levels should be evaluated and appropriately replaced. If total thyroidectomy or extensive paratracheal dissection was performed, then calcium levels should be monitored and appropriately replaced and thyroid replacement should be initiated.

To mitigate the effects of reflux on the pharyngeal reconstruction, the head of the bed is maintained in an elevated position and proton-pump inhibitors are administered. Tube feedings are initiated on the first postoperative day and slowly advanced to goal volumes. They should be held for signs of ileus and symptoms of nausea to prevent vomiting.

Wounds and drains are monitored for early signs of fistula. If there are none, we initiate an oral feeding trial at 7 days and delay it to 10–14 days in cases of previous irradiation. An esophagram is not routinely obtained prior to oral feeding but can be considered if a specific concern exists. Ideally, speech and language pathology is involved in care preoperatively and therapy should continue in the early postoperative period to assist with all aspects of total laryngectomy rehabilitation.

Complications

Early complications of total laryngectomy include wound infection, dehiscence, hematoma, and pharyngocutaneous fistula. Later complications include stomal stenosis and dysphagia, usually due to pharyngeal stenosis. Fistula can also present as a late complication but persistent or recurrent disease should be ruled out. Other complications of total laryngectomy are similar to those of other major surgeries and include stroke, myocardial infarction, pulmonary complications, and death. In the salvage setting patients are at significantly higher risk of wound-related complications, and postoperative fistula rates following salvage total laryngectomy are estimated to be 30–50%[11,12] and are even higher in some series.

Frequently, small fistulae can be managed successfully with conservative measures and tend to resolve over the course of weeks. Patients remain NPO and fistula tracts can be packed with wet gauze or formalized with drain placement to divert a small tract away from the carotid artery and jugular vein, reducing the risk of vascular rupture. In the case of a separate stoma, a fistula manifesting within the neck incision can often be managed and closed more quickly with a vacuum-assisted wound closure system, which can be more easily applied away from the stoma. Larger fistulae with extensive wound breakdown and persistent fistulae may require revision surgery with pectoralis major or free-flap reconstruction.

REFERENCES

1. Kirchner JA. A historical and histological view of partial laryngectomy. Bull N Y Acad Med. 1986;62(8):808-17.
2. Wolf G, Hong K, Fisher S, et al. The Department of Veterans Affairs Laryngeal Cancer Study Group. Induction chemotherapy plus radiation compared with surgery plus radiation in patients with advanced laryngeal cancer. N Engl J Med. 1991;324(24):1685-90.
3. Forastiere AA, Goepfert H, Maor M, et al. Concurrent chemotherapy and radiotherapy for organ preservation in advanced laryngeal cancer. N Engl J Med. 2003;349(22):2091-8.
4. Hoffman HT, Porter K, Karnell LH, et al. Laryngeal cancer in the United States: changes in demographics, patterns of care, and survival. Laryngoscope. 2006;116(9)(Suppl 111):1-13.
5. Machtay M, Moughan J, Trotti A, et al. Factors associated with severe late toxicity after concurrent chemoradiation for locally advanced head and neck cancer: an RTOG analysis. J Clin Oncol. 2008;26(21):3582-9.
6. Pfister DG, Laurie SA, Weinstein GS, et al. American Society of Clinical Oncology. American Society of Clinical Oncology clinical practice guideline for the use of larynx-preservation strategies in the treatment of laryngeal cancer. J Clin Oncol. 2006;24(22):3693-704.
7. Weinstein GS, Laccourreye O. Vertical partial laryngectomies. In: Weinstein GS, Laccourreye O, Brasnu D, Laccourreye H (Eds). Organ Preservation Surgery for Laryngeal Cancer. San Diego: Singular Publishing Group; 2000.
8. Succo G, Peretti G, Piazza C, et al. Open partial horizontal laryngectomies: a proposal for classification by the working committee on nomenclature of the European Laryngological Society. Eur Arch Otorhinolaryngol. 2014;271(9):2489-96.
9. Laccourreye O, Laccourrreye H, El-Sawy M, Weinstein GS. Supracricoid partial laryngectomy with cricohyoidoepiglottopexy. In: Weinstein GS, Laccourreye O, Brasnu D, Laccourreye H (Eds). Organ Preservation Surgery for Laryngeal Cancer. San Diego: Singular Publishing Group; 2000.
10. Holsinger FC, Jantharapattana K, Weinstein GS. Supracricoid partial laryngectomy with cricohyoidopexy or cricohyoidoepiglottopexy. In: Cohen JI, Clayman GL (eds). Atlas of Head and Neck Surgery. Philadelphia: Elsevier Saunders; 2011.
11. Patel UA, Moore BA, Wax M, et al. Impact of pharyngeal closure technique on fistula after salvage laryngectomy. JAMA Otolaryngol Head Neck Surg. 2013;139(11):1156-62.
12. Sassler AM, Esclamado RM, Wolf GT. Surgery after organ preservation therapy: analysis of wound complications. Arch Otolaryngol Head Neck Surg. 1995:121(2);162-5.

CHAPTER

13

Surgery for Hypopharyngeal Cancer

Kim Atiyeh, David Myssiorek

ANATOMY

The hypopharynx is a mucosally lined tube that is divided into four subsites: the posterior pharyngeal wall, two pyriform sinuses, and the postcricoid region (Fig. 13.1). The inferior border of the hypopharynx is the cricopharyngeus muscle, a condensation of the inferior constrictor muscle. The pyriform sinuses have a medial wall and a lateral wall. The superior limit of the pyriform sinus is the pharyngoepiglottic fold. The lateral border is the thyroid ala and thyrohyoid membrane. The medial wall is bounded superiorly by the aryepiglottic fold and inferomedially by the postcricoid mucosa. It lies posterior to the paraglottic and glottic spaces. The postcricoid region is the mucosa over the posterior cricoid lamina and the mucosa within the circumference of the cricopharyngeus. The posterior hypopharyngeal wall is bounded superiorly by an imaginary line at the level of the tip of the epiglottis and inferiorly by the cricopharyngeus muscle. The posterior hypopharynx is arbitrarily delineated by the lateral pyriform sinus mucosa. The relationship of the posterior pharyngeal wall to the underlying prevertebral musculature is critical. Tumors of the posterior pharyngeal wall can traverse the retropharyngeal space to involve the prevertebral muscles.

The pharyngeal wall consists of four layers. The mucosal layer is composed of stratified squamous epithelium. Deep to this is the fibrous pharyngeal aponeurosis. The pharyngeal muscular layer is next and consists of the cricopharyngeus, inferior constrictors, and middle constrictors. Finally, the buccopharyngeal fascia envelops these muscles.

The arterial blood supply to the hypopharynx is from the ascending pharyngeal, lingual, and superior thyroid arteries. Sensory innervation is predominantly via cranial nerves IX and X. The internal branch of the superior laryngeal nerve lies deep to the mucosa of the lateral wall of the pyriform sinus and is vulnerable to damage at this level. It then exits the thyrohyoid membrane and ascends to the vagus nerve. After entering the larynx, the recurrent laryngeal nerve lies at the apex of the pyriform sinus. Tumors involving the apex can cause vocal fold immobility by direct muscle invasion, cricoarytenoid fixation, or recurrent laryngeal nerve involvement.

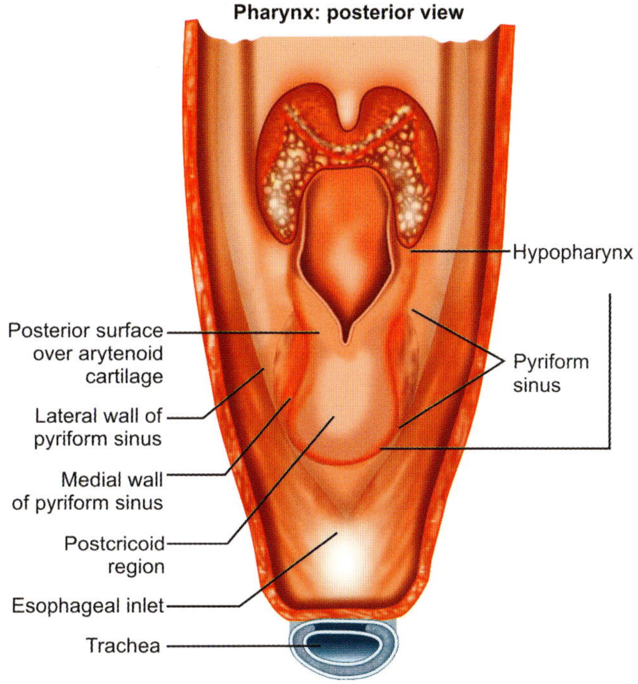

Fig. 13.1: The hypopharynx is a mucosally lined tube that is divided into four subsites: the posterior pharyngeal wall (not shown), two pyriform sinuses, and the postcricoid region.

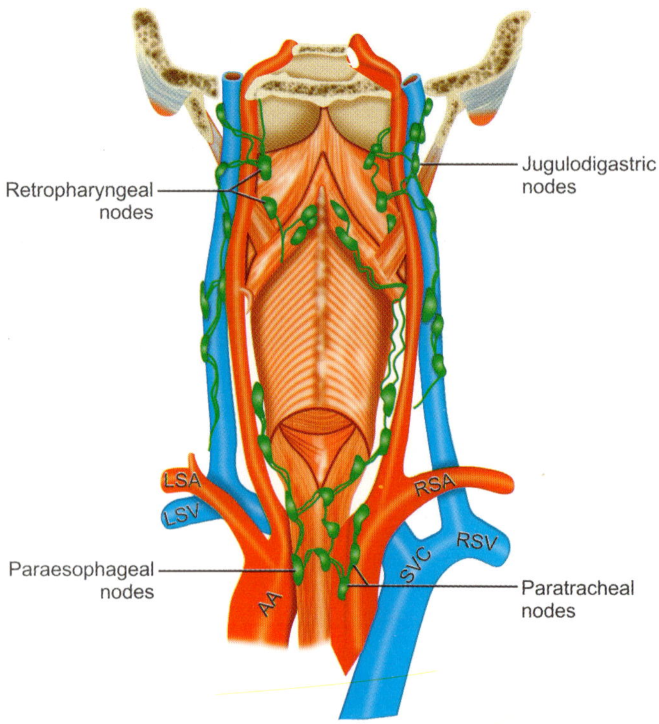

Fig. 13.2: Posterior hypopharyngeal lymphatic drainage includes the jugulodigastric nodes. Retropharyngeal, paraesophageal, and paratracheal nodes are at risk, in addition to level V lymph nodes (not pictured).

Knowledge of the lymphatics of the hypopharynx is important in determining patterns of spread of disease and setting forth a strategy for treatment. The lymphatic drainage from the pyriform sinuses follows the superior laryngeal artery through the thyrohyoid membrane and drains to the level II, III, and IV nodes. The inferior hypopharynx and the postcricoid region lymphatics drain into the paratracheal and paraesophageal nodes, less commonly into the supraclavicular fossa lymph nodes. Tumors of the posterior pharyngeal wall will have ready access to the retropharyngeal lymphatics (Fig. 13.2).

PATHOLOGY

Hypopharyngeal cancer is not common, representing approximately 10% of head and neck malignancies. In Northern Europe, postcricoid cancer is more prevalent than pyriform sinus cancer, but in the United States, pyriform sinus cancer predominates. Ninety-five percent of hypopharyngeal cancers are squamous cell carcinoma or a variant and will be the assumed pathology of the techniques described. They tend to be less well differentiated than their laryngeal counterparts. Minor salivary gland tumors make up the majority of the remaining cancers.

BEHAVIOR OF HYPOPHARYNGEAL CANCER

Pyriform Sinus

The pyriform sinus medial wall abuts the paraglottic space and thus allows spread of cancer into the larynx. Medial extension frequently fixes the vocal fold by muscle invasion, not recurrent laryngeal nerve involvement, or cricoarytenoid joint involvement. Lateral extension can occur and involve the thyroid ala or thyrohyoid membrane. Larger tumors can involve the posterior hypopharyngeal wall. Tumors of the pyriform sinus remain relatively asymptomatic until the tumor is large, at which point the epicenter may be difficult to identify. Submucosal extension beyond the visible lesion is common.

Pyriform sinus cancers spread predominantly into jugular lymph nodes. Levels I and V are involved very infrequently.[1,2] Paratracheal nodes are found in 8.3% of dissected patients.[3]

Posterior Hypopharyngeal Wall

These tumors usually attain large size before detection. These tumors tend to spread submucosally superiorly into the oropharynx and inferiorly toward the esophagus. As with pyriform tumors, submucosal spread is the rule. Deep extension into the prevertebral muscles may not be detected until targeted examination under anesthesia. Cervical adenopathy is frequent, as is retropharyngeal adenopathy. The jugular chain is a first echelon site for regional disease.

Postcricoid Carcinoma

These tumors are uncommon in the United States and tend to occur in women. These tumors are diagnosed late in their course. Cricoid cartilage and posterior cricoarytenoid muscle invasion is common with vocal fold paralysis as a presenting sign. Lymph node spread is usually to the paratracheal nodes and lower jugular nodes.

TREATMENT OF HYPOPHARYNGEAL CANCERS

Surgery as the primary modality of treatment for hypopharyngeal tumors is dependent on several factors. These tumors tend to reveal themselves late with cervical adenopathy as the initial presenting complaint. The tendency to spread submucosally must be acknowledged when considering resectability. Organ preservation protocols are also critical in determining if a tumor should be resected at all. The following treatments are surgical options for hypopharyngeal cancers.

Indications for surgery are not codified in most textbooks. Separating these tumors into early (T1, T2) and late presentations (T3, T4) is a reasonable way to guide the surgical approach. T1 and T2 lesions are more amenable to organ sparing surgery, whereas the larger tumors tend to require more radical resection. Despite aggressive treatment, overall survival rates have not improved much over the last few decades. Laryngeal preservation therefore is an important goal. The frequency of open procedures for hypopharyngeal carcinoma has diminished with the advent of organ sparing protocols and transoral laser procedures. Effectively, surgical procedures for hypopharyngeal cancer consist of conservation procedures or operations that require laryngectomy.

Laryngeal preservation may be achieved by several techniques, whether from one of several types of open external approaches or from endoscopic techniques. Each of the external approaches is generally limited toward a particular subsite or subsites. The approach follows a relatively standardized sequence of steps that will be described. On the other hand, the endoscopic approach as described is a technique that is adaptable toward all subsites of the hypopharynx and its limitations are primarily based on surgical skill and tumor extent. The precise steps of extirpation are unique for each tumor, but strategies for this approach and style of extirpation will be described.

Transhyoid Pharyngectomy

Indications: There are few indications for a transhyoid pharyngectomy. Primarily T1 and T2 tumors of the posterior inferior pharyngeal wall that cannot be accessed via other routes (transoral, lateral pharyngotomy, or other) are best suited for this approach.

Contraindications: This approach should not be performed if there is invasion of the prevertebral fascia that may be evaluated by direct palpation or less commonly by barium pharyngoesophagram. Temporary aspiration is expected, and thus functional status preoperatively is an important consideration.

Surgical technique: The patient is placed in extension and a tracheotomy is performed to provide an uninhibited view of the posterior pharynx and protect the airway in the context of significant tongue edema. Preoperative antibiotics are given. A curvilinear incision is created in a natural skin crease slightly below the hyoid from mid-sternocleidomastoid muscle to mid-sternocleidomastoid muscle (Fig. 13.3A). Subplatysmal flaps are elevated superiorly and inferiorly. The hyoid and strap muscles are exposed. The suprahyoid musculature is separated from the hyoid bone taking care to spare the hypoglossal nerves and lingual arteries in addition to the superior laryngeal nerves. This step may be assisted by grasping the hyoid and lifting it anteriorly. The dissection is carried to the pharyngeal mucosa, at which point a curved metal instrument may be placed transorally into the vallecula to guide entrance into the pharynx with electrocautery or sharp dissection. Once the pharynx is entered, large curved retractors are placed to retract the tongue base superiorly and the larynx inferiorly to provide access to the posterior pharyngeal wall (Fig. 13.3C). For additional access, the hyoid may be transected or the middle third may be resected (Fig. 13.3B). The tumor is resected down to and through the prevertebral fascia (Fig. 13.3D). Resection margins should be confirmed intraoperatively. Smaller defects may be closed by secondary intention with suturing of the remaining mucosa to the prevertebral fascia, while larger defects may require a skin graft, tongue flap, or radial forearm free flap depending on the size (Fig. 13.3E). A nasogastric tube is placed under direct visualization. The mucosa is approximated with running or interrupted Connell-type sutures (refer to Figure 13.17). Zero vicryl sutures are used to approximate the base of the tongue to the hyoid bone or strap muscles. If divided, the hyoid may be wired together. Drains are placed in the neck. Postoperatively, the patient is kept NPO for 5–7 days with decannulation in 4–7 days.

As with all open approaches, care must be taken to avoid pharyngocutaneous fistulae. Closure should be meticulous. Radiated patients are at risk of wound breakdown, especially after combined chemotherapy and radiation therapy. In the nonradiated patient, wounds usually heal rapidly and the tracheotomy can be reversed promptly. Dysphagia is common after the procedure, secondary to an insensate posterior pharyngeal wall and disruption of the pharyngeal musculature.

Lateral Pharyngotomy

Indications: This approach can be used for tumors of the lateral and posterior pharyngeal walls as well as the pyriform sinus.

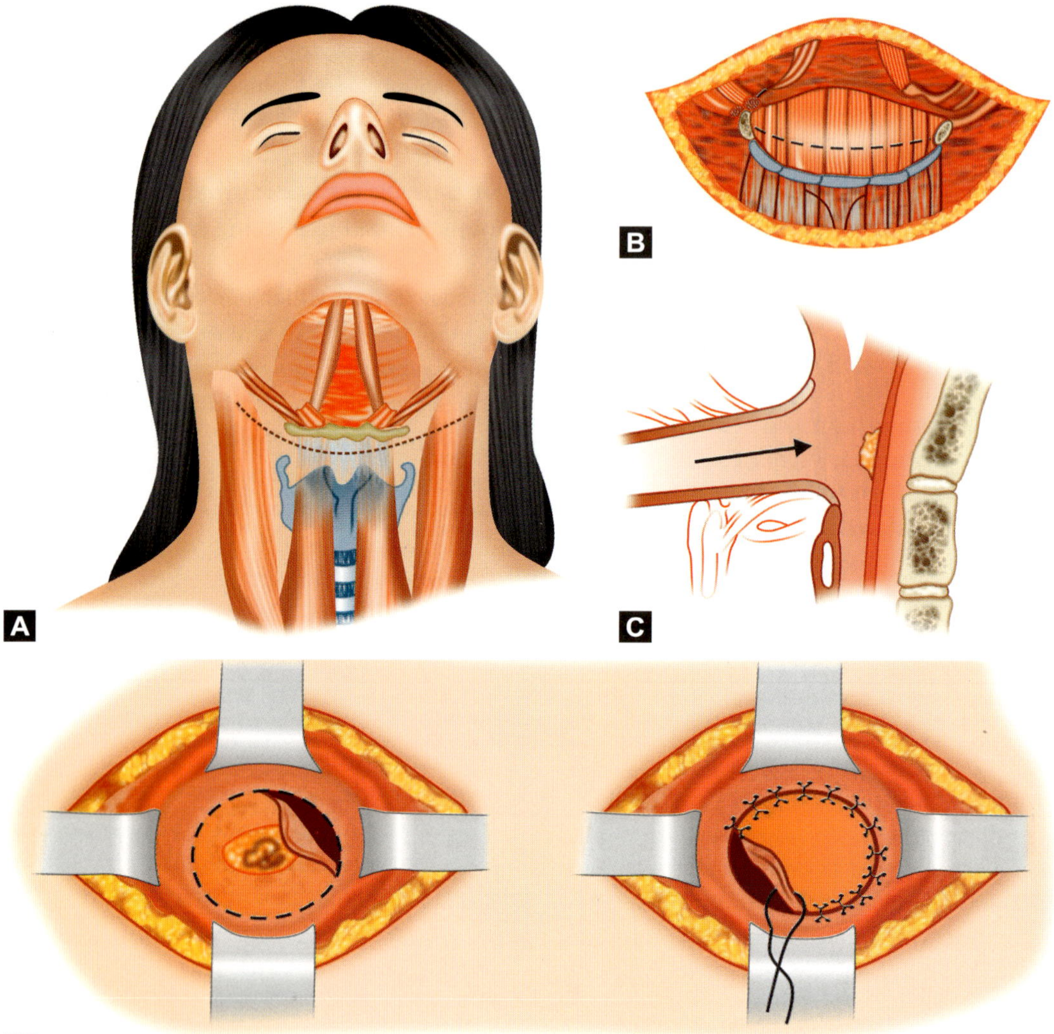

Figs. 13.3A to E: Transhyoid pharyngectomy. (A) A curvilinear incision is created slightly below the hyoid from mid-sternocleidomastoid muscle to mid-sternocleidomastoid muscle. (B) For additional access, the hyoid may be transected or the middle third may be resected. (C) Large curved retractors are placed to retract the tongue superiorly and the larynx inferiorly to provide access to the posterior pharyngeal wall. (D) The tumor is resected down to and through the prevertebral fascia. (E) Smaller defects may be closed by secondary intention with suturing of the remaining mucosa to the prevertebral fascia, while larger defects may require a skin graft, tongue flap, or radial forearm free flap depending on the size.

Contraindications: This approach is inadequate for tumors that involve more than a third of the pharyngeal circumference.[4] Tumors that include more than one wall of the pyriform, extend to the pyriform apex, or involve the larynx in any way cannot be resected adequately by this approach.

Surgical technique: A tracheotomy is performed in anticipation of pharyngeal edema and dysphagia. A horizontal incision is made around the level of the thyrohyoid membrane, ideally within an existing skin crease (Fig. 13.4A). Subplatysmal flaps are raised. The marginal mandibular nerve is protected in the usual fashion by carrying the superior flap dissection deep to the submandibular gland, identifying and ligating the facial vein, and retracting it superiorly with the cervical flap. The sternocleidomastoid is separated from the strap muscles; the carotid sheath is exposed and retracted laterally to expose the inferior constrictor muscle and the superior pole of the thyroid gland (Figs. 13.4B and C). The thyroid cartilage is retracted anteriorly to facilitate dissection. Identification and cephalic retraction of the superior laryngeal neurovascular bundle and hypoglossal nerve

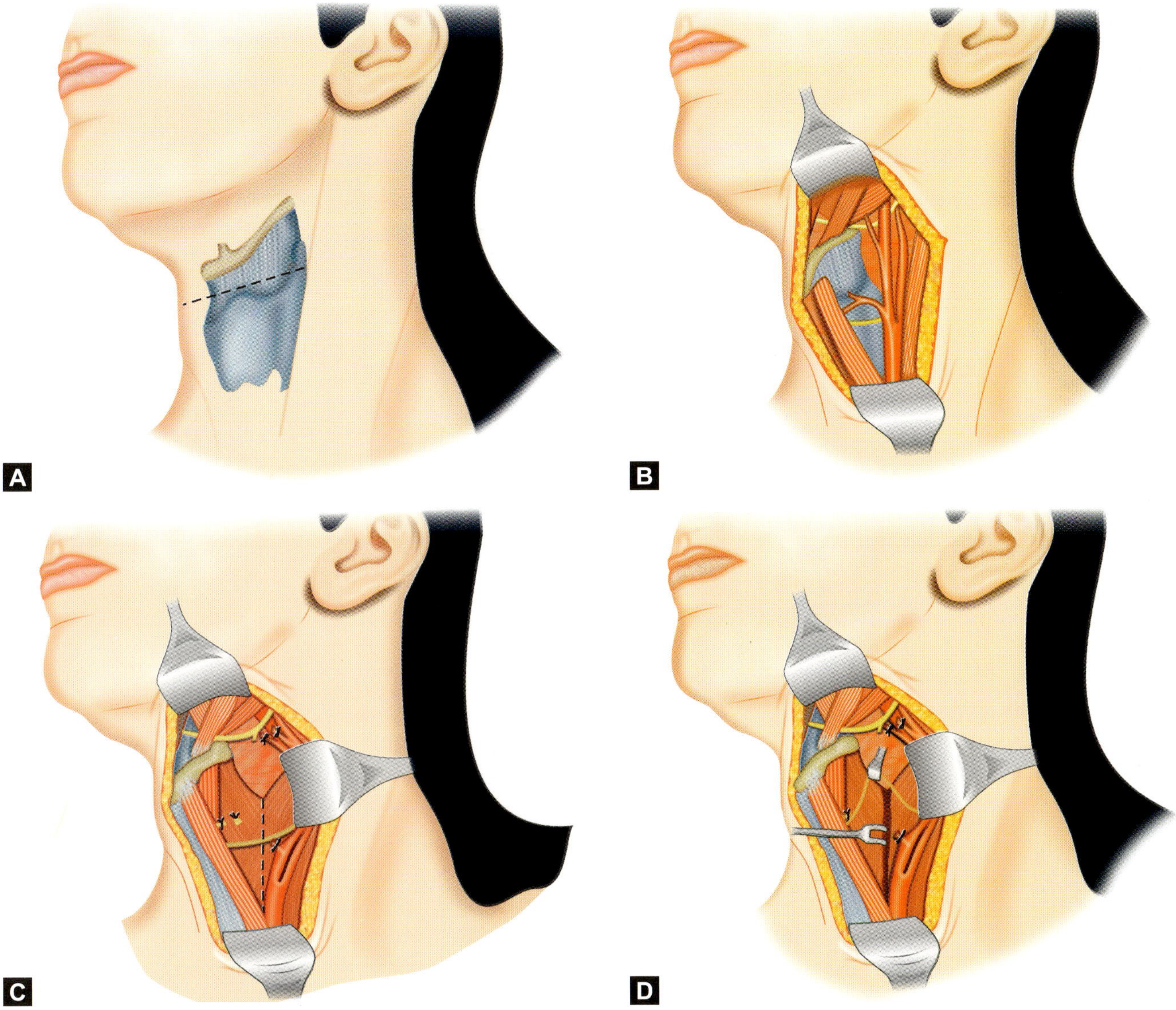

A B C D

Figs. 13.4A to D: Lateral pharyngotomy. (A) A curvilinear incision is made around the level of the thyrohyoid membrane. (B) After the sternocleidomastoid is dissected laterally and the strap muscles are dissected medially, the carotid sheath is exposed. (C) The superior thyroid vasculature may be ligated and the superior laryngeal nerve retracted superiorly. The carotid sheath contents are retracted laterally. (D) The inferior constrictor myotomy is performed at the posterior edge of the thyroid cartilage ala.

facilitates superior extension of this approach. The inferior constrictor muscle is transected off of the posterior limit of the thyroid ala, exposing the mucosa of the pyriform sinus. The mucosa is dissected from the medial aspect of the thyroid ala (Fig. 13.4D). The pharyngotomy is performed sharply or with electrocautery under tension, ideally at the resection margin. The extirpation is performed with appropriate margins and a nasogastric tube is placed. The mucosa is closed with an inverting stitch, the constrictor muscle is reapproximated, a hemovac drain is placed, and the neck is closed using layer-by-layer technique.

Lateral Transthyroid Pharyngotomy

This approach is an extension of the lateral pharyngotomy approach that is used for tumors that more extensively involve the lateral hypopharyngeal wall. The same initial steps are taken, but rather than entering the pharynx through the pyriform, the mucosal incision is initiated in the vallecula. In this technique, once the thyroid cartilage is identified, an inferomedially based perichondrial flap is raised. The hyoid bone is dissected laterally and a cut is made through the lesser cornu. The posterior one third

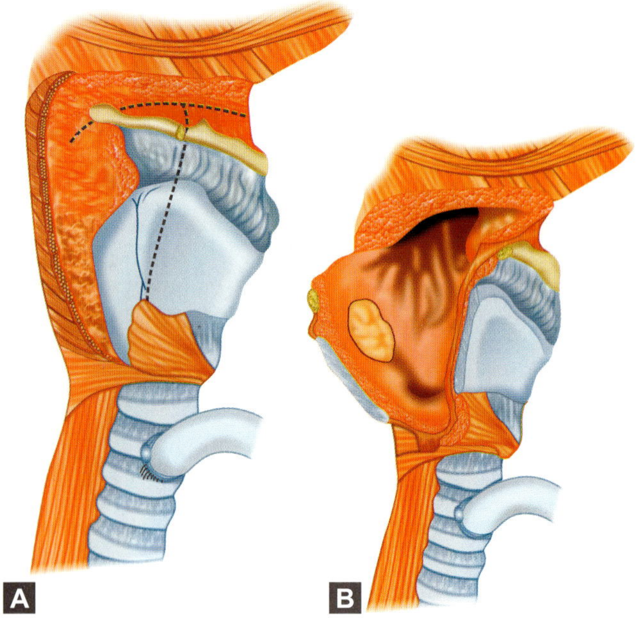

Figs. 13.5A and B: Partial pharyngectomy via the lateral pharyngotomy. (A) Dotted lines show cuts on the thyroid cartilage, hyoid, and vallecula. (B) After entry into the hypopharynx, the specimen is reflected laterally and final cuts are made.

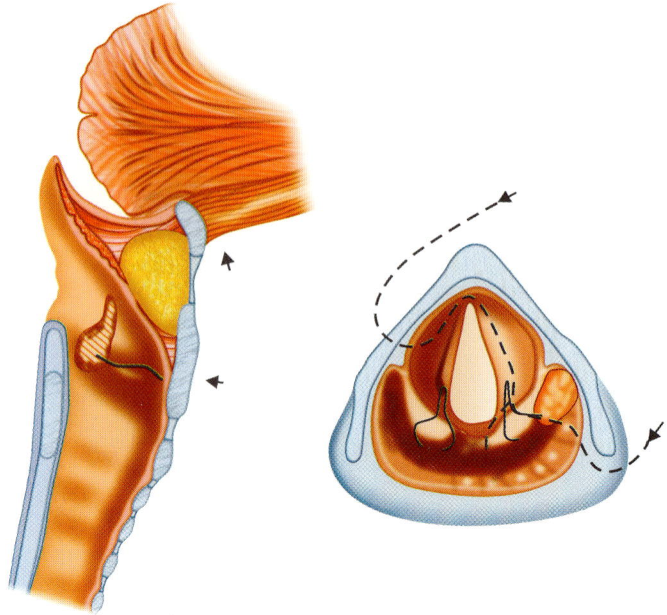

Fig. 13.6: Partial laryngopharyngectomy. The surgical technique is similar to supraglottic laryngectomy and extends to include the hypopharyngeal lesion.

of the thyroid cartilage is cut vertically (Fig. 13.5A). The pharynx is entered through the vallecula and retractors enable direct visualization of the tumor and necessary margins. The incision is extended inferiorly through the cartilaginous cut, the lesion is retracted laterally, and circumferential dissection of the tumor is completed (Fig. 13.5B). Once the tumor is extirpated, closure is performed with inverted sutures of the mucosa and the perichondrium approximated as the second layer.

Median Labiomandibular Glossotomy

The median labiomandibular glossotomy, otherwise known as the Trotter procedure, is seldom performed and is mentioned largely for historical purposes. This approach is preceded by a tracheostomy. Successive midline divisions are made of the lip, gingival, mandible, floor of mouth, tongue, and base of tongue, taking advantage of the lateral locations of neurovascular bundles. Direct access to the pharynx is gained, but at the expensive of significant morbidity.

Partial Laryngopharyngectomy

Indications: Tumors limited to the aryepiglottic fold, medial wall of the pyriform sinus, and anterior wall of the pyriform sinus may be candidates for the partial laryngopharyngectomy. Tumors may include extension into the base of tongue, lateral pyriform sinus, and vallecula.

Contraindications: Extension into the apex of the pyriform sinus (this is caudal to the plane of the laryngeal ventricle, which may result in persistence of disease), extension to the postcricoid region, ipsilateral true vocal fold paralysis, encroachment into the cricopharyngeus, and inadequate pulmonary function are considered contraindications to partial laryngopharyngectomy.

General approach: The general principle is that these tumors are embryologically similar to those arising in the supraglottic larynx. The surgical technique is similar to supraglottic laryngectomy and extends to include the hypopharyngeal lesion (Fig. 13.6).

An apron incision is made and a subplatysmal flap is elevated superiorly. In most cases, a bilateral neck dissection is performed. A tracheotomy is performed in a separate skin incision. The hyoid bone is skeletonized superiorly, taking care to preserve the hypoglossal nerves and lingual arteries. The infrahyoid musculature is released approximately 2 cm inferiorly to the inferior edge of the hyoid, which enables en bloc resection of the pre-epiglottic space. The external perichondrium of the thyroid cartilage is incised sharply at its superior-most extent and

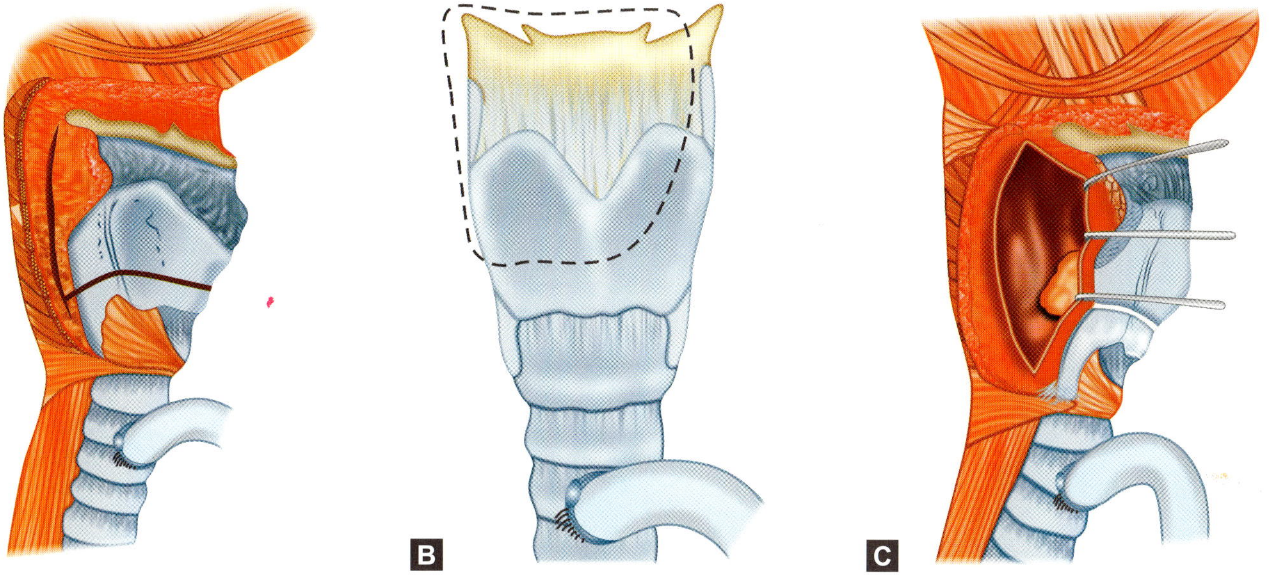

A B C

Figs. 13.7A to C: Partial laryngopharyngectomy. (A) The constrictor muscles are dissected off of the thyroid cartilage. The horizontal cartilaginous cut is made after raising inferiorly based perichondrial flaps. (B) The contralateral cartilaginous cut may rise superolaterally. (C) The pharynx is entered in the vallecula. Once the tumor is visualized, it may be excised circumferentially with margins.

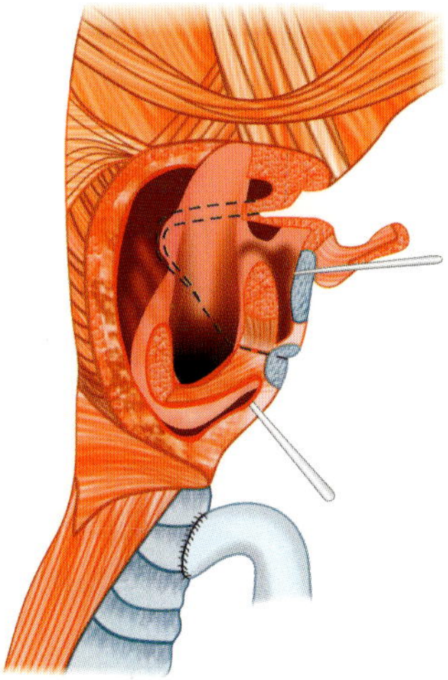

Fig. 13.8: Extirpation continues with cuts through the ventricle to meet the contralateral cartilaginous cut at the anterior commissure.

carefully reflected inferiorly, bearing in mind its eventual use as a layer of closure after extirpation is complete. Once the perichondrium is brought inferiorly, an oscillating saw is used to divide the cartilage horizontally (Fig. 13.7A). In the midline, this division should be halfway between the thyroid notch and the inferior border of the thyroid cartilage. On the ipsilateral side, the superior constrictor is separated from the lateral aspect of the thyroid cartilage. The entire superior quadrant of the thyroid cartilage will be removed on this side and thus the cartilaginous cut is horizontal. On the contralateral side, the superior cornu may be spared, so the cartilaginous cut rises superolaterally (Fig. 13.7B). The pharynx is entered on the side of the lesion superior to the hyoid into the vallecula and carried to the contralateral vallecula (Fig. 13.7C). The epiglottis may be grasped and retracted to assist in direct visualization of the tumor such that an appropriate margin is maintained and healthy mucosa is preserved. On the contralateral side, the incision is carried along the aryepiglottic fold, then transects the aryepiglottic fold just anterior to but sparing the cricoarytenoid unit, and along the ventricle to the anterior commissure. On the ipsilateral side, the incision is carried from the vallecula and includes the medial, anterior, and lateral walls of the pyriform as indicated. A vertical incision is made between the arytenoids down to the level of the cricoid, the vocal process is transected keeping a majority of the ipsilateral arytenoid with the specimen. The incision is likewise progressed through the ventricle and meets the contralateral cut at the anterior commissure. These incisions are followed through to meet the external cartilaginous cuts (Fig. 13.8). Reconstruction of the defect is begun by suturing the vocal process remnant to the cricoid cartilage, tacking the vocal fold in the midline (Fig. 13.9). The tongue base is then sutured to the flap of thyroid perichondrium and reinforced by closure of the overlying strap muscles.

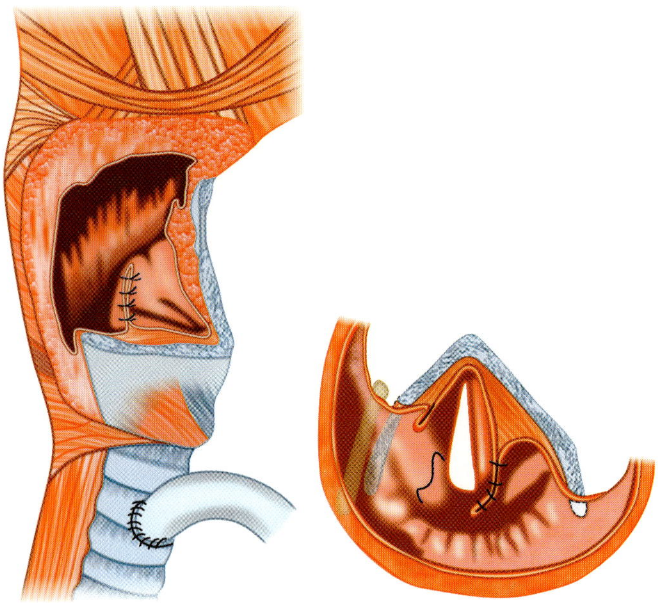

Fig. 13.9: Closure of the defect. The remnant of the vocal process is sutured to the cricoid cartilage, effectively tacking the vocal fold in the midline.

TRANSORAL APPROACH TO THE HYPOPHARYNX

Indications: While there are no fixed guidelines for when to approach the hypopharynx open versus endoscopic, there are several evolving principles that will help the physician in this decision. There are several advantages to the endoscopic approach: (1) tracheotomy is less frequently required, (2) suprahyoid musculature and its associated contribution to the swallow is preserved, (3) reconstruction is frequently not required, and (4) hospital stay is significantly reduced with return to an oral diet as early as postoperative day 1.[5] Furthermore, this approach does not limit further treatment of any kind including adjuvant radiotherapy, transoral retreatment, or salvage surgery.[6] The low incidence of permanent gastrostomy tubes and tracheostomies, and high rate of preservation of larynx function and sensation, contribute to the overall low morbidity and mortality rates and a higher quality of life.[7,8]

Patient factors: In order to gain adequate exposure of the tumor, there are several patient factors that affect patient selection. Short, stiff necks; prominent tongue bases; long protruding maxillary teeth or other permanent implants, or a class I overbite; trismus with an interincisor opening <2.5–3 cm; a short mental-hyoid distance; and a narrow mandibular arch can significantly limit exposure and jeopardize the success of the surgery.[9,10]

Tumor factors: In general, superficially infiltrative lesions are the best for the endoscopic approach. The bulk of endoscopically resected tumors are T1-2. Although not commonly used for large tumors, acceptable outcomes have been described for all size tumors except T4b.[8] At least one mobile arytenoid must be preserved to avoid aspiration.[8,11] Lateral pharyngeal wall tumors are generally easily accessed. Postcricoid region tumors are only suitable without cartilage involvement, and without involvement of the arytenoid joints.[11] Exophytic and narrow-based tumors of the postcricoid region are most suitable.[12] Lack of anatomical barriers between the medial wall and fornix of the pyriform and the supraglottis and paraglottic space allows rapid invasion, which may be included in the resection specimen. However, invasion of the paraglottic space lateral to the true vocal fold usually precludes the use of the transoral approach.[11] Transregional tumors may be included if they are not deeply infiltrating, including pyriform tumors involving the pharyngoepiglottic fold and marginal zone tumors involving the supraglottis or pyriform.[12]

Contraindications: There are relatively few strict contraindications. The extent of the tumor is the main limitation and endoscopic techniques should not be employed if the lesion involves great vessels of the neck, the cricopharyngeal sphincter, or structures that would put the patient at an unacceptable risk of aspiration such as bilateral arytenoids.[7,12] Notably absent in the contraindications for this approach are age criteria, overall health, and pulmonary status. Thus, elderly patients or those with a moderate degree of COPD may be candidates for this approach, whereas they would not be eligible for other voice-preserving treatment options. Additionally, prior treatment does not exclude a patient from this approach as a salvage strategy.[7]

Surgical technique: Although the approach is different, the resection of hypopharyngeal tumors transorally follows the same principles. Once a decision is made that a partial pharyngectomy is appropriate, the approach (transoral versus open) is determined primarily by patient factors and ability to achieve adequate exposure and access to the tumor. Equipment and setup are critical. Aside from an operating microscope, CO_2 laser, and the usual laryngeal instruments, setup should also include distending laryngoscopes, insulated laryngeal suction cautery, tissue holding forceps with suction channel, and a smoke evacuator.[12] A tooth guard is placed and the laryngoscope inserted. In order to utilize the distension laryngopharyngoscope, the tongue may be

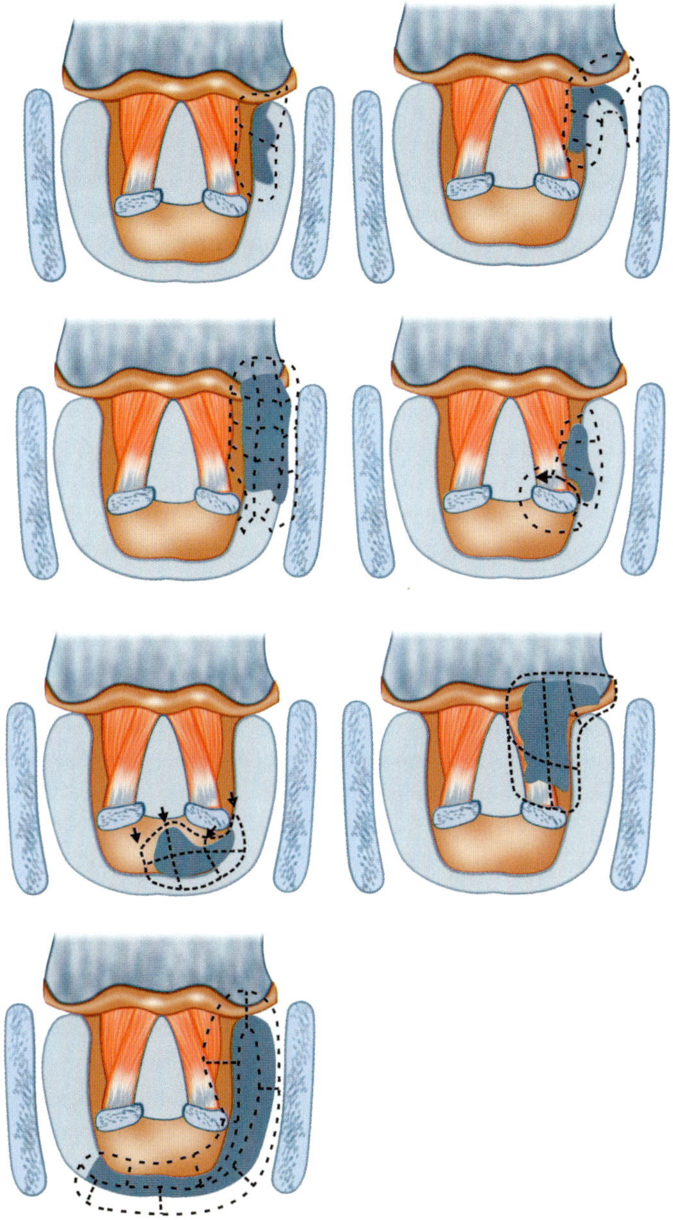

Fig. 13.10: Margins may be delineated with the laser to guide further resection and are modified based on exact location and extent of the tumor.

pulled anteriorly. Gauze may be placed over the mandibular dentition and the tongue retracted outward. The laryngopharyngoscope should be inserted into the uninvolved hypopharynx to avoid trauma to a potentially friable tumor. While select small tumors may be adequately visualized with initial positioning, the surgeon should expect to reposition the laryngopharyngoscope multiple times for adequate exposure and resection of the tumor margins.

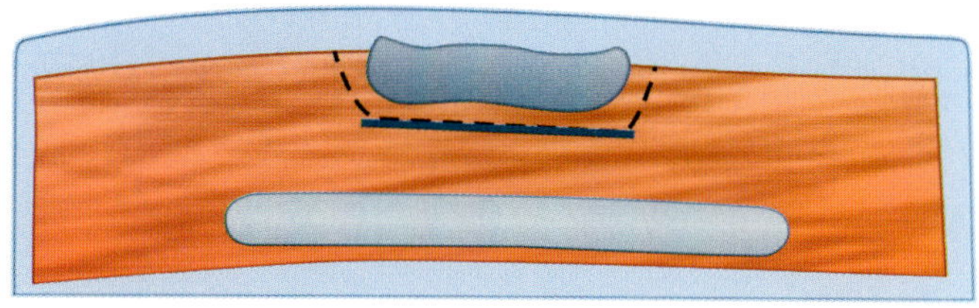

Fig. 13.11: For smaller and well-circumscribed lesions of the hypopharynx, resection may be performed en bloc.

The risk of airway fire should be acknowledged and minimized. "Laser safe" endotracheal tubes exist but are not 100% effective in preventing airway fires. The most vulnerable parts of the endotracheal tube are the tip and the cuff. The cuff may be inflated with saline or methylene blue-impregnated saline rather than air, and moist neurosurgical patties may be placed over the cuff and exposed endotracheal tube to decrease the likelihood of ignition. All exposed surfaces of the face and anesthesia circuits are covered with wet towels as well.

After appropriate setup is achieved, thorough examination may be performed to assess tumor extent and fixation. Margins may be delineated with the laser to guide further resection and are modified based on exact location and extent of the tumor (Fig. 13.10).

Extirpation then proceeds in one of two styles. For smaller, well-circumscribed lesions of the hypopharynx, resection may be performed en bloc (Fig. 13.11). The surgeon identifies the cranial-most border and, using the laser to identify the deep resection margin, resects the tumor with a combination of laser cutting and blunt dissection with forceps and laryngeal suction. When the main specimen is resected, it should be oriented, including marking of the deep margin of the tumor. Additional margins should be made by making cuts parallel to the margin of the tumor.

The en bloc technique is more difficult in the typical hypopharyngeal lesion—one that is large and infiltrating with submucosal extension. Another technique that may be more apt for these types of lesions was described by Steiner and utilizes the unique features of the transoral laser resection approach. Due to the lack of bleeding with the laser, the boundary between tumor and healthy tumor can be easily assessed with the optic power of the operating microscope. With the eye of an experienced surgeon, the degree of carbonization will assist in delineation of normal tissue versus tumor tissue. Tumor tissue will show a greater degree of carbonization and furthermore will cut with more resistance than normal healthy tissue.

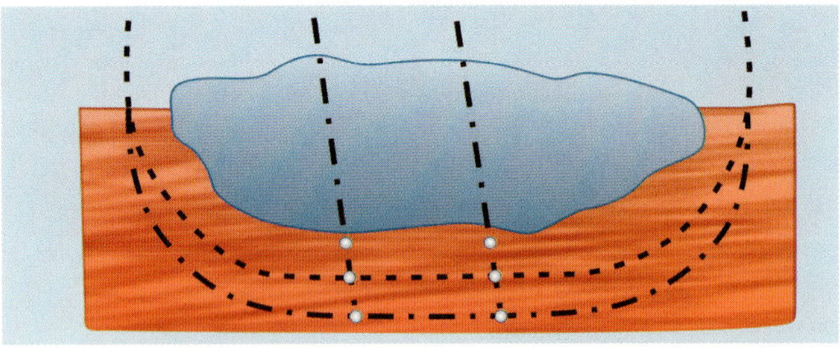

Fig. 13.12: Resection may proceed in a piecemeal systematic fashion ensuring an adequate oncologic procedure while avoiding over-resection and sparing deep structures when appropriate.

When the lesion is large or not well circumscribed, the tumor may be intentionally bisected, allowing for visualization of the deep margin. After initial incision through the mucosa and submucosa, the free edge may be grasped and retracted, providing more effective laser technique. The surgeon must be diligent not to transect tissue tangentially, resulting in unintentionally close or positive margins. Once the deep margin of the tumor has been identified, a rim of healthy tissue is resected as well. Resection may proceed in a piecemeal systematic fashion ensuring an adequate oncologic procedure while avoiding over-resection and sparing deep structures when appropriate (Fig. 13.12). Generally, the resection is started cranially and proceeds caudally, laterally, or medially. The laryngopharyngoscope may need to be tilted or advanced to ensure adequate visualization of the tumor. When tumors are large, debulking may be performed first, in which case an obvious margin of tumor should be intentionally left to assist with the oncologic resection. The remaining rim of tumor should then be resected piecemeal, with clear labeling and diagramming of the site of resection. As the resection proceeds from block to block, the margins of the pieces of resection should intentionally overlap so as to clear all tumors.

Tumors of the Posterior Pharyngeal Wall

These tumors are relatively straightforward to excise using the above techniques. The pharyngeal tissue is removed to the level of the prevertebral fascia. Unlike open approaches to this type of tumor, reconstruction is not mandatory and although the open wound may be painful, the defect can heal by secondary intention. A feeding tube is placed, often only for a few days postoperatively until a diet is commenced.

Lateral Wall of Pyriform Sinus

Careful preoperative radiologic evaluation must be ensured to assess the deep extent of lateral pyriform sinus wall tumors. Large vessels may be encountered at the deep margin of the tumor and may result in catastrophic bleeding. If hemorrhage is encountered, the hypopharynx is packed and the neck is opened to ligate the vessel.

Medial Wall of Pyriform Sinus

If the tumor is not deeply infiltrating, these tumors may be resected akin to an extended mucosectomy, sparing the underlying laryngeal cartilages. A narrow margin may be necessary to preserve arytenoid function; however, unilateral arytenoidectomy usually results in only temporary aspiration and should not be avoided if needed for oncologic resection. If a deeper tumor is suspected by preoperative imaging, decreased vocal cord mobility, or intraoperative findings, the technique should be modified. An exploratory incision should be made anterior to the arytenoid to determine extent of infiltration. If the arytenoid is involved, it should be resected and cuts may be carried to and include the cricoid.

Apex of the Pyriform Sinus

The concern with tumors of the apex of the pyriform sinus is extension into the esophagus. Resection of the esophageal inlet to obtain margins risks entry into the mediastinum and the associated risks of infection. Steiner recommends vaporization of this tissue rather than resection in an attempt to circumvent this issue.[9] If a significant portion of the esophageal circumference is involved, this may result in stricture with healing. Stents may be placed to avoid stenosis and feeding tubes should be carefully placed under direct visualization.

TOTAL LARYNGECTOMY WITH PARTIAL PHARYNGECTOMY

Lesions that are not amenable to conservation surgical techniques may require total laryngectomy with partial pharyngectomy. This procedure is being performed for failure, as well as therapy that results in chondronecrosis of the laryngopharyngeal unit. Functional laryngectomy may also be necessitated if intractable aspiration is predicted. Submucosal spread frequently results in excessive hypopharyngeal mucosal loss during surgery. Primary closure can be performed but risks stenosis and fistula. Regional or microvascular free flaps provide the neopharynx with a healthy blood supply and decrease the likelihood of stenosis and fistula. As lesions descend in the hypopharynx, the possibility of a total (circumferential or "sleeve") hypopharyngectomy increases. Despite maximal efforts, the survival rate for these patients remains low. Five-year survival rates for patients treated with radiation or with chemotherapy for stage III–IV hypopharyngeal cancer are 20–35%.[13] When patients undergo total laryngectomy with partial pharyngectomy as a salvage procedure for higher staged lesions, the results are usually poor, with disease-free survival rates of 11%. In many cases, by the time the persistent or recurrent disease is detected, patients are inoperable.[14]

When the cervical esophagus or cricopharyngeal region is involved by hypopharyngeal cancer, total laryngopharyngoesophagectomy may be necessary. Skip lesions may occur with postcricoid tumors. As such, Harrison advocates for total laryngopharyngoesophagectomy in these cases.[15] The main advantages of this procedure are a negative inferior margin of resection and the creation of only one anastomosis. When any procedure less than this is performed, there are multiple anastomoses needed for reconstructive efforts. The disadvantage of this operation is increased operative mortality. Five to twenty percent of patients undergoing this operation died from the procedure, according to Wei et al.[16]

Hypopharyngeal tumors that would necessitate removal of the larynx can be treated with total laryngo-partial pharyngectomy. One third of the circumference of the hypopharynx should remain after this procedure is performed with adequate margins. If more resection is anticipated, a total laryngopharyngectomy is indicated. Tumors <3 cm are amenable to conservation surgery. Larger tumors will require resection of much of the hypopharynx mucosa, resulting in near total loss. Additionally, large tumors tend to invade the larynx, making conservation surgery very unlikely. Prior to undertaking a total laryngo-partial pharyngectomy, direct laryngoscopy should be performed to assess whether a flap will be necessary and if there is posterior penetration into the prevertebral fascia. The initial steps are identical to those in total laryngectomy. The pharynx is entered either through the contralateral pyriform sinus or through the vallecula. As much hypopharyngeal mucosa as possible should be spared during this maneuver. If the entry is through the vallecula, it allows visualization of the tumor and maximal sparing of contralateral pyriform mucosa (Fig. 13.13).

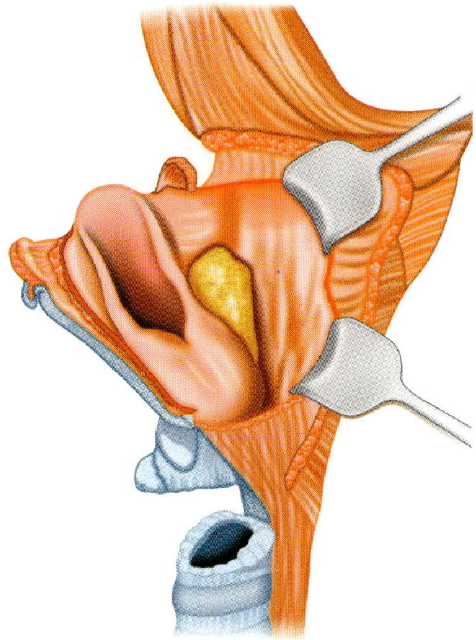

Fig. 13.13: Entry into the hypopharynx through the vallecula allows for maximal sparing of mucosa and excellent resection margin assessment.

The tumor is excised by obtaining a wide margin around the cancer. Bearing in mind that there may be extensive submucosal spread, this step should not be dictated by the potential need for repair with a flap. The author prefers a pair of Metzenbaum scissors for this step (Fig. 13.14A).

The defect can be closed primarily if more than half of the pharyngeal mucosa remains. This is not usually possible, and proper preoperative planning with CT scanning and laryngoscopy are useful predictors of this probability. In radiated patients, flaps should always be used. Cricopharyngeal myotomy may be considered (Fig. 13.15). A typical defect is shown in Figure 13.14B.

An estimate of where to begin the closure is made by selecting a point laterally along the cut mucosa that roughly equally divides the remnant mucosa in two halves (Fig. 13.16). Connell sutures are placed with a slowly absorbed suture such as a 3-0 Vicryl. The cadence "far near near far" may be used in teaching this technique, whereby far indicates approximately 5 mm from the mucosal edge and near is 2-3 mm from the mucosal edge, starting outside the lumen and ending outside the contralateral lumen (Fig. 13.17). The Connell suture can be performed continuously or interrupted. This type of stitch inverts the mucosal edge and in effect is a two-layer closure. The knots remain on the outside of the closure. Care should be taken to not overly tighten these knots as they may strangulate the blood supply of the mucosa (Figs. 13.18A and B).

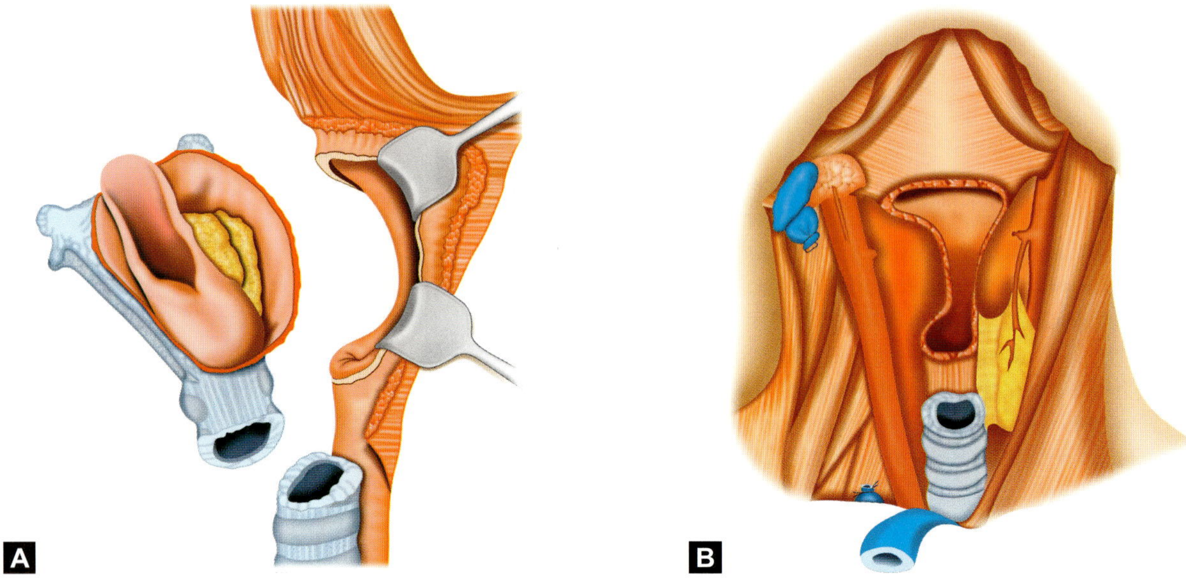

Figs. 13.14A and B: Typical defect following total laryngo-partial pharyngectomy.

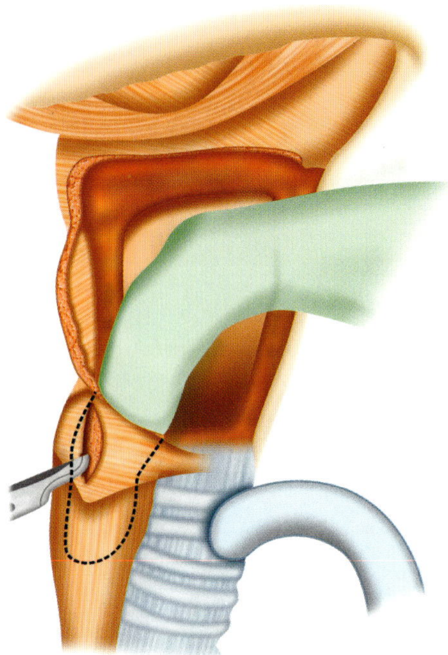

Fig. 13.15: In radiated patients, flaps should always be used. The author always performs a cricopharyngeal myotomy.

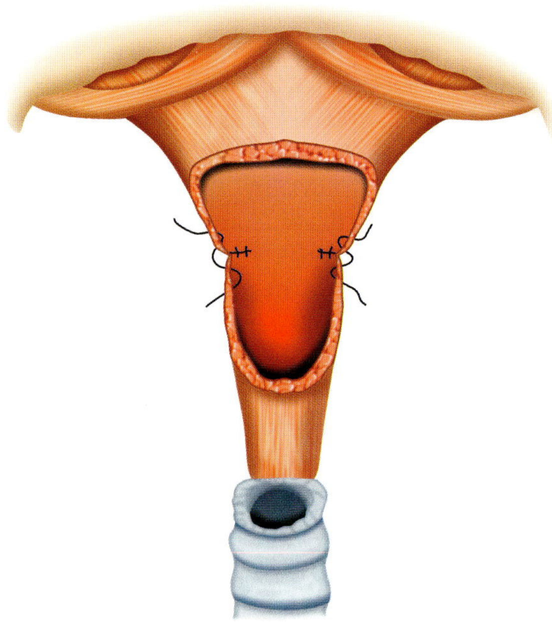

Fig. 13.16: For primary closures, an estimate of where to begin the closure is made by selecting a point laterally along the cut mucosa that roughly equally divides the remnant mucosa into two halves.

It is possible to perform a horizontal closure. Frequently, a T type closure is required, which is more prone to break down. Neck flexure is important to decrease tension during this step. Stoma creation and wound closure are once again identical to that performed in total laryngectomy.

TREATMENT OF THE NECK

Neck treatment depends on several factors, including presence or lack of clinical nodal disease at initiation of treatment and location of the primary tumor. Most authors agree that if a surgical approach is contemplated

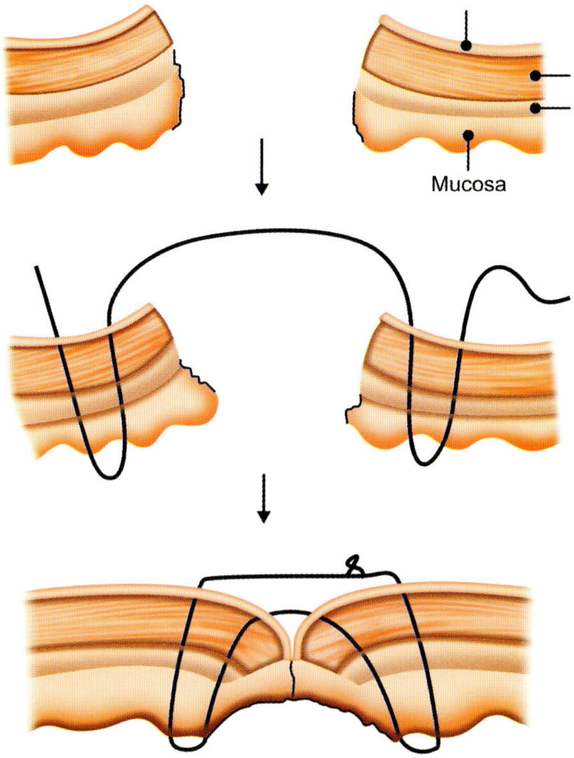

Fig. 13.17: The cadence "far near near far" may be used in teaching this technique, whereby far indicates 3–4 mm from the mucosal edge and near is 2 mm from the mucosal edge, starting outside the lumen and ending outside the lumen on the other side.

for hypopharyngeal cancer, then the neck should be surgically addressed as well. Besides harvesting lymph nodes, it allows for easier access to the hypopharynx and access to vasculature if a microvascular free flap is employed.

Most patients present with adenopathy because of the lack of symptoms associated with early hypopharyngeal cancer. Candela et al. demonstrated that for those with clinical N0 disease, 41% were found to have metastases to the neck.[17] The main lymph node basins for hypopharyngeal cancer are cervical node levels II and III. The more caudal a lesion is in the hypopharynx, the more likely level IV will be involved. Additionally, 8.3% of Weber's patients had metastases to level VI.[3] As such, at least levels II–IV should be dissected and level VI when appropriate.

Management of the neck differs in patients with clinically N+ disease, which is the majority of hypopharyngeal cancer patients. In Lefebvre et al.'s study of hypopharyngeal cancer, 70% presented with palpable adenopathy.[18] For these patients, a comprehensive neck dissection is indicated, sparing uninvolved major structures and nerves.

Retropharyngeal nodes are very difficult to approach through standard neck incisions. Amatsu et al. discovered

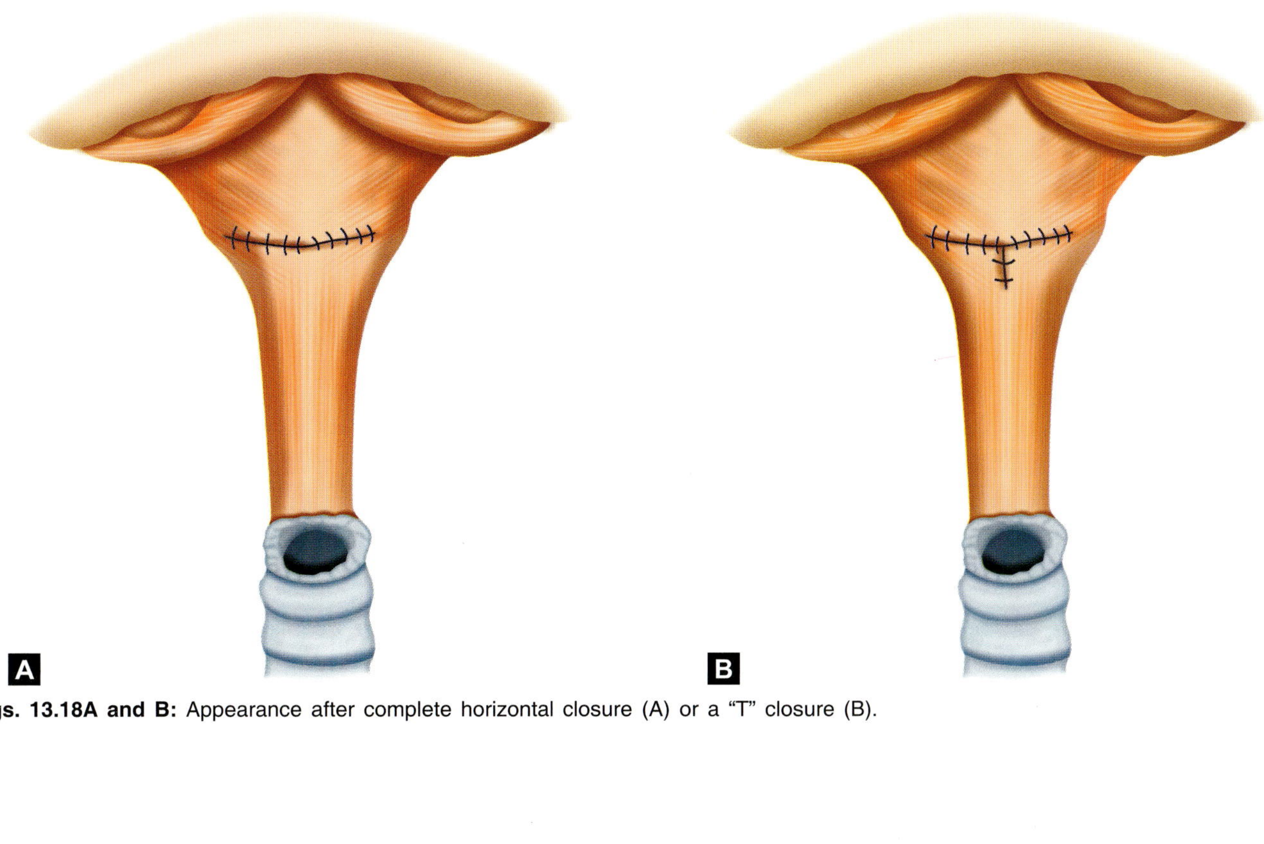

Figs. 13.18A and B: Appearance after complete horizontal closure (A) or a "T" closure (B).

retropharyngeal adenopathy in 20% of their patients with hypopharyngeal cancer.[19] Despite this, most authors do not address these nodes in neck dissection for hypopharyngeal cancer, even in comprehensive dissections. There are very little data regarding the survival of patients with retropharyngeal nodes.

The subsite of the primary may influence election to treat the contralateral neck. Lateral pyriform sinus wall cancers tend to metastasize ipsilaterally. In select cases, unilateral selective neck dissection for these cancers is adequate. Tumors of the medial pyriform sinus wall, postcricoid wall, and posterior wall tend to involve bilateral lymph nodes.[20] As such, bilateral neck dissections are recommended.

Selective Neck Dissection

Skin flaps are raised subplatysmally. The great auricular nerve and marginal mandibular nerve are identified and preserved.

The superficial cervical fascia is divided along the lateral surface of the sternocleidomastoid muscle and reflected forward. The external jugular vein is divided and included in the specimen.

The medial surface of the sternocleidomastoid muscle is further dissected. This fascia is divided along the submandibular gland and inferior parotid gland.

The spinal accessory nerve is identified and dissected inferiorly. The overlying fascia is divided and tissue is divided down to the levator scapulae muscle. This tissue is reflected forward up to the jugular vein.

The nodal bearing tissue is reflected forward using a scalpel or pair of tenotomy scissors to skeletonize the internal jugular vein. Usually, the facial vein is divided and contained in the specimen.

The remaining attachments of the nodal tissue are divided. The spinal accessory nerve, great auricular nerve, marginal mandibular nerve, and internal jugular vein are preserved. Levels II, III, and IV are included in the specimen.

REFERENCES

1. Wenig BL, Applebaum EL. The submandibular triangle in squamous cell carcinoma of the larynx and hypopharynx. Laryngoscope. 1991;101:516-8
2. Davidson BJ, Kulkarny V, Delacure MD, et al. Posterior triangle metastases of squamous cell carcinoma of the upper aerodigestive tract. Am J Surg. 1993;166:395-8.
3. Weber RS, Marvel J, Smith P, et al. Paratracheal lymph node dissection for carcinoma of the larynx, hypopharynx, and cervical esophagus. Otolaryngol Head Neck Surg. 1993;108:11-17.
4. Myers EN, Eibling DE. Operative Otolaryngology: Head and Neck Surgery. Philadelphia, PA: Saunders Elsevier; 2008.
5. Flint PW, Haughey BH, Lund VJ, et al. Cummings Otolaryngology—Head and Neck Surgery. Philadelphia, PA: Elsevier, 2010.
6. Leong SC, Kathan C, Mortimore S. Early outcomes after transoral CO_2 laser resection of laryngeal and hypopharyngeal squamous cell carcinoma: one centre's experience. J Laryngol Otol. 2010;124:185-93.
7. Grant DG, Salassa JR, Hinni ML, et al. Transoral laser microsurgery for recurrent laryngeal and pharyngeal cancer. Otolaryngol Head Neck Surg. 2008;138:606-13.
8. Martin A, Jackel M, Christiansen H, et al. Organ Preserving transoral laser microsurgery for cancer of the hypopharynx. Laryngoscope. 2008;118:398-402.
9. Steiner W, Ambrosch P. Endoscopic laser surgery of the upper aerodigestive tract: with special emphasis on cancer surgery. New York, NY: Georg Thieme Verlag; 2000.
10. Cohen JI, Clayman GL. Atlas of Head and Neck Surgery. Philadelphia, PA: Saunders Elsevier; 2011.
11. Suarez C, Rodrigo JP. Transoral microsurgery for treatment of laryngeal and pharyngeal cancers. Curr Oncol Rep. 2013; 15:134-41.
12. Pradhan S, Mehta M, Hakeem A, et al. Transoral resection of laryngeal and hypopharyngeal cancers. Indian J Surg Oncol. 2010;1(2):207-11.
13. Ambrosch P, Fazel A. Functional organ preservation in laryngeal and hypopharyngeal cancer. GMS Curr Top Otorhinolaryngol Head Neck Surg. 2011;10:Doc02. Epub 2012 Apr 26.
14. Taki S, Homma A, Oridate N, et al. Salvage surgery for local recurrence after chemoradiotherapy or radiotherapy in hypopharyngeal cancer patients. Eur Arch Otorhinolaryngol. 2010;267:1765-9.
15. Harrison DF, Thompson AE. Pharyngolaryngoesophagectomy with pharyngogastric anastomosis for cancer of the hypopharynx: review of 101 operations. Head Neck Surg. 1986;8:418-28.
16. Wei WI, Lam LK, Yuen PW, et al. Current status of pharyngolaryngoesophagectomy and pharyngogastric anastomosis. Head Neck 1998; 20: 240
17. Candela FC, Kothari K, Shah JP. Patterns of cervical node metastases from squamous carcinoma of the oropharynx and hypopharynx. Head Neck 1990; 12:197-203.
18. Lefebvre JL, Chevalier D, Luboinski B, et al. Larynx preservation in pyriform sinus cancer: preliminary results of a European Organization for Research and Treatment of Cancer phase III trial. EORTC Head and Neck Cancer Cooperative Group. J Natl Cancer Inst. 1996;88:890-99.
19. Amatsu M, Mohri M, Kinishi M. Significance of retropharyngeal node dissection at radical surgery for carcinoma of the hypopharynx and cervical esophagus. Laryngoscope. 2001;111:1099-103.
20. Johnson JT, Bacon GW, Myers EN, et al. Medial vs lateral wall pyriform sinus carcinoma: implications for management of regional lymphatics. Head Neck. 1994;16:401-5.

CHAPTER 14

Microlaryngoscopic Laser Excision of Glottic Malignancies

Garret W Choby, Robert L. Ferris

INTRODUCTION

Laryngeal cancer is the second most common malignancy of the upper aerodigestive system and accounts for 3,000 deaths annually. The overall 5-year survival rate for laryngeal squamous cell carcinoma, which accounts for 95% of laryngeal malignancies, is 64%.[1-3] Traditional risk factors for laryngeal cancer include tobacco and alcohol use.[4] Other potential contributing factors include laryngopharyngeal reflux and asbestos.[1,5]

A variety of techniques have been used to treat laryngeal malignancies, including laser resection. A wide array of lasers is available for use in otolaryngology; the selection of the appropriate laser is based upon its wavelength and appropriate interaction with targeted tissues. The CO_2 laser has a wavelength of 10,600 nm and has a strong predilection for water contained within tissues. This has been the traditional workhorse for laryngeal surgery and thus will be focused upon in this chapter. The CO_2 laser has the ability to be emitted in pulsed or continuous waves and makes use of a micromanipulator coupled to the microscope to accurately guide its beam. The beam is delivered along the axis of the microscope. As a general rule, the CO_2 laser is maintained at low settings (3 to 10 watts) using an intermittent or superpulse mode. The spot size is kept quite small to allow for tissue cutting, typically 0.27 mm in diameter. In certain situations, this may be defocused to allow for control of bleeding during the surgery.[1,6-9]

Advantages of the CO_2 laser include avoidance of external incisions, improved ability to make accurate tumor cuts in an area with limited exposure, simultaneous hemostasis while cutting, and the ability to vaporize tissue. Disadvantages of the CO_2 laser include added cost and personnel staffing, incompatibility with fiberoptic guide, concern for thermal injury to surrounding tissues, and potential risk of airway fire.

INDICATIONS

Indications for microscopic laser resection parallel those for traditional open conservation surgery. For beginning surgeons, ideal candidates for microscopic laser resection have unilateral tumors, including Tis and T1a. As experience and confidence is gained, selected T1b and T2 tumors may also be considered for laser resection. This technique may also be used to debulk large laryngeal tumors to avoid tracheostomy in certain patients.

Contraindications include cartilaginous invasion, extralaryngeal tumor spread, subglottic extension of tumor, invasion of the pyriform sinus, and indadequate endoscopic access (trismus, inability to extend the neck, severe retrognathia, or tongue hypertrophy).[6-7] If there is any question regarding thyroid cartilage invasion, a fine-cut laryngeal computed tomographic scan or magnetic resonance imaging can be useful. Moreover, patients with compromised pulmonary function may be poor candidates due to decreased tolerance of postoperative microaspiration, which may compromise their swallowing and functional outcomes.

SURGICAL TECHNIQUE

Preoperative Considerations

Communication with the anesthesia team is critical in transoral laser cases. Specifications regarding intubation technique, inhaled oxygen concentration, and postoperative airway management should be addressed. In general

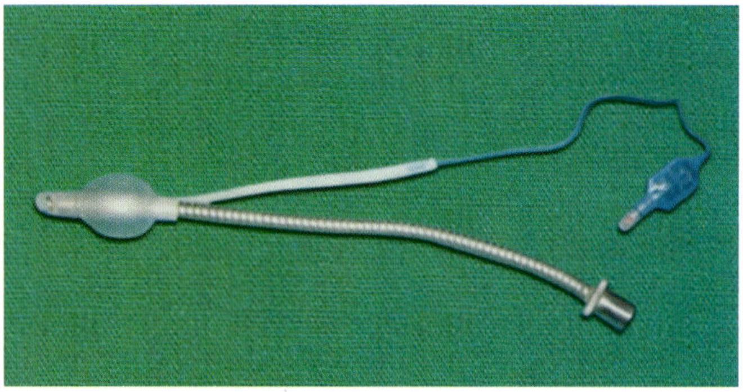

Fig. 14.1: Laser-safe metal endotracheal tube.

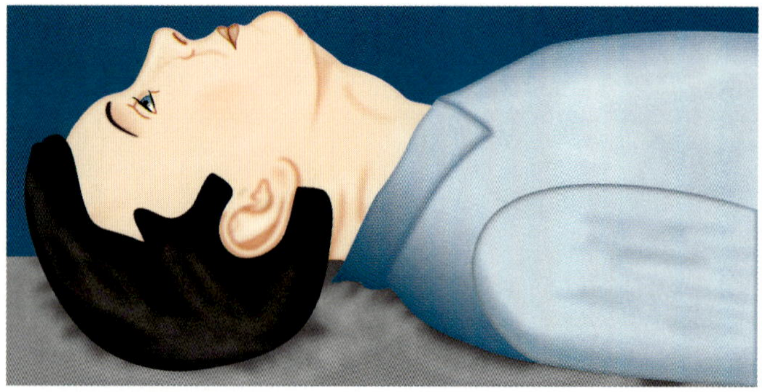

Fig. 14.2: Flexion-extension position: the patient's neck is flexed and the head is slightly extended at the atlanto–occipital joint.

terms, the anesthesia and otolaryngology teams share the airway during the case. However, the otolaryngologist is often more adept at navigating difficult laryngeal anatomy and should be prepared to personally perform the intubation if the anatomy dictates.

Laser safety should be emphasized in any operating room utilizing this technique. Signs placed on the operating room doors should alert visitors to the use of the laser and allow placement of laser-safe goggles prior to entrance. The patient's eyes are taped shut, covered in goggles, and moist gauze is placed over the goggles. Moistened towels are applied to the patient's face, eyes, and neck. Moreover, a laser-safe endotracheal tube (ETT) must be utilized. A variety of these tubes are available commercially, including metal tubes and specially coated plastic tubes (Fig. 14.1). Moreover, the ETT balloon should be filled with colored saline to alert the surgeon if a breach of the balloon has occurred. To further help prevent airway fire, a moist cottonoid should be placed in the subglottis and O_2 concentration should be kept <30%. A basin of saline should always be available on the scrub technician's Mayo stand to place in the larynx should an airway fire arise. If an airway fire should arise, the ETT should be immediately removed, supplemental oxygen shut off, saline flushed into the airway, and reintubation performed.

Positioning

The patient is intubated with the laser-safe ETT in a supine position on the operating room table. To allow adequate working space, the ETT should be the smallest size possible with the ability to adequately ventilate the patient. The optimal patient position is usually with some degree of neck flexion and head extension (Fig. 14.2). It is often helpful to place a piece of 3-inch tape or Velcro strap over the thyroid cartilage to more adequately expose the anterior commissure. A standard tooth guard is used to protect the upper dentition; a moist gauze or sponge is used in the edentulous patient. Many authors advocate a full laryngoscopic examination utilizing 0°, 30°, and 70° endoscopes to fully appreciate the tumor extent.[6-8]

Operative Steps

A laryngoscope is then introduced by the surgeon, typically the largest scope that is able to adequately display the anatomy of interest. For supraglottic tumors, the Lindholm laryngoscope is often useful (Fig. 14.3A). For glottic tumors as addressed in this chapter, a Jako–Dedo type IV laryngoscope is most frequently utilized (Fig. 14.3B). In some cases, an anterior commissure scope may be required to visualize anterior lesions (Fig. 14.3C). After the desired view has been obtained, the laryngoscope is suspended using a Gallows system or a traditional fulcrum system with the Mayo stand. The entirety of the glottis should be visualized, including the anterior commissure (Fig. 14.4).

At this juncture, an operating binocular microscope is introduced for magnified visualization (Figs. 14.5A and B). A moist cottonoid pledget is placed in the subglottis to protect the trachea and ETT from errant laser strikes. As stated above, the patient's eyes, face, and chest should be covered in moist towels. The laser size and orientation are tested on a moist wooden tongue depressor. The laser may be set on traditional single spot size or may be utilized as a pulsed beam in several different computer

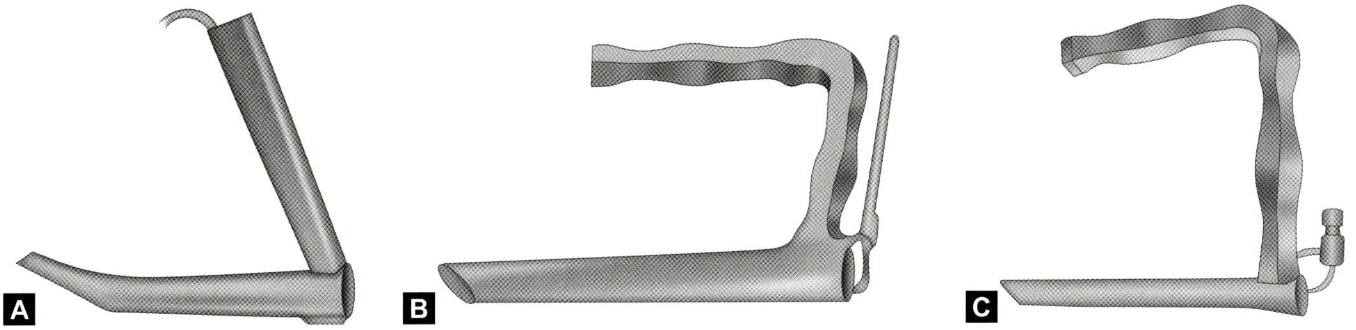

Figs. 14.3A to C: (A) Lindholm laryngoscope. (B) Jako–Dedo Type IV laryngoscope. (C) Anterior commissure laryngoscope.

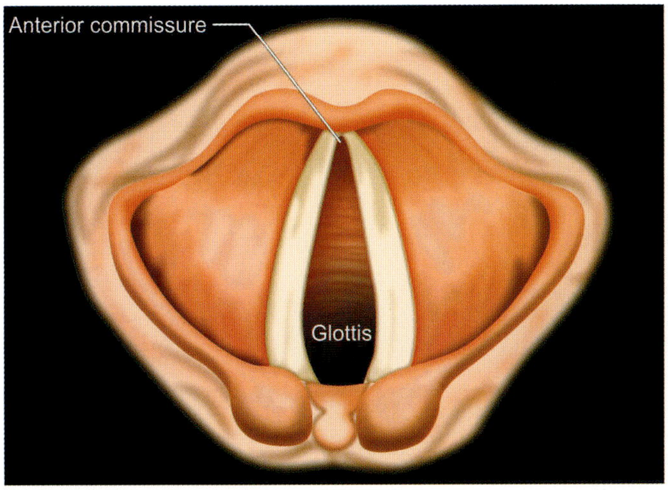

Fig. 14.4: Endoscopic view of the glottis. The entirety of the glottis should be visualized, including the anterior commissure.

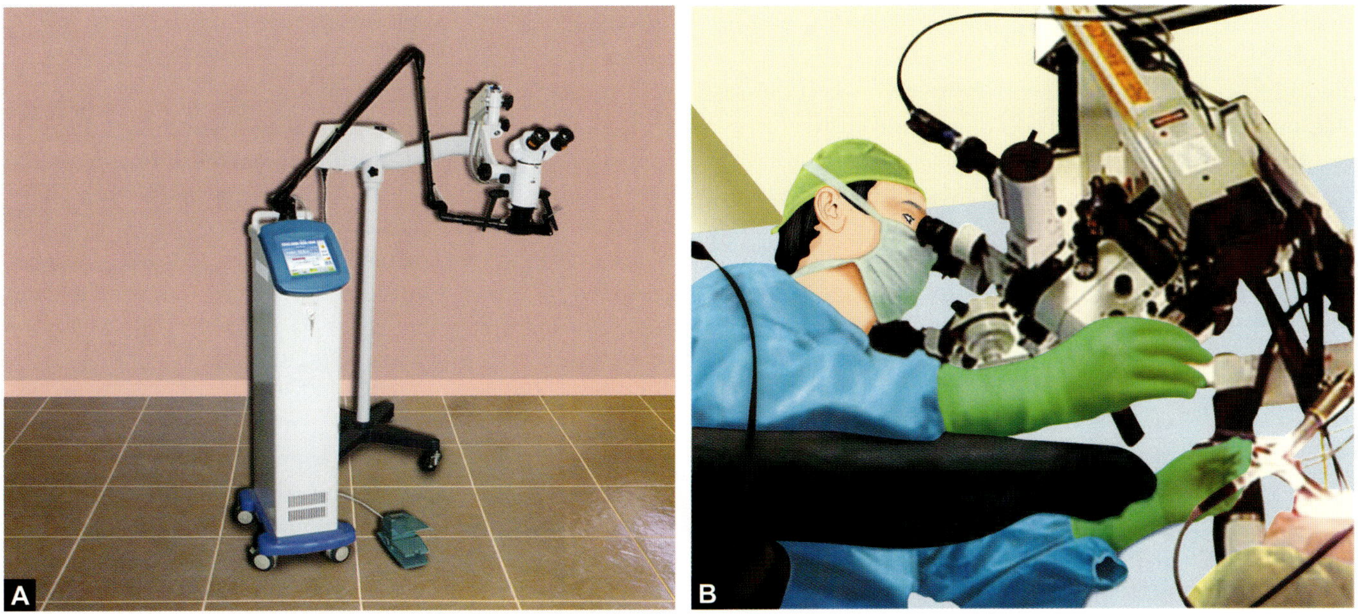

Figs. 14.5A and B: Operating microscope with CO_2 laser. (A) CO_2 laser connected to microscope. (B) Microscope positioning at the head of the patient.

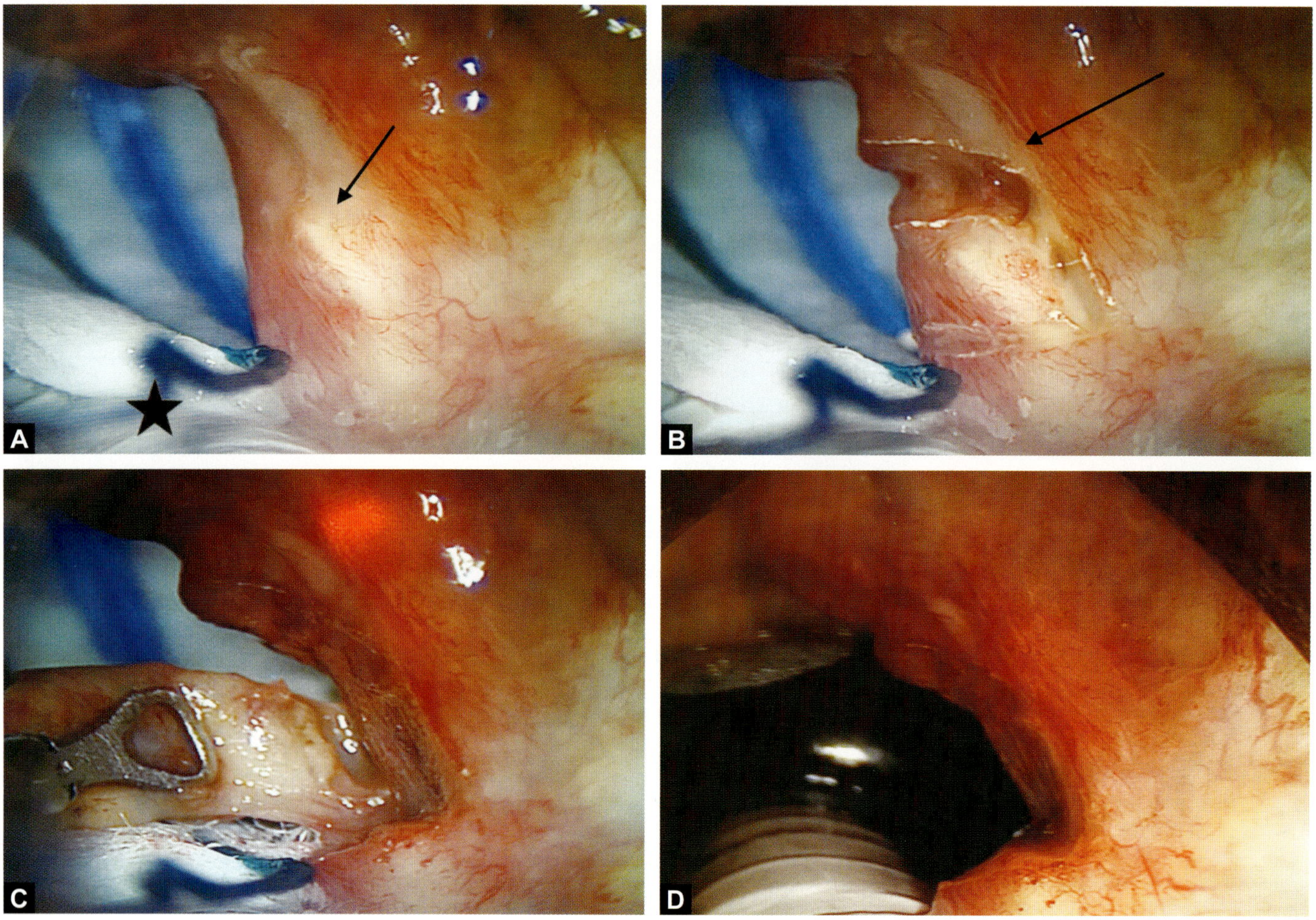

Figs. 14.6A to D: (A) Right true vocal fold subepithelial tumor (arrow). For orientation, the ETT is at the bottom of the photo (marked with a star). Notice the moist cottonoid in the subglottis. (B) Initial incision at the most anterior extent of the tumor (arrow). (C) Tumor is dissected from lateral to medial with the assistance of a grasping triangle forceps. (D) Tumor removal completed.

algorithm-based shapes. In certain tumors, the generated shapes may help with precision of planned cuts.

After the laser has been properly tested, planned resection margins should be marked out on the tumor with single-pulsed laser emissions. We generally advocate resection margins of 1–3 mm. In previously radiated patients, it may be prudent to allow a wider resection margin due to the infiltrative nature of these recurrences. A butterfly needle may be utilized to inject a saline–epinephrine mixture in a subepithelial plane. This will help determine the depth of tumor invasion and allow for a heat-dissipated buffer to protect the vocal ligament. For larger tumors, the surgeon may first need to perform an incision of the false vocal fold in the infrapetiole region and bring this posteriorly toward the level of the vocal process of the arytenoids. Bleeding may be controlled with a combination of defocused laser and afrin-soaked pledgets.

Dissection of the glottic lesion may proceed with the assistance of a grasping endoscopic forceps to provide countertraction as the tumor is excised. For superficial lesions, dissection is carried out in a subepithelial plane. For more invasive tumors, subligamental cordectomy, or transmuscular cordectomy may be necessary. Preoperative and intraoperative assessment of depth of invasion should guide the depth of dissection. As a general rule, dissection proceeds in a lateral to medial direction to allow for adequate visualization of tissue planes (Figs. 14.6A to D).

During the procedure, it is crucial to maintain three-dimensional special orientation of the tumor to ensure negative margins. Close communication and orientation of the specimen with the consulting frozen section pathologist is crucial to ensure that no confusion regarding the specimen occurs. If possible, the pathologist should come to the operating room to receive the specimen and

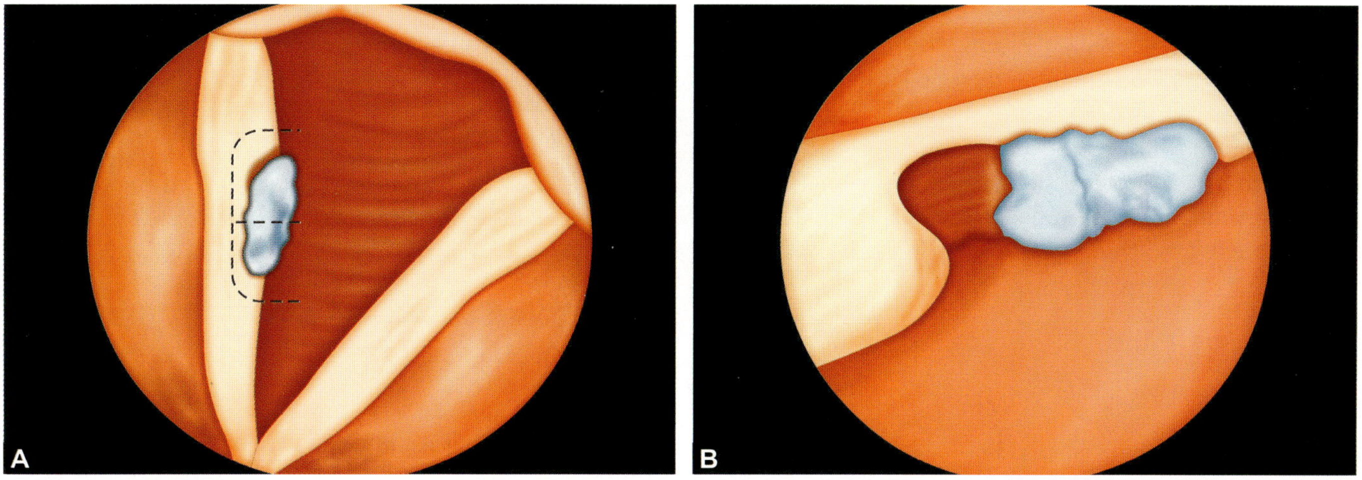

Figs. 14.7A and B: Tumor bisection. Certain tumors may require bisection to determine depth of invasion to ensure complete tumor resection. (A) Planned resection planes. (B) Depth of invasion displayed after tumor bisection.

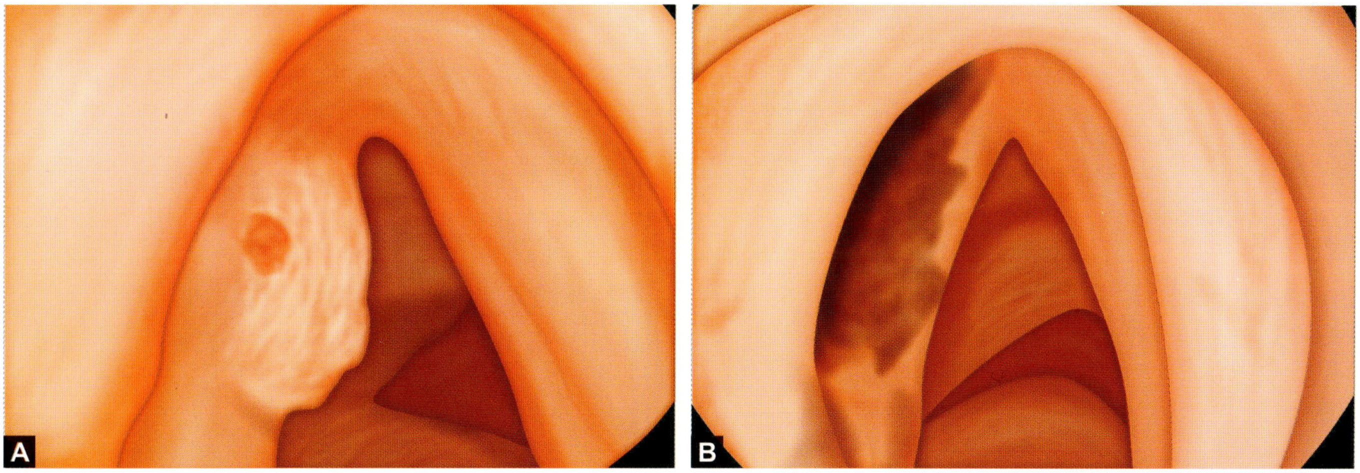

Figs. 14.8A and B: Pre- (A) and postoperative (B) views of T1a lesion of right true vocal fold after frozen margins were obtained.

ensure its proper orientation. By definition, transoral laser microsurgery depends on narrow margins, thus necessitating meticulous attention to proper orientation of the main specimen and frozen section margins. In larger or invasive tumors, the tumor may be removed in multiple sections. The tumor may need to be bisected to determine it depth of invasion and adequate depth of dissection (Figs. 14.7A and B). Frozen sections are then paramount to ensure complete removal (Figs. 14.8A and B).

Postoperative Considerations

Postoperative care is dictated by the individual patient and extent of resection. The majorities of patients do not require tracheotomy and are able to be extubated at the end of the case. The surgeon should always be in the room upon extubation in case issues with bleeding or airway edema are evident after ETT removal. Perioperative corticosteroids are often given to prevent airway edema, and broad spectrum antibiotics may be indicated if exposed cartilage is present at the end of the case. Many physicians also advocate prophylactic treatment for laryngopharyngeal reflux for 6–8 weeks postoperatively with a proton pump inhibitor or H2-blocker.[7]

Of paramount concern is the development of airway bleeding in the postoperative period. For larger resections, the patient may be observed in an ICU setting for 24–48 hours. If significant bleeding arises, the recommended immediate intervention is intubation or, in rare cases, tracheotomy.

Postoperative feeding should also be evaluated by a speech-language pathologist. A bedside swallow test is often performed to ensure that the patient has no signs or symptoms of aspiration. Swallowing management techniques may be introduced if clinically suspected aspiration occurs. The effects of postoperative voice rest on phonation outcomes have not been well studied. We do not routinely advocate voice rest in the majority of our patients.

REFERENCES

1. Rubinstein M, Armstrong WB. Transoral laser microsurgery for laryngeal cancer: a primer and review of laser dosimetry. Lasers Med Sci. 2011;26(1):113-24.
2. Jemal A, Siegel R, Ward E, et al. Cancer statistics, 2008. CA Cancer J Clin. 2008;58(2):71-96.
3. Hoffman HT, Porter K, Karnell LH, et al. Laryngeal cancer in the United States: changes in demographics, patterns of care, and survival. Laryngoscope. 2006;116(9 Pt 2 Suppl 111): 1-13.
4. Altieri A, Garavello W, Bosetti C, et al. Alcohol consumption and risk of laryngeal cancer. Oral Oncol. 2005;41(10): 956-65.
5. Menvielle G, Luce D, Goldberg P, et al. Smoking, alcohol drinking, occupational exposures and social inequalities in hypopharyngeal and laryngeal cancer. Int J Epidemiol. 2004;33(4):799-806.
6. Ferris RL, Simental A. Endoscopic surgery for early glottic carcinoma. Oper Tech Otolaryngol Head Neck Surg. 2003; 14:49-54.
7. Christopoulos A, Holsinger FC, Ferris RL. Transoral laser resection of glottic tumors. In: Cohen JI, Clayman GL (Eds). Atlas of Head and Neck Surgery. Philadelphia, PA: Elsevier Saunders; 2011. pp. 397-408.
8. Ferris RL. Endoscopic laser excision of laryngeal carcinoma. In: Myers E (Ed). Operative Otolaryngology: Head and Neck Surgery. Philadelphia, PA: Elsevier Saunders; 2008. pp. 397-402.
9. Rosen CA. Principles of laser microlaryngoscopy. In: Rosen CA, Simpson B (Ed). Operative Techniques in Laryngology. Berlin: Saunders; 2008. pp. 81-9.

CHAPTER

15 Transoral Robotic Surgery of the Larynx

J Kenneth Byrd, Robert L Ferris

INTRODUCTION

Early laryngeal cancer may be treated with either resurgery or radiation therapy with roughly equivalent outcomes. However, the relative contraindication to reradiation more than once and long-term sequelae of treatment favor surgery when the preservation of laryngeal function is possible. Although open conservation laryngeal surgery is associated with satisfactory oncologic outcomes and function, there is significant perioperative morbidity. Voice and swallowing outcomes are always better when laryngeal reconstruction is not required. As a result, transoral laser microsurgical approaches have been the mainstay for partial laryngeal surgery. However, the recent introduction and widespread adoption of robotics into head and neck surgery for oropharyngeal cancer has led some to expand indications of transoral robotic surgery (TORS) to laryngeal carcinoma due to the excellent visualization and improved dexterity over traditional laryngeal instruments.

Because the standard 5-mm robotic instruments are not well suited for endolaryngeal work, and because a laryngoscope that allows freedom of motion with these instruments has not been developed, TORS for glottic cancer has not been widely adopted, despite a promising animal feasibility study.[1] There are several case series reporting the use of the spatula tip monopolar cautery and Feyh-Kastenbauer (FK) retractor for early glottic cancer,[2-4] and other groups have experimented with the CO_2 laser for TORS cases due to less thermal spread and resultant edema.[5,6]

Ultimately, current robotic technology is too cumbersome for routine endolaryngeal work, in our opinion, and awaits in-line laser technology and flexible robot optics for better exposure.

Transoral robotic total laryngectomy has recently been proposed as an alternative to standard oral laryngectomy for patients who do not require a neck dissection. The authors use a small incision for tracheostomal management and use a modification of the techniques for TORS supraglottic laryngectomy and pharyngectomy to remove the entire larynx.[7] One of three patients required conversion to open laryngectomy, and two were completed successfully and had subsequent secondary tracheoesophageal puncture.[8] The procedure may have potential for patients who develop a nonfunctional larynx due to chemoradiation, but neck dissection cannot be performed concurrently, and the authors did not address surgical margin control. Therefore, the role of this procedure for recurrent or persistent disease is unclear.

Although the aforementioned techniques are under development and may prove useful after further study, this chapter will focus on the most common use of transoral robotic laryngeal surgery, TORS supraglottic partial laryngectomy (SGPL). TORS SGPL was first reported in three patients by Weinstein et al. in 2007.[9] Since then several other groups have reported favorable short-term outcomes using the technique.[4,10-13] In a retrospective comparison of a small group of patients, Park et al. found that TORS SGPL was associated with significantly shorter operating times, length of hospitalization, and time to decannulation and oral diet compared with open SGPL, with an equivalent rate of negative margins and disease control.[14]

Although the TORS operative techniques reported by different groups are similar, perioperative management of airway and feeding varies by institution and series. In a description of their early experience with TORS SGPL, Olsen et al. reported a series of nine T1–T3 patients who underwent TORS SGPL and neck dissection. Seven patients required tracheotomy at the time of surgery, and four required gastrostomy due to postoperative dysphagia. At last follow-up, 78% of patients were free from tracheostomy and gastrostomy, and 77% were disease free (mean 26 months). The authors noted that TORS was technically difficult in one patient who had undergone prior bilateral neck dissection due to airway edema.[10] Similarly, in Lallemant's series of glottic and supraglottic TORS, 3/10 patients required tracheotomy and 8/10 required enteral feeding, including one who was gastrostomy dependent for 2 years.[4] In contrast, Mendelsohn et al. describe 18 patients with T1–T4 supraglottic tumors in whom no patients required tracheotomy or gastrostomy. The authors noted a mean time to oral intake of thin liquids of 5.5 days (range 2–45). Ozer et al. routinely start an oral diet on postoperative day 1, and report that 11 of 13 patients were able to avoid nasogastric or gastrostomy feeding. One patient required tracheotomy and gastrostomy due to delayed postoperative edema.[11]

LIMITATIONS

There are limitations to TORS for supraglottic carcinoma. First of all, the FK retractor does not expose the supraglottic larynx sufficiently in all patients. In addition, as the surgeon is manipulating tissue deep in the larynx, increasingly acute angles of the robotic arms in relation to the endoscope are required, which can restrict movement and ability to clear submucosal disease.[10] In our experience, the infrahyoid supraglottis is difficult to resect using TORS, and may be better approached with transoral laser microsurgery (TLM). In a retrospective comparison of ten early TORS cases to ten early TLM cases by Ansarin et al., a higher rate of positive margins and longer postoperative dysphagia was found in the TORS group. There were also 2 patients in whom TORS was planned but converted to TLM and open supraglottic laryngectomy due to inadequate exposure. Of the patients not undergoing simultaneous neck dissection (six in each group), operating times were significantly shorter in the TORS group by approximately 90 minutes. The authors concluded that the available retractors for TORS SGPL were not optimal for every patient, but that TORS may be associated with shorter operative times, although the surgeons' previous experience with TLM may have confounded this finding.[15] Although strong conclusions about the superiority of one procedure over another cannot be drawn, it is likely that TORS and TLM are complementary procedures, and that patient anatomy and tumor size and location should be considered when choosing the optimal approach.

PREOPERATIVE PLANNING

All patients who are candidates for TORS supraglottic laryngectomy should undergo preoperative imaging with contrasted computed tomography (fine cuts through the larynx) to evaluate for pre- and paraglottic space involvement, extralaryngeal spread, and nodal metastasis. In addition, preoperative fiberoptic endoscopy, using angled rigid telescopes, should be performed in the office to assess for tongue base extension, translaryngeal spread, and glottic motion impairment. Operative laryngoscopy may be performed at a separate time prior to TORS or at the beginning of the procedure, although the surgical plan is subject to change depending on findings at the time of endoscopy.

CONTRAINDICATIONS

Contraindications to TORS SGPL include extralaryngeal involvement, invasion of the tongue base, or thyroid cartilage. Extensive preepiglottic and/or paraglottic space involvement is a relative contraindication. Tumors with glottic extension may be better approached with TLM, in our experience. Furthermore, anterior or bilateral involvement of the glottis may be better approached with the supracricoid partial laryngectomy so that the arytenoids and hypopharynx can be repositioned to aid in airway protection and swallowing. Advanced neck stage should be considered a relative contraindication as well, as postoperative (chemo)radiotherapy will significantly worsen the patient's function. Finally, cardiopulmonary function should be considered in patients when choosing operative versus nonoperative treatment, because many patients will have postoperative transient aspiration.

TORS SUPRAGLOTTIC LARYNGECTOMY: SURGICAL PROCEDURE

Step 1: General anesthesia is used for orotracheal or nasotracheal intubation, depending on surgeon's preference. Nasotracheal intubation may allow for a more posteriorly placed tube and more working room, but we find orotracheal intubation satisfactory. The tube should be secured in place with a suture to the mucosal gingiva or lip, or through the patient's nasal septum.

Step 2: After rotating the operating table to 180° from anesthesia and sliding the table on its base toward the

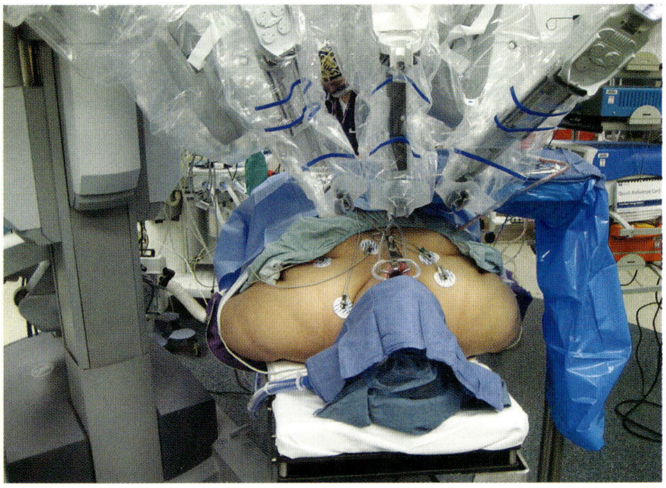

Fig. 15.1: The robot is docked at a 30° to the head of the bed.

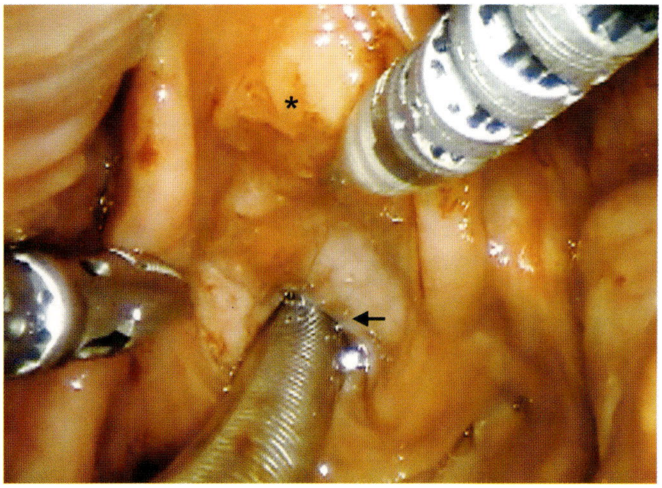

Fig. 15.2: Exposure of the epiglottis and vallecula with 30° endoscope. The tumor is marked by an asterisk, and the edematous false cords are shown with an arrow.

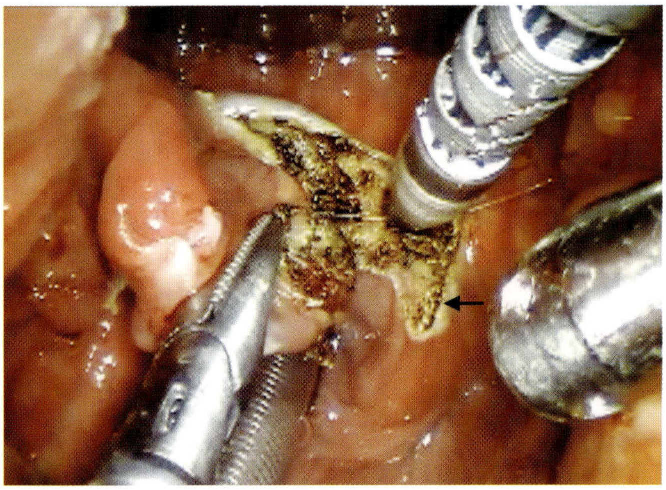

Fig. 15.3: The vallecular incision (arrow) is then made while retracting the epiglottis.

patient's head, direct laryngoscopy is performed to fully map the tumor and ensure that there is no contraindication to the procedure.

Step 3: The teeth are protected with a tooth guard and a suture is placed through the tongue to retract anteriorly with a hemostat, exposing and exteriorizing the vallecula and supraglottic structures.

Step 4: The FK retractor is inserted through the oral cavity and into the vallecula. The retractor is adjusted so that the tongue base is retracted anteriorly and the larynx is exposed sufficiently to allow for use of a 30° endoscope directed anterosuperiorly. The mouth should be opened as widely as possible without damaging the teeth or oral tongue.

Step 5: The base of the Da Vinci robot is brought in at 30° to the operating table (Fig. 15.1). The camera/endoscope is introduced into the oral cavity with the operating arms on each side entering at 30–45° angles. A Maryland retractor and the monopolar cautery are used for robotic arms 1 and 2. A Lisa laser can also be used. The FK should provide adequate visualization of the vallecula and epiglottis (Fig. 15.2).

Step 6: The epiglottis is grasped with the Maryland in an area uninvolved by tumor and rotated, while the cautery is used on cut to incise the mucosa. If visualization is limited by the patient's anatomy or tumor, the epiglottis may be bisected prior to the vallecular incision. This aids in determining tumor depth and preepiglottic and/or vallecula extension. Splitting the epiglottis is preferred to measure depth of the tumor extent as well as to retain sufficient vallecula for optimal swallowing.

Step 7: Rotating the portion of the epiglottis to be removed carefully, the vallecular incision is made (Fig. 15.3), maintaining at least 1-cm margin from the tumor, but preserving as much normal tissue as possible. The superior laryngeal arterial supply should be positively identified and clipped twice. If concurrent neck dissection is performed, it may alternatively be ligated proximally in the neck.

Step 8: The inferior incision is made after the epiglottis has been otherwise circumferentially dissected. The false vocal folds may be excised if necessary, but this will cause increased postoperative swallowing dysfunction.

Step 9: Margins are taken from the specimen, in close direct consultation with the pathologist, with additional margins taken where close (Fig. 15.4). At our institution,

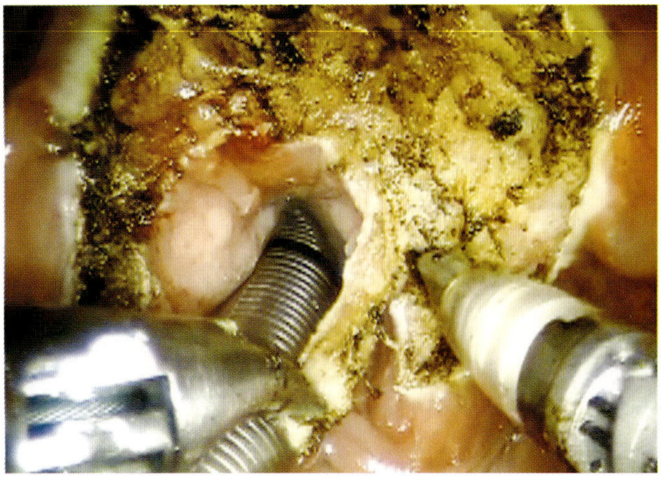

Fig. 15.4: Circumferential margins are then sent for frozen section pathologic analysis.

if the margin is closer than 3 mm on pathological examination, additional tissue is taken.

Step 10: A hemostatic agent, such as thrombin, is applied to the wound bed and packed with tonsil balls. The wound is irrigated and inspected for bleeding. Tracheotomy is not necessary but airway observation is crucial to monitor for postoperative edema or catastrophic hemorrhage.

Step 11: Patient selection is key to avoid dual or three-modality therapy, which reduces outcome and obviates the benefit of surgical therapy. The philosophy is to provide single modality therapy, and thus N0-N1 disease, confirmed pathologically at simultaneous or delayed neck dissection, is the goal. If simultaneous neck dissection is performed, efforts should be made to preserve venous outflow from the larynx to prevent severe postoperative edema.

REFERENCES

1. O'Malley BW, Jr., Weinstein GS, Hockstein NG. Transoral robotic surgery (TORS): glottic microsurgery in a canine model. J Voice. 2006;20(2):263-8.
2. Park YM, Lee WJ, Lee JG, et al. Transoral robotic surgery (TORS) in laryngeal and hypopharyngeal cancer. J Laparoendosc Adv Surg Techn. Part A. 2009;19(3):361-8.
3. Kayhan FT, Kaya KH, Sayin I. Transoral robotic cordectomy for early glottic carcinoma. Ann Otol Rhinol Laryngol. 2012;121(8):497-502.
4. Lallemant B, Chambon G, Garrel R, et al. Transoral robotic surgery for the treatment of T1-T2 carcinoma of the larynx: preliminary study. Laryngoscope. 2013;123(10):2485-90.
5. Blanco RG, Ha PK, Califano JA, Saunders JM. Transoral robotic surgery of the vocal cord. J Laparoendos Adv Surg Techn Part A. 2011;21(2):157-9.
6. Remacle M, Matar N, Lawson G, et al. Combining a new CO_2 laser wave guide with transoral robotic surgery: a feasibility study on four patients with malignant tumors. Eur Arch Otorhinolaryngol. 2012;269(7):1833-7.
7. Lawson G, Mendelsohn AH, Van Der Vorst S, et al. Transoral robotic surgery total laryngectomy. Laryngoscope. 2013;123(1):193-6.
8. Dowthwaite S, Nichols AC, Yoo J, et al. Transoral robotic total laryngectomy: report of 3 cases. Head Neck. 2013; 35(11):E338-42.
9. Weinstein GS, O'Malley BW, Jr., Snyder W, et al. Transoral robotic surgery: supraglottic partial laryngectomy. Ann Otol Rhinol Laryngol. 2007;116(1):19-23.
10. Olsen SM, Moore EJ, Koch CA, et al. Transoral robotic surgery for supraglottic squamous cell carcinoma. Am J Otolaryngol. 2012;33(4):379-84.
11. Ozer E, Alvarez B, Kakarala K, et al. Clinical outcomes of transoral robotic supraglottic laryngectomy. Head Neck. 2013;35(8):1158-61.
12. Park YM, Kim WS, Byeon HK, et al. Surgical techniques and treatment outcomes of transoral robotic supraglottic partial laryngectomy. Laryngoscope. 2013;123(3):670-7.
13. Mendelsohn AH, Remacle M, Van Der Vorst S, et al. Outcomes following transoral robotic surgery: supraglottic laryngectomy. Laryngoscope. 2013;123(1):208-14.
14. Park YM, Byeon HK, Chung HP, et al. Comparison of treatment outcomes after transoral robotic surgery and supraglottic partial laryngectomy: our experience with seventeen and seventeen patients respectively. Clin Otolaryngol. 2013;38(3):270-4.
15. Ansarin M, Zorzi S, Massaro MA, et al. Transoral robotic surgery vs transoral laser microsurgery for resection of supraglottic cancer: a pilot surgery. Int J Med Robot Comput Assist Surg: MRCAS. 2014;10(1):107-12. Epub Nov 28, 2013.

Section 4

Neck Dissections

Section Editor: ***Neerav Goyal***

Chapters

CHAPTER

16

Radical Neck Dissection

Ali Khaku, David Goldenberg, Frank G Garritano

INTRODUCTION

The radical neck dissection (RND) was first described in 1906 by Crile, based on Halsted's concept of en bloc resection. The purpose was to effectively remove all of the ipsilateral cervical lymph nodes and interconnected lymphatic drainage channels present in the neck extending from the inferior border of the mandible to the clavicle, from the lateral border of the sternohyoid muscle, hyoid bone, and contralateral anterior belly of the digastric muscle medially, to the anterior border of the trapezius posteriorly.[1] This essentially removes all of the nodes included in levels I–V in addition to the sternocleidomastoid muscle (SCM), the submandibular gland, the tail of the parotid gland, the internal and external jugular veins, the cervical sensory nerves, and the spinal accessory nerve (cranial nerve XI). Later, fascial coverings of the submandibular gland, carotid sheath, and deep cervical muscles and nerves were also incorporated into the RND. The majority of the morbidity of an RND is a consequence of the removal of these additional structures, particularly the spinal accessory nerve, SCM, and internal jugular vein, rather than the removal of the lymph nodes. The RND stands in comparison to the extended neck dissection (END), which refers to the removal of one or more additional lymph node groups and/or nonlymphatic structures due to the extent of nodal metastases, not encompassed by the RND. An END may include the removal, for instance, of the mediastinal nodes, or carotid artery, or hypoglossal nerve.[1] The END can also include the removal of the postauricular and suboccipital nodes, the periparotid nodes (with the exception of a minimal number of nodes found in the tail of the parotid gland), the perifacial and buccinators nodes, the retropharyngeal nodes, or the paratracheal nodes, which are only removed in certain types of END.[2] In 1967, Ferlito, Bocca, and Pignataro described what is now called the "modified neck dissection", which removes all of the lymphatics but preserves the nonlymphatic-containing structures. Hence, anything less than the classical RND is considered a "modified" neck dissection.

CLASSIFICATION, PERTINENT ANATOMY, AND SURGICAL LANDMARKS BY LEVEL

Originally described by the Memorial Sloan-Kettering Group in 1981, the seven cervical lymph node groups have been further delineated in 2001 and again in 2008 by the American Head and Neck Society's Neck Dissection Committee's recommendation on the use of sublevels for further defining selected lymph node groups within levels I through VII on the basis of biologic significance.[3] Surgical landmarks are outlined in Table 16.1 and Figure 16.1.

Level $I_{(A/B)}$

The submental triangle corresponds to sublevel I_A, while the submandibular triangle corresponds to sublevel I_B. The submental triangle is the region bounded by (1) the symphysis superiorly, (2) the anterior bellies of the digastric muscle bilaterally, and (3) the hyoid bone inferiorly. The submandibular triangle is bordered by (1) the mandible superiorly, (2) the posterior belly of the digastric muscle and the stylohyoid muscle posteroinferiorly, and (3) the anterior belly of the digastric muscle anteroinferiorly. It includes the submandibular gland as well as the pre- and postvascular nodes that are related to the facial artery (Fig. 16.2).

Table 16.1: Anatomic and radiographic boundaries of each lymph node level.

	Boundary							
	Superior		*Inferior*		*Lateral*		*Medial*	
Sublevel	Anatomic	Radiographic	Anatomic	Radiographic	Anatomic	Radiographic	Anatomic	Radiographic
I_A	Mandibular symphysis	Geniohyoid muscle	Hyoid body		Digastric muscle (anterior belly)			
I_B	Mandibular body	Mylohyoid muscle	Hyoid body		Submandibular gland (posterior edge)		Digastric muscle (anterior belly)	
II_A	Skull base	Transverse process C1	Carotid bifurcation	Hyoid bone	SAN	IJV	Submandibular gland (posterior edge)	
II_B	Skull base	Transverse process C1	Carotid bifurcation	Hyoid bone	SCM (posterior edge)		SAN	Paraspinal muscles
III	Carotid bifurcation	Hyoid bone	Omohyoid muscle	Cricoid cartilage	Cervical rootlets	SCM (posterior edge)	Sternohyoid muscle	Paraspinal muscles
IV	Omohyoid muscle	Cricoid cartilage	Clavicle	Sternoclavicular joint	Cervical rootlets	SCM (posterior edge)	Sternohyoid muscle	Paraspinal muscles
V_A	SCM and trapezius muscle		Cricoid cartilage		Trapezius muscle (anterior edge)		Cervical plexus	SCM (posterior edge)
V_B	Cricoid cartilage		Clavicle		Trapezius muscle (anterior edge)		Cervical plexus	SCM (posterior edge)
VI	Hyoid bone		Sternal manubrium (superior)		Common carotid artery			
VII	Sternal manubrium (superior edge)		Innominate artery		Innominate artery (right) Common carotid artery (left)			

(IJV: Internal jugular vein; SAN: Spinal accessory nerve; SCM: Sternocleidomastoid muscle).

Significant local anatomical structures include the marginal branch of the facial nerve, the facial artery, the submental artery, the lingual artery and nerve, Wharton's duct, and the hypoglossal nerve.

Level $II_{(A/B)}$

Level II, also known as the upper jugular or jugulodigastric region, contains two zones, levels II_A and II_B. The boundaries between these two zones are defined in terms of their relationship to the spinal accessory nerve. Level II_A is defined by (1) the skull base superiorly, (2) inferiorly by the carotid bifurcation (surgically) and hyoid bone (radiographically), (3) the stylohyoid muscle anteriorly, (4) the vertical plane defined by the spinal accessory nerve *posteriorly*, (5) the posterior border of the SCM laterally, and (6) the lateral border of the sternohyoid and stylohyoid muscles medially. Level II_B is defined by (1) the skull base superiorly, (2) inferiorly by the carotid bifurcation (surgically) and hyoid bone (radiographically), (3) the vertical plane defined by the spinal accessory nerve *anteriorly*, and (4) the lateral aspect of the sternocleidomastoid posteriorly. A subsection of level II_B, the submuscular triangle (recess), includes the most superior aspect of this zone and lies laterally to the spinal accessory nerve at the skull base. Level II contains the upper jugular lymph nodes that surround the upper third of the internal jugular vein, the spinal accessory nerve, and the jugulodigastric node (the principal node of Kuttner). The principal node of Kuttner is the most common node containing metastases in oral malignancy (Fig. 16.2).

Significant local anatomical structures include the common trunk of the spinal accessory nerve, the cervical plexus, the carotid arteries, the internal jugular vein, the vagus nerve, the hypoglossal nerve, and the phrenic nerve.

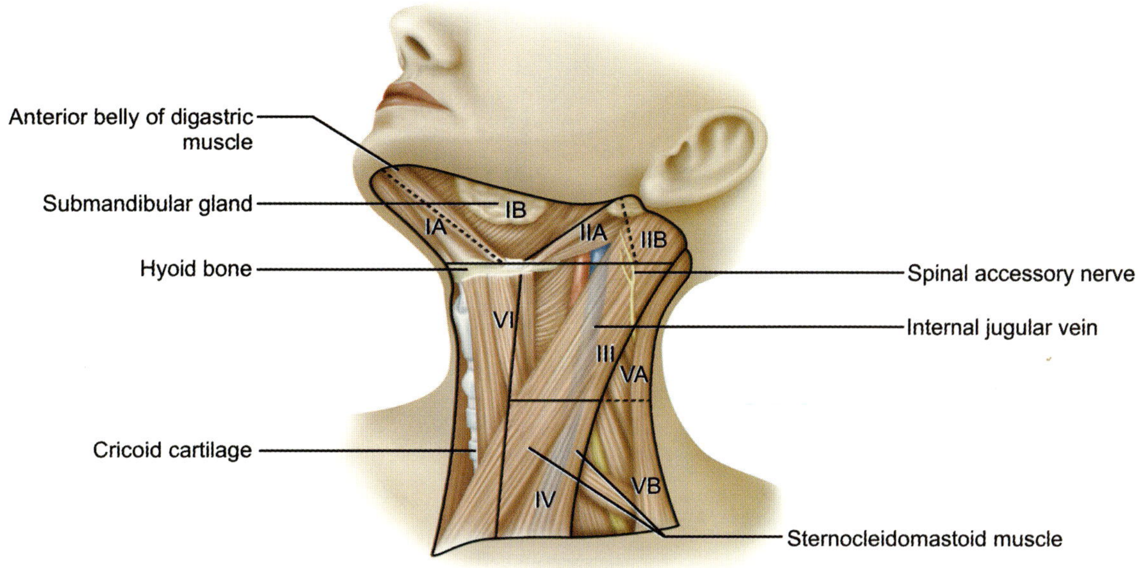

Fig. 16.1: Cervical lymph node levels. Level system for describing the location of nodes.

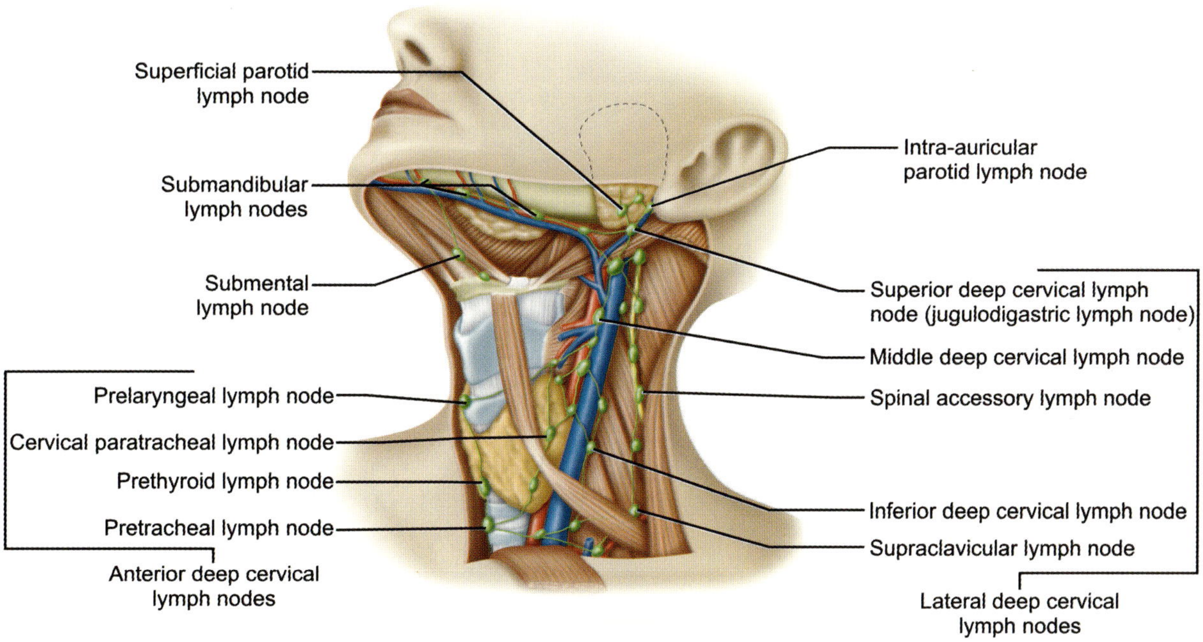

Fig. 16.2: Deep lymph nodes of the neck, including lateral deep and anterior deep cervical node.

Level III

Level III, also known as the middle jugular region, is bounded by (1) the carotid bifurcation (surgically) and the hyoid bone (radiographically) superiorly, (2) the junction of the omohyoid muscle and the internal jugular vein (surgically), and the cricoid cartilage (radiographically) inferiorly, (3) the lateral border of sternohyoid muscle anteriorly, and (4) the lateral border of the SCM posteriorly.

Significant local anatomical structures include the cervical plexus, the carotid artery, the internal jugular vein, the vagus nerve, and the phrenic nerve.

Level IV

Level IV, also known as the lower jugular region, is bounded by (1) the omohyoid superiorly, (2) the clavicle inferiorly, (3) the lateral border of the sternohyoid muscle anteriorly, and (4) extends to the posterior border of the SCM posteriorly.

Significant local anatomical structures include the cervical plexus, the carotid artery, the internal jugular vein, the vagus nerve, and phrenic nerve, the thoracic duct and the subclavian artery.

Level $V_{(A/B)}$

Level V, also known as the posterior triangle and the supraclavicular region, is subdivided by a plane defined by the inferior border of the cricoid cartilage into level V_A superiorly and level V_B inferiorly. Level V_A begins at the apex formed by the intersection of the SCM and the trapezius and bound by a horizontal line defined by (1) the hyoid bone superiorly, (2) the spinal accessory nerve inferiorly, (3) the posterior edge of the SCM anteriorly, (4) the anterolateral edge of the trapezius muscle posteriorly, (5) the skin and platysma laterally, and (6) the deep paraspinal muscles medially. Level V_B is defined by (1) the spinal accessory nerve superiorly, (2) the transverse cervical artery inferiorly, (3) the posterior edge of the SCM anteriorly, (4) the anterolateral trapezius muscle posteriorly, (5) the skin and platysma laterally, and (6) the deep paraspinal muscles medially. Level V_A contains the nodes associated with the spinal accessory nerve, and level V_B contains the transverse cervical and supraclavicular nodes.

Significant local anatomical structures include Erb's point (punctum nervosum), the external jugular vein, the spinal accessory nerve, the great auricular nerve, the brachial plexus, the scalene muscles, the phrenic nerve, the transverse cervical artery, and the subclavian artery.

Level VI

Level VI, also known as the anterior or central compartment, is bounded by (1) the hyoid bone superiorly, (2) the suprasternal notch inferiorly, and (3) the common carotid arteries laterally. Level VI is typically dissected only in conjunction with laryngectomy and thyroidectomy. The anterior compartment lymph node group is of minimal importance in primary tumors originating from the oral cavity or oropharynx. It consists of lymph node bearing tissue that occupies the visceral space, comprising the paratracheal and thyroidal basins. These lymph nodes can contain metastases from primary thyroid, piriform sinus, and subglottic cancers.

Significant local anatomical structures include the infrahyoid muscles, the larynx, the quadrangular membrane, the conus elasticus, the hypopharynx, the trachea, the cervical esophagus, the thyroid gland, the parathyroid glands, the superior and recurrent laryngeal nerves, the vagus nerve, Galen's loop, the anterior jugular veins, the superior and inferior thyroid artery, the cricothyroid artery, the brachiocephalic artery (innominate artery), the subclavian artery, the thyrocervical trunk, and vertebral artery.

Posterior Neck

The posterior neck contains two groups of lymph nodes: the suboccipital lymph nodes and retroauricular lymph nodes. The suboccipital lymph nodes can be divided into three groups: the superficial occipital nodes, the deep occipital nodes, and a sole lymph node found along the splenius segment of the occipital artery. The superficial occipital nodes are located close to cutaneous branch of the occipital artery and greater occipital nerve at the insertion of the trapezius muscle to the superior nuchal line. The deep occipital nodes are located beneath the superficial layer of the deep cervical fascia. The additional sole lymph node is found along the splenius segment of the occipital artery. The retroauricular lymph nodes can be found on or behind the mastoid process. Both the suboccipital and retroauricular lymph nodes drain primarily into the spinal accessory lymph node chain and secondarily into level II (*see* Fig. 16.2).

Significant local anatomical structures include the occipital artery, trapezius muscle, the splenius capitis muscle, the levator scapulae, anterior scalene muscle, middle scalene muscle, posterior scalene muscle, and the brachial plexus.

INDICATIONS

Current indications for a classic radical neck dissection generally include patients with widely metastatic cervical disease: (1) N3 neck disease in the upper part of the neck, (2) extensive lymph node metastases with extension beyond the capsule or to nodes involving the accessory nerve and/or internal jugular vein, (3) recurrent tumor after previous irradiation, (4) recurrent disease in the neck after previous neck dissection, (4) salvage surgery in patients after chemoirradiation, (5) gross extranodal spread of disease, and (6) involvement of the platysma or skin, requiring sacrifice of a portion of skin in the upper neck.[4]

CONTRAINDICATIONS

Contraindications to RND include frank invasion or encasement of the internal carotid artery, invasion of the deep prevertebral musculature, or skull base involvement by metastatic disease. However, occasionally such extensive disease cannot be viewed radiologically and can only be apparent during intraoperative exploration.[5]

TREATMENT

Preoperative Evaluation

Patient selection is a critical portion of preoperative planning. A basic assessment of the patient's disease, comorbidities, and treatment goals is required.[6] Patients who have been irradiated are particularly problematic due to impaired wound healing and are at significantly higher risk for complications.[7] A basic assessment of a patient's nutritional status should also be explored, particularly in the presence of red flags such as significant weight loss or hypoalbuminemia. Preoperative evaluation includes contrast-enhanced computed tomography scan and fine-needle aspiration cytology for confirmation of tissue diagnosis.[4] The use of positron emission tomography in conjunction with a fluorodeoxyglucose radiotracer (FDG-PET) has more recently been found to improve the accuracy of preoperative staging and is commonly used.[8] If there is evidence of extensive disease surrounding the carotid artery and one is considering carotid resection, preoperative evaluation of the carotid and cerebral blood flow, including four-vessel cerebral angiography and carotid balloon test occlusion, is highly recommended.[9]

Antibiotics

Operations on the neck alone are considered to be "clean," whereas operations that also involve the oral cavity are considered "clean contaminated." Perioperative antibiotics are indicated for both circumstances. Several well-controlled studies have demonstrated that antibiotics started before the incision and continued for no more than 24 hours serve to minimize perioperative infections and the emergence of resistant bacterial strains.[10] Continuation beyond 24 hours should be considered in patients at increased risk for infection or those with ongoing contamination. First-generation cephalosporins and clindamycin represent the most commonly used prophylactic antibiotics in cervical and oral cancer surgery. However, amoxicillin-clavulanate, clindamycin plus gentamicin, and cefazolin seem to have similar efficacy when administered prophylactically.[10] Topical antimicrobials, such as chlorhexidine and clindamycin rinses, have also been shown to successfully reduce the incidence of infections.[1,11-13]

Anesthesia and Positioning

The radical neck dissection is performed under general endotracheal anesthesia with the patient in the supine position. The neck is optimally hyperextended with the use of a shoulder roll and turned to the contralateral side with the endotracheal tube position in the corner of the mouth contralateral to the operative field. The skin should be prepped and draped to allowed clear visualization of the surrounding landmarks (the mentum, mastoid processes, earlobes, the clavicles, and suprasternal notch inferiorly). Estimated blood loss is roughly 150 mL and the need for transfusion is rare.[2] Identify the angle of the jaw, the mastoid tip, the midline of the neck, anterior and posterior borders of the SCM, and the clavicles.

Surgical Technique

In general, neck skin flaps should be broadly based and raised either superiorly or inferiorly. Hence, trifurcation incisions, particularly those overlying the carotid sheath, should be avoided. Three common incisions used are the Lahey incision, the Schobinger incision, and the MacFee incision. In patients undergoing bilateral neck dissections, the apron incision, which is a bilateral "hockey stick" incision, is often used (Figs. 16.3A to G). The Lahey incision is made in the skin creases of the neck beginning in the low neck and extending to the mastoid tip. The Schobinger incision, which may be better suited for oral lesions, uses a high horizontal incision from the hyoid to the mastoid tip and a long curving descending limb. The MacFee incision, which is useful in postradiation patients where the risk of skin flap necrosis is higher, consists of two parallel horizontal incisions. Figures 16.4A to C provide a diagrammatic overview of the RND.

The initial incision is carried through the skin, and if there is no evidence of gross disease extending through the skin or the platysma muscle, then the incision is carried through the platysma. The posterior skin flap is elevated in the subplatysmal plane and should not include the cervical plexus nerves (the greater auricular nerves) or external jugular veins. However, if there is gross pathologic evidence of tumor invasion and extension

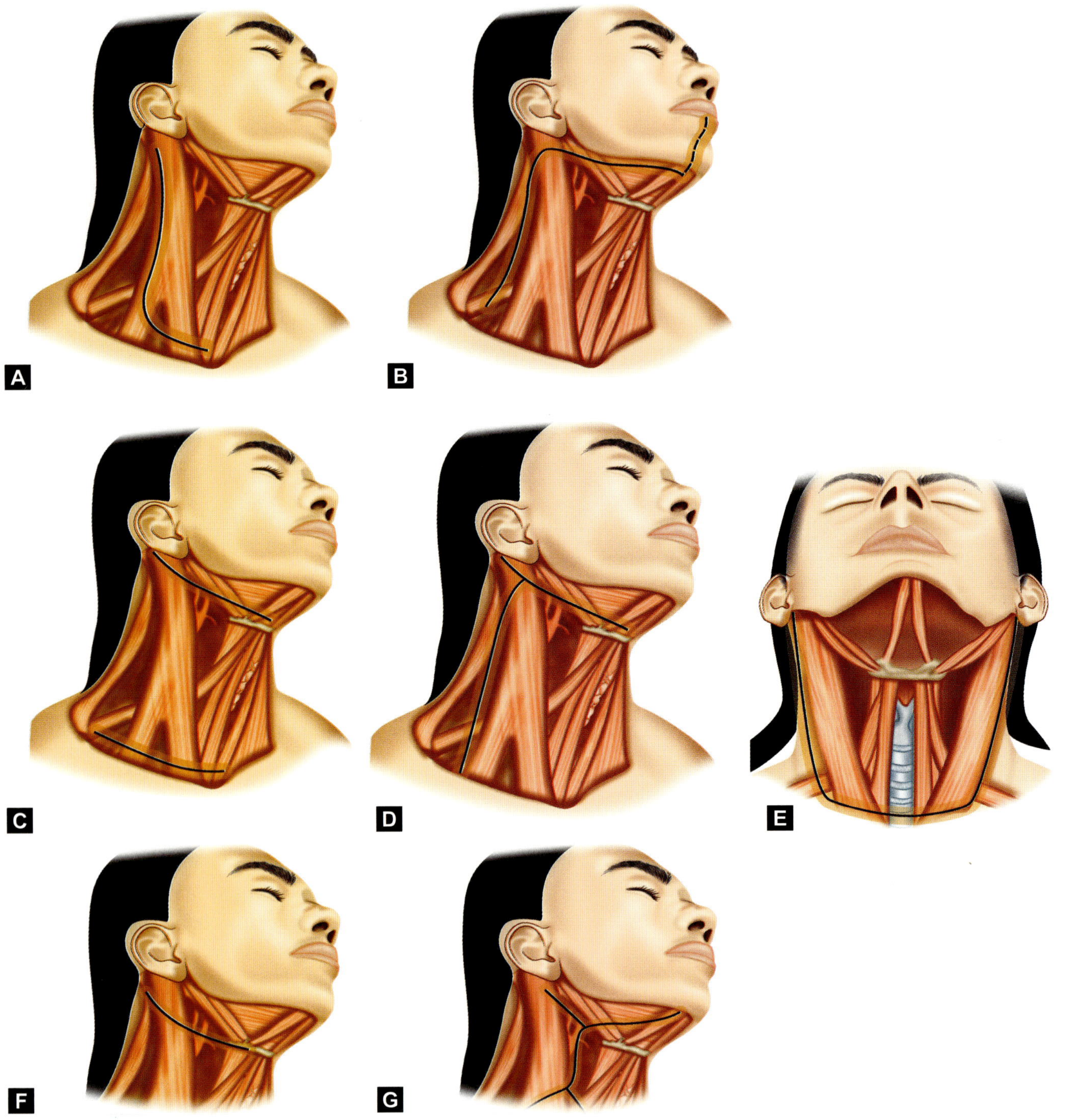

Figs. 16.3A to G: Surgical incisions used for radical neck dissection: the three most common incisions used for a radical neck dissection consist of the Lahey incision, the Schobinger incision, and the MacFee incision. (A) Lahey (hockey stick). (B) Boomerang. (C) MacFee. (D) Modified Schobinger. (E) Apron or bilateral hockey stick. (F) Gluck. (G) Martin double-Y.

into the platysma, then one should consider resecting the overlying muscle and skin. The posterior skin flap is elevated to the level of the anterior border of the trapezius muscle. The superior limit of the skin flap is the hyoid bone, the submandibular gland, and the tail of the parotid gland. Lateral (or posterior) to the platysma it is important

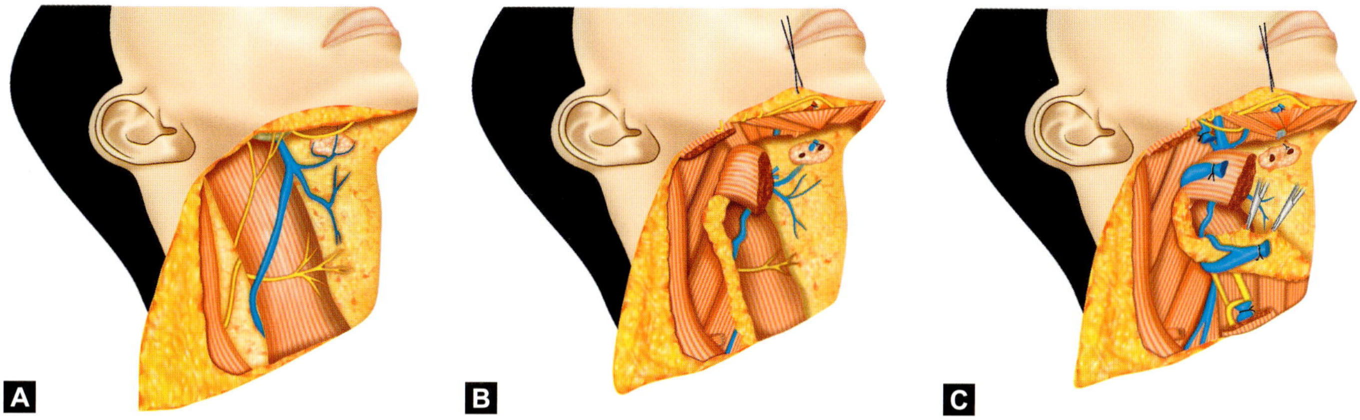

Figs. 16.4A to C: (A) Elevation of subplatysmal skin flaps allows broad visualization of relevant anatomy and identification of the marginal mandibular nerve where it crosses over the facial artery and vein. (B) Incision of the fascial packet at the anterior border of the trapezius dividing the spinal accessory nerve along with the division of the sternocleidomastroid muscle allows for the fascial packet to be rolled anteriorly to be removed en bloc. (C) The jugular vein is divided at both its proximal and distal attachments to allow for its inclusion in the final specimen.

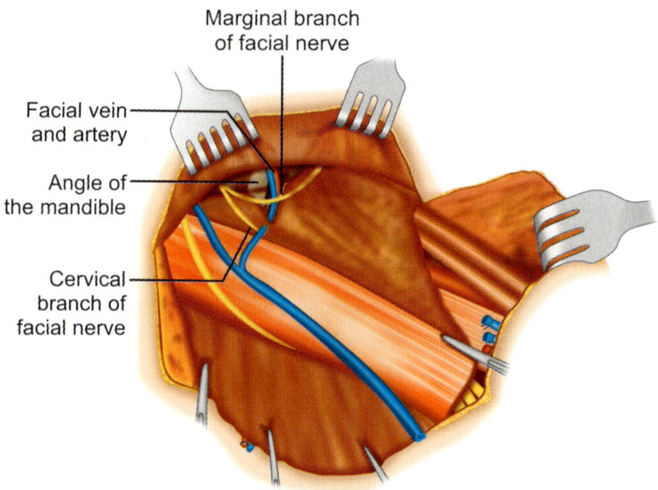

Fig. 16.5: The marginal mandibular branch of the facial nerve is identified as it crosses superficial to the facial artery and vein. The cervical branch of the facial nerve may be divided.

to stay in a superficial plane as the spinal accessory nerve can be found relatively superficially within the posterior neck nodal packet. The anteromedial limit of dissection is the anterior border of the sternohyoid and thyroid strap muscles while the inferior limit is the clavicle. It is important to remain in the proper subplatysmal plane in order to maintain uniform thickness of the skin flap and to prevent complications such as skin flap necrosis.

At this point there are many variations on how to proceed. Some surgeons prefer a posterior to anterior (or lateral to medial) approach, others prefer a superior to inferior approach or an inferior to superior approach. Some surgeons prefer to begin the dissection in the region where there is the least amount of pathologic lymphadenopathy, whereas others prefer to address these areas first. We will first discuss the dissection performed in level I and will then proceed from posterior to anterior by discussing the dissection of level V followed by levels II–IV. In cases where there is concern or suspicion of carotid involvement or unresectability, these areas should be addressed or evaluated first before proceeding with the surgery.

Excision of level I lymph nodes is begun by identifying the submandibular gland. In order to facilitate identification of the submandibular gland palpate for the greater horn of the hyoid bone. The bottom of the gland typically overlies this portion of the hyoid bone.[14] The fascia over the gland is incised, and the facial vein is ligated and divided while elevated off the gland. Leaving a long tie attached to the vein and retracting this with a hemostat allows one to keep the fascia elevated and avoid injury to the marginal mandibular branch of the facial nerve (Hayes-Martin maneuver) (Fig. 16.5). The deep inferior portion of the gland can be elevated off the muscle by inserting an index finger under the gland and sweeping the finger anteriorly and then posteriorly, bringing the anterior belly of the digastric muscle and tendon into view. Delineate the boundaries of the submental triangle using the anterior bellies of the ipsilateral and contralateral digastric muscles. Dissection of the submental triangle, level Ia, is performed by incising the fascia overlying the ipsilateral anterior tendon of the digastric muscle. The fascial packet is elevated off of the mylohyoid muscle and divided from its attachments superiorly at the mandibular symphysis and inferiorly at the hyoid bone. Dissection continues along the mylohyoid muscle until the contralateral anterior belly of the digastric tendon is reached. The fascial packet can then be transpositioned and removed in continuity with the remainder of the lymph node specimen.

The contents of the submandibular triangle, level I_B, are dissected in a medial to lateral direction and the use of the digastric tunnel can facilitate this dissection. Using the tendinous attachment of the digastric to the hyoid bone, pass a hemostat adjacent to the lateral aspect of the tendon along the posterior belly. By opening the clamp it will create a pocket large enough to admit the index finger, which is passed over the digastric muscle inferior to the submandibular gland and toward the anterior border of the SCM. An imaginary line between the digastric tendon and the mastoid tip is used to orient the surgeon's index finger when creating the tunnel. Note that in a previously irradiated patient, the fascia overlying the digastric muscle can become significantly fibrotic and scarred, becoming resistant to finger dissection. If this is the case, create a smaller tunnel with the hemostat. Use the Bovie cautery to cut through the fascia overlying the tunnel. Pay particular attention not to inadvertently follow the stylohyoid muscle rather than the posterior belly of the digastric muscle because this could lead to the anterior aspect of the parotid tail and result in significant risk of damaging the marginal mandibular nerve (*see* Fig. 16.5). As part of an RNO the dissection extends posteriorly toward the tail of the parotid gland and the greater auricular nerve may be sacrificed.

Once the ascending portion of the hypoglossal nerve has been identified, the surgeon can determine where the horizontal portion of the nerve is located by dissecting with a fine clamp inferior to the border of the digastric muscle. Once identified the nerve is dissected posterosuperiorly, with the removal of the overlying fascia. Note that often there are moderate-sized veins, the vena comitans of the hypoglossal nerve (*ranine veins*), that cross the horizontal aspect of the hypoglossal nerve and that will need to be avoided or suture ligated. Unexpected bleeding at this stage places the nerve at a higher risk for accidental thermal or clamp injury. Therefore, if bleeding is encountered pressure should be applied with a finger and then, with an assistant suctioning the bleed, the finger is removed and a clamp is carefully applied to the bleeding vessel while avoiding damage to the nerve. Next, the hypoglossal nerve can be tracked superiorly and posteriorly leading to the occipital artery proper, which is usually left intact. Retraction of the posterior belly of the digastric muscle with an Army-Navy retractor or Richardson retractor should be carried out firmly but gently in order to avoid excessive pressure applied to the parotid gland and the facial nerve. Dissect the fascia immediately posterior to the hypoglossal nerve to identify the jugular vein. Once the fascia is removed from the jugular, dissect posterolateral to the internal jugular vein to identify the superior extent of the spinal accessory nerve.

Next, the contents of the anterior portion of the submandibular triangle are dissected from the overlying cervical fascia and from its attachments to the underlying mylohyoid muscle until the lateral border of the mylohyoid can be identified. The lateral border of the muscle is then retracted anteriorly, exposing the deep contents of the submandibular triangle. This allows for visualization of the lingual nerve and the submandibular duct. The submandibular duct is isolated, divided, and ligated. Next, the submandibular ganglion should be divided, thus allowing the lingual nerve to retract superiorly away from the area of dissection. The last attachment of the contents of the submandibular triangle is the proximal end of the facial artery as it courses deep to the submandibular gland. The facial artery is divided a second time at the posterior aspect of the gland. The specimen is rolled off the posterior belly of the digastric muscle and may be kept pedicled to the Level II neck contents or removed separately. It is, however, important to remember that complete excision of all contents of the submandibular triangle within its muscular boundaries—and not just the submandibular gland—is required.

The next step is to expose the anterior border of the trapezius muscle extending from its superior aspect, where it converges with the posterior border of the SCM, to its inferior aspect where it approaches the clavicle. The fibrofatty tissue of the fascial packet is then incised, exposing the muscular floor of the posterior triangle (Fig. 16.6). While dissecting free the fascial packet in the lower aspect of the posterior triangle, the spinal accessory nerve will be transected at the point at which it enters the trapezius muscle. The inferior aspect of the posterior triangle can be exposed by incising through the inferior belly of the omohyoid muscle and the fibrofatty tissue overlying the brachial plexus. At this point, take care to preserve the transverse facial artery, as it will be encountered immediately overlying the muscular floor

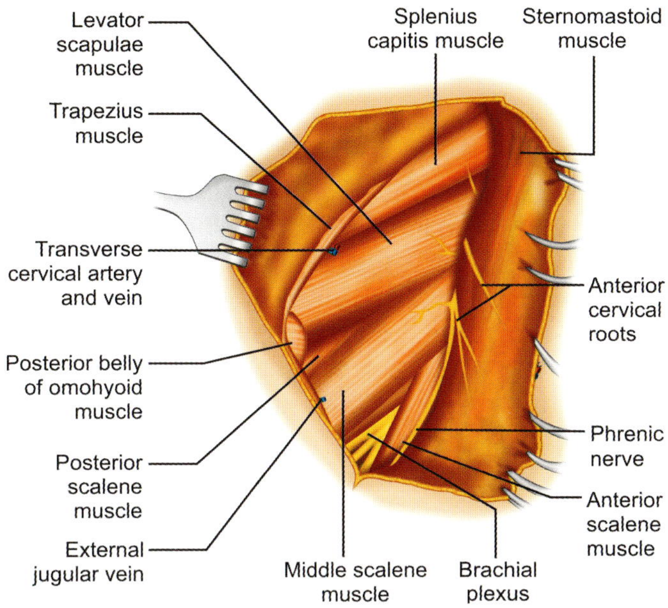

Fig. 16.6: Elevation of the fibrofatty and lymphatic tissue off the floor of the posterior triangle reveals the phrenic nerve and its cervical nerve rootlets on the surface of the anterior scalene muscle, and the brachial plexus between the middle and anterior scalene muscles.

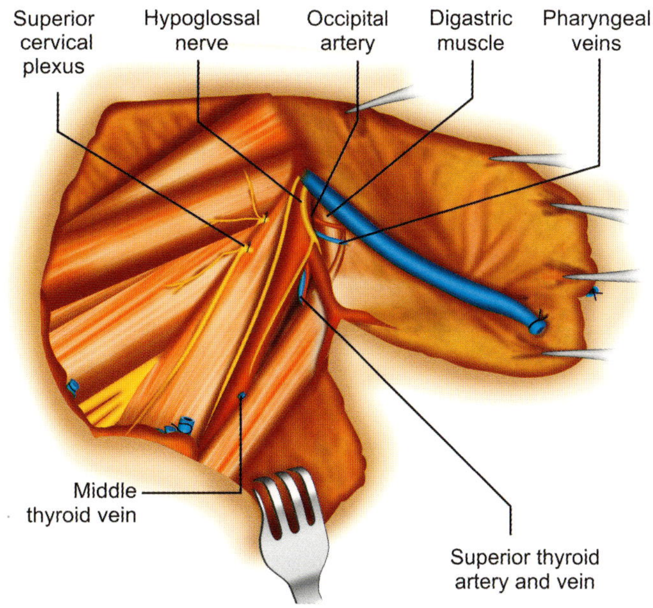

Fig. 16.7: The cervical nerve rootlets are divided leaving small stumps on the phrenic nerve to assure its preservation. The pharyngeal venous plexus and occipital artery are divided between clamps and ligated.

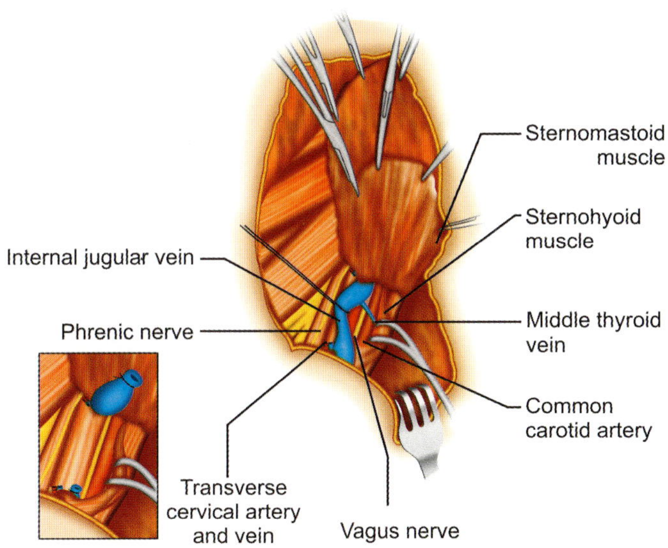

Fig. 16.8: With the sternocleidomastoid muscle retracted superiorly and the strap muscles retracted medially, the carotid sheath is entered. The internal jugular vein is divided and doubly ligated after the vagus nerve has been identified and protected.

of the posterior triangle. However, if there is evidence of gross disease infiltration of the artery it should be resected. At this point, it becomes critically important to remain superficial to the deep fascia overlying the deep cervical musculature in order to avoid damage to the phrenic nerve and brachial plexus (Fig. 16.7). The SCM can be transected roughly 2 cm above the clavicle with an electrocautery or harmonic device aided with traction and counter-traction as well as at its attachment to the mastoid bone. This allows dissection to continue anteriorly toward the carotid sheath. As the cutaneous nerve rootlets are encountered along the floor of the neck, they are transected high adjacent to the specimen in order to prevent injury to the phrenic nerve (Fig. 16.7).

Careful attention should be paid after the carotid sheath is exposed, allowing for identification of the common carotid artery and vagus nerve (Fig. 16.8). Furthermore, careful attention should be paid to the cervical sympathetic chain, which is in close relationship with the prevertebral fascia deep to the carotid sheath. Next, attention is turned toward skeletonizing and ligating the internal jugular vein. In order to ligate the internal jugular vein, it must be mobilized from the skull base superiorly (Fig. 16.9) and from the clavicle inferiorly. Use 2-0 silk ties, performing first a stick-tie followed by a standard tie immediately adjacent to the transected portion of the vein in order to minimize the risk of tie slippage and inadvertent bleeding. Using this method, two ties are placed superiorly and two inferiorly and the internal jugular vein is able to be transected and freely mobilized. At this point in the lower

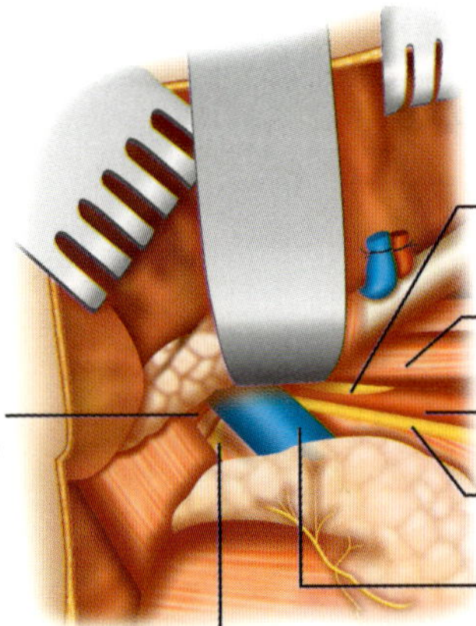

Fig. 16.9: Skeletonizing and ligation of the internal jugular vein. At the skull base, the spinal accessory nerve and occipital artery and vein are identified to aid in visualization and skeletonization of the upper end of the jugular vein.

medial aspect of the anterior triangle, lymphatic channels will commonly be encountered, particularly but not exclusively in the left neck. The thoracic duct is most commonly located behind the left common carotid artery and the vagus nerve, where it arches superiorly, anteriorly and laterally, passing deep to the internal jugular vein and superficial to the anterior scalene muscle and phrenic nerve. The thoracic duct is anterior to the thyrocervical trunk and the transverse cervical artery. Keeping the level of dissection approximately 2 cm above the clavicle may help prevent a chyle leak. Note that the thoracic duct may be in the form of multiple ducts in its upper end and that, at the base of the neck, it usually receives the jugular trunk, a subclavian trunk, and maybe other minor lymphatic trunks that should be individually divided and ligated or clipped to minimize the risk of chylous fistula.

After ligation of the inferior aspect of the internal jugular vein, retract the specimen superiorly and medially and continue to carry the dissection medially to the sternohyoid muscle. Continued elevation of the specimen will expose the carotid bifurcation and along the way will also expose additional branches of the internal jugular vein (the middle and superior thyroid veins and the retromandibular vein) which will require ligation. Further superior elevation of the fibrofatty contents away from the upper part of the carotid sheath will expose the hypoglossal nerve that lies lateral to the external carotid artery and the spinal accessory nerve. The ansa cervicalis branches are ligated as they exit cranial nerve XII near the carotid. The specimen should be divided anteriorly at the level of the sternohyoid and thyroid strap muscles. At this point, the contents of the radical neck dissection specimen should be freely mobile and can be removed en bloc and sent off to pathology.

The wound should be carefully inspected for any bleeding and this should be carefully controlled with pressure and appropriate ligature, via either suture or clips. The use of several Valsalva maneuvers in order to increase the central venous pressure may be helpful in order to identify any areas of concern. Note that the risk of intraoperative hemorrhage is increased when performing dissection in a previously irradiated patient because fibrotic tissue prevents collapse of the veins as well as the normal retraction and constriction of arteries. The wound should be thoroughly irrigated with normal saline and suctioned clear. Neck drains are inserted and brought through separate stab incisions through the most dependent areas of the dead space. Closure of the incisions is usually performed in two to three layers, including approximation of the platysma, the subcutaneous tissue, and the skin.

RISK FACTORS AND COMPLICATIONS

Preoperative chemoradiation therapy is a risk factor for major wound complications such as wound dehiscence, hematoma, or a chylous fistula. The higher complication rate observed in previously chemoirradiated patients is attributable to normal tissue reaction to radiation. Radiotherapy activates a different wound-healing process, causing an excessive deposition of the extracellular matrix and collagen that is characteristic of radiation fibrosis. Furthermore, radiation also induces vascular damage that increases the risk of tissue hypoxia and perpetuates a fibrogenic response, which leads to delayed and altered wound-healing after surgery.[7]

Early Postoperative Complications

- *Hematoma*: Hematomas are at the highest risk of occurring immediately during the postoperative period and may rarely present as a life-threatening situation. Immediate exploration and control of the bleeding vessel in the operating room is indicated.[15]
- *Seroma*: Seromas appear at a slightly later stage postoperatively and are less dramatic and, depending on size, may resolve spontaneously. Seromas are more

frequently caused by overenthusiastic early drain removal rather than drain failure. Larger seromas may need drainage and the application of a pressure bandage. However, the use of long-term suction drains, until evidence of minimal drainage is noted, lowers the incidence of seromas.

- *Infection*: Wound infections and abscesses are rare and treated, depending on size, with surgically incision and drainage and antibiotics.
- *Chyle leak*: Chyle leaks are caused by injury to the thoracic duct or to one of its tributaries, occurring most often during manipulation of the internal jugular vein deep in the left neck. The thoracic duct lies on the anterior scalene muscle and phrenic nerve. The duct terminates most commonly in the left internal jugular vein and less commonly it may enter the left subclavian, left external jugular, left innominate vein or the right internal jugular vein. The injury is manifest by the appearance of clear or milky fluid in the surgical field. The key to treatment is prevention, which demands knowledge of the relevant anatomy.[13] In rare situations, chyle leaks can lead to severe fluid and electrolyte imbalances, causing death if not treated.[16] A chyle leak can be confirmed by testing the triglyceride content of the drainage and comparing them to the serum values.[1] If a chyle leak is identified intraoperatively, the leaking vessel should be repaired by oversewing the tissue around the duct with multiple nonabsorbable sutures. A Valsalva maneuver may help localize the leak and improve outcomes. Postoperatively, low output fistulas < 500 mL can be managed conservatively with the use of pressure bandages, suction drainage, and nutritional support restricting diet to a high protein and medium triglyceride diet or a non-fat diet, as well as with pharmacological therapy (such as sclerosing agents).[13] However, high output fistulas (> 500–1,000 mL per 24 hours or leaks of 300–400 mL persisting for > 4–5 days) may require intraoperative repair with clamping of the leaking vessel[15] or interventional radiologic coiling of the duct.
- *Cerebrovascular incident*: Cerebrovascular incidents are rare; however, careful preoperative examination including auscultation or ultrasonographic examination of the carotid arteries is warranted. If a significant degree of carotid stenosis is present, it should be studied and potentially repaired prior to the neck dissection.
- *Facial lymphedema*: Bilateral radical neck dissection can result in significant facial lymphedema, which dissipates slowly[17] and can cause prolonged problems for patients. Lymphedema massage therapy may be helpful for some patients.

Neurologic Injuries

- *Shoulder syndrome (winging of the scapula)*: Shoulder syndrome occurs after sacrifice of the spinal accessory nerve and subsequent loss of trapezius muscle function. This can cause limitation of shoulder movement (most prominently abduction of the shoulder to < 90°), asymmetry of the scapula (dropped inferiorly on the ipsilateral side), and in some cases, severe pain.[15] Most of the modifications to neck dissections have been made in an attempt to prevent the morbidity of the painful shoulder syndrome associated with the sacrifice of the spinal accessory nerve. Shoulder syndrome has led many clinicians to preserve the spinal accessory, hence leading to the modified neck dissection. However, not all patients in whom the nerve is intentionally sacrificed develop shoulder syndrome. Furthermore, while preservation of the accessory nerve decreases the incidence, it does not completely eliminate the risk of shoulder syndrome. A review by Kraus et al. suggests that a level IIB dissection is low yield in the N0 neck, with a 1.6% incidence of metastasis in the area. They recommend dissection in the presence of bulky level IIA nodal disease on gross examination.[18]
- *Facial nerve injury*: Injury to the marginal mandibular branch of the facial nerve during radical neck dissection is not uncommon and dysfunction can result from prolonged retraction of the nerve. While the majority will recover, some may not. Although relatively rare, dissection in the area of the tail of the parotid gland, in order to remove bulky disease, can result in injury to the cervicofacial division of the facial nerve or even the main trunk. If the injury in recognized intraoperatively, every attempt at repair should be made.[1,13]
- *Hypoglossal nerve injury*: The hypoglossal nerve is especially at risk in patients who have undergone chemoradiation therapy prior to surgery. A confluence of scarring, fibrosis, and veins surrounding the nerve just anterior to the carotid artery can lead to troublesome bleeding and inadvertent injury to the nerve. Furthermore, bulky disease can result in nerve transection while obtaining adequate margins. Immediate repair should be considered; however, in most cases, results are unsatisfying.[1,13]

- *Phrenic nerve injury*: The phrenic nerve lies deep to the cervical fascia over the anterior scalene muscles. Difficulty primarily results from dissecting in the postirradiated field or in the setting of bulky disease. Phrenic nerve injury manifests by elevation of the hemidiaphragm noted on postoperative chest radiographs. Bilateral injury can lead to respiratory failure requiring prolonged mechanical ventilation. Nonetheless, pulmonary complications arising from unilateral phrenic nerve injury are typically limited in patients without evidence of pulmonary co-morbidities or pulmonary compromise as evident by pulmonary function testing.[1,13]
- *Brachial plexus injury*: Although the brachial plexus is not commonly encountered in the traditional RND, it may be visualized in an extended RND or due to extensive gross pathologic disease. Futhermore, devastating injury to the brachial plexus can occur when the dissection is inadvertently performed deep to the prevertebral fascia in the lower neck. Early recognition of brachial plexus injury should lead to early consultation and consideration of repair. However, most repairs do not result in satisfactory results.[1,13]
- *Cervical sympathetic trunk injury*: Injury to the cervical sympathetic trunk (which lies posterior to the carotid sheath) can result in Horner's syndrome (ptosis, miosis, and anhidrosis). The incidence of Horner's syndrome following a neck dissection is increased when the dissection is carried posterior to the carotid.[1,13]
- *Vagus nerve injury*: The vagus nerve is at the greatest risk during ligation of the internal jugular vein, particularly when dividing the IJV in the inferior portion of the neck. Unilateral injury results in unilateral vocal cord paralysis, which is manifested clinically by a "breathy, weak" voice. If the vagus nerve is injured proximally and above the branch of the superior laryngeal nerve, then laryngeal sensation can be compromised, which may result in a significantly higher risk of aspiration.[1,13]
- *Lingual nerve injury*: Injury to the lingual nerve can occur during the dissection of the submandibular triangle. Lingual nerve injury can occur due to aggressive mobilization of the nerve when removing gross pathologic disease or due to blind clamping of the lingual vessels. Therefore, in order to reduce the risk of injury to the lingual nerve, attachments between the nerve and the submandibular gland should be carefully transected while keeping the nerve in view.[1,13]

Vascular Injury

- *Carotid sinus sensitivity*: Carotid sinus sensitivity results from manipulation of the carotid body and manifests as acute bradycardia and decreased cardiac output.
- *Carotid blowout*: Carotid blowout is a late hemorrhagic event typically occurring in a previously irradiated surgical field. Carotid blowouts can occur as a result of tissue breakdown secondary to radiation and occasionally secondary to infection. While carotid blowout was a common complication in the 1970s and 1980s, its incidence has significantly decreased with improved surgical and radiation techniques. The use of pedicled flaps (such as the pectoralis myocutaneous flap) or a free flap protects the carotid artery with extensive soft tissue coverage and has contributed to the decreasing incidence of this complication.[19] However, the risk of a salivary fistula or flap failure is increased in the setting of malnutrition, diabetes, and compromised vascular flow to the pedicle or free flap. Hence, particular emphasis should be placed on ensuring adequate closure of the oral cavity and pharynx in order to prevent a communication to the neck and nidus for fistula formation.[13] The loss of free tissue transfers with avulsion of the arterial pedicle can also result in late hemorrhage.[13]

POSTOPERATIVE CARE

Early hypertension following RND is thought to possibly be related to carotid sinus denervation or secondary to increased intracranial hypertension (Cushing's reflex).[20] Some also suggest a prolonged QT interval following right-sided neck dissection; this should be monitored, and serum potassium levels should be followed.[21] Aggressive respiratory support and inspiratory spirometry is mandatory and helps to clear secretions, which is especially important in the tracheotomized individual. Early mobilization should be encouraged as it further decreases morbidity. Due to likely shoulder function impairment, proactive treatment with physiotherapy is also recommended.[22]

Radiation therapy is a vital aspect of management in head and neck oncology. There is a body of evidence that confirms low cervical recurrence rates when RND was combined with radiation therapy. For instance, Strong et al. in a prospective study reported the recurrence rate in the neck was 28.7% versus 17.6% in patients with N1 disease without radiation therapy compared to those with radiation therapy, respectively. Indications for radiation therapy include disease involvement of two or more nodes and nodal involvement at multiple levels. However, there are conflicting data on the postoperative versus preoperative use of radiation therapy.[23,24] Postoperative radiation therapy has various advantages, including maintaining a radiation-naive surgical field and the ability to evaluate tumor margins, the histology of the tumor, the location of the involved nodes, and the presence or absence of extracapsular spread in the resected specimens.[25]

CONCLUSION

The classic radical neck dissection is unfortunately associated with significant morbidity and aesthetic deformity as discussed in the complications section of this chapter. Much of this morbidity is due to the sacrifice of the spinal accessory nerve and subsequent loss of function of the trapezius muscle and the removal of sternocleidomastoid musculature, leading to drooping of the shoulder and winging of the scapula. Complication rates are much higher in patients who have previously undergone chemoradiation therapy. However, there is a strong body of evidence that confirms low cervical recurrence rates when RND was combined with radiation therapy. Therefore, the importance of radiation therapy in the treatment plan of head and neck cancer with involved nodes has been emphasized by most authors.[25]

With the advent of the selective neck dissection, which spares some of the morbidity and aesthetic deformity associated with RND, and a growing body of evidence showing similar outcomes compared to the RND and MND[26], the RND is reserved for extreme and extensive cases. The indications for RND are becoming increasingly limited to more advanced cervical disease states.

REFERENCES

1. Holmes JD. Neck dissection: nomenclature, classification, and technique. Oral Maxillofac Surg Clin North Am. 2008; 20(3):459-75.
2. Cummings CW, Flint PW. Cummings Otolaryngology Head and Neck Surgery, Vol. 1. Philadelphia: Mosby Elsevier; 2010.
3. Deschler DG, Day T (eds.), Head and Neck Surgery Committee of the American Academy of Otolaryngology—Head and Neck Surgery, Neck Dissection Classification Committee of the American Head and Neck Society. Pocket Guide to Neck Dissection Classification and TNM Staging of Head and Neck Cancer, 3rd edn. Alexandria, VA: American Academy of Otolaryngology—Head and Neck Surgery Foundation; 2008.
4. McCammon SD, Shah JP. Radical neck dissection. Oper Tech Otolaryngol Head Neck Surg. 2004;15(3):152-9.
5. Righi PD, Kelley DJ, Ernst R, et al. Evaluation of prevertebral muscle invasion by squamous cell carcinoma. Can computed tomography replace open neck exploration? Arch Otolaryngol Head Neck Surg. 1996;122(6):660-3.
6. Myers E, Carrau R. Operative Otolaryngology: Head and Neck Surgery. Philadelphia: Saunders/Elsevier; 2008.
7. Pellini R, Mercante G, Marchese C, et al. Predictive factors for postoperative wound complications after neck dissection. Acta Otorhinolaryngol Ital. 2013;33(1):16-22.
8. Menda Y, Graham MM. FDG PET imaging of head and neck cancers. Methods Mol Biol. 2011;727:21-31.
9. Krause HR. Reinnervation of the trapezius muscle after radical neck dissection. J Craniomaxillofac Surg. 1994;22(6):323-9.
10. Rodrigo JP, Alvarez JC, Gómez JR, et al. Comparison of three prophylactic antibiotic regimens in clean-contaminated head and neck surgery. Head Neck. 1997;19(3):188-93.
11. Becker GD, Parell GJ. Cefazolin prophylaxis in head and neck cancer surgery. Ann Otol Rhinol Laryngol. 1979;88(2 Pt 1): 183-6.
12. Mombelli G, Coppens L, Dor P, et al. Antibiotic prophylaxis in surgery for head and neck cancer. Comparative study of short and prolonged administration of carbenicillin. J Antimicrob Chemother. 1981;7(6):665-71.
13. Kerawala CJ, Heliotos M. Prevention of complications in neck dissection. Head Neck Oncol. 2009;1:35.
14. Wein RO, Weinstein GS. The anterolateral neck dissection with special reference to the digastric and hypoglossal tunnels. Oper Tech Otolaryngol Head Neck Surg. 2003;14(2):129-49.
15. Khafif A. Lateral neck dissection. Oper Tech Otolaryngol Head Neck Surg. 2004;15(3):160-67.
16. Santaolalla F, Anta JA, Zabala A, et al. Management of chylous fistula as a complication of neck dissection: a 10-year retrospective review. Eur J Cancer Care (Engl). 2010;19(4):510-15.
17. Razack MS, Baffi R, Sako K. Bilateral radical neck dissection. Cancer. 1981;47(1):197-9.
18. Kraus DH, Rosenberg DB, Davidson BJ, et al. Supraspinal accessory lymph node metastases in supraomohyoid neck dissection. Am J Surg. 1996;172(6):646-9.
19. Shaha AR. Extended neck dissection. J Surg Oncol. 1990; 45(4):229-33.
20. Celikkanat S, Akyol MU, Koç C, et al. Postoperative hypertension after radical neck dissection. Otolaryngol Head Neck Surg. 1997;117(1):91-2.
21. Otteni JC, Pottecher T, Bronner G, et al. Prolongation of the Q-T interval and sudden cardiac arrest following right radical neck dissection. Anesthesiology. 1983;59(4):358-61.
22. Lauchlan DT, McCaul JA, McCarron T. Neck dissection and the clinical appearance of post-operative shoulder disability: the post-operative role of physiotherapy. Eur J Cancer Care (Engl). 2008;17(6):542-8.
23. Stenson KM, Haraf DJ, Pelzer H, et al. The role of cervical lymphadenectomy after aggressive concomitant chemoradiotherapy: the feasibility of selective neck dissection. Arch Otolaryngol Head Neck Surg. 2000;126(8):950-6.
24. Clayman GL, Johnson CJ 2nd, Morrison W, et al. The role of neck dissection after chemoradiotherapy for oropharyngeal cancer with advanced nodal disease. Arch Otolaryngol Head Neck Surg. 2001;127(2):135-9.
25. Muzaffar K. Therapeutic selective neck dissection: a 25-year review. Laryngoscope. 2003;113(9):1460-65.
26. Ferlito A, Silver CE, Rinaldo A. Selective neck dissection (IIA, III): a rational replacement for complete functional neck dissection in patients with N0 supraglottic and glottic squamous carcinoma. Laryngoscope. 2008;118(4):676-9.

CHAPTER 17

Modified Radical Neck Dissection

Darrin V Bann, Benjamin Oberman, David Goldenberg

INTRODUCTION

The first successful radical en bloc neck dissection was performed on January 17, 1888 by Franciszek Jawdyński and included removal of all ipsilateral lymphatic structures, the internal jugular vein, the internal and external carotid arteries, and the sternocleidomastoid muscle (SCM).[1] Although the technique was used only sporadically until the mid-20th century, radical neck dissections gained widespread use after Martin et al. published the results of 665 procedures performed on 599 patients in 1951.[2] This technique included removal of all cervical lymphatics plus the SCM, omohyoid muscle, spinal accessory nerve, internal jugular vein, and submandibular salivary gland, and for several years was considered the only truly curative treatment for head and neck cancers involving regional lymph nodes.[3,4] However, in 1963 Suárez published a technique based on 1318 cases that preserved the SCM and omohyoid muscles, the submandibular gland, the internal jugular vein, and the spinal accessory nerve.[4] In 1978 Jesse et al. popularized Suarez's technique by publishing a series of 310 patients showing that procedures sparing the accessory spinal nerve or removing only the lymph nodes at highest risk for metastasis produced outcomes equivalent to the classical neck dissection.[4,5] Their technique, which was identical to that of Suárez, became known as the modified radical neck dissection (MRND).[4]

The modern definition of the MRND is based on the 2008 American Head and Neck Society (AHNS) Committee for Neck Dissection Classification (Table 17.1).[6] Compared to a radical neck dissection, the MRND includes the removal of all lymph nodes in levels I through V (see Anatomy below) with preservation of one or more of the following structures: the SCM, the internal jugular vein, or the spinal accessory nerve.[6,7] The AHNS stipulates that all structures preserved during MRND should be named in the procedure,[7] resulting in six potential variations. In this chapter, we define the surgical anatomy relevant to the MRND, discuss indications for the procedure, and outline the surgical technique and potential complications.

Table 17.1: Definitions of neck dissections

Procedure	*Definition*
Radical	Removal of lymph nodes levels I–V, sternocleidomastoid muscle, spinal accessory nerve, and internal jugular vein
Modified	Removal of lymph nodes levels I–V with preservation of at least one of the following structures: Sternocleidomastoid muscle Spinal accessory nerve Internal jugular vein
Selective	Preservation of one or more lymph node levels I–V
Extended	Removal of an additional lymph node level or group or nonlymphatic structures relative to a radical neck dissection. Additional lymphatic structures include superior mediastinal, retropharyngeal, periparotid, postauricular, suboccipital, or buccinator lymph nodes. Nonlymphatic structures may include the external carotid artery, hypoglossal nerve, or vagus nerve

ANATOMY

With respect to the MRND the major anatomic considerations are the cervical lymph nodes and the distinct

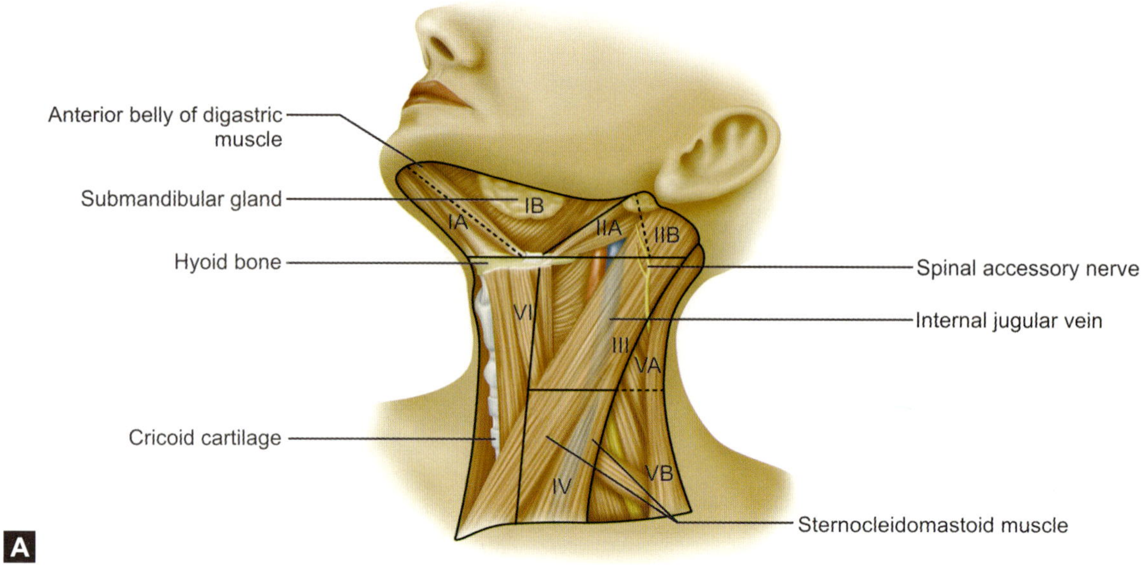

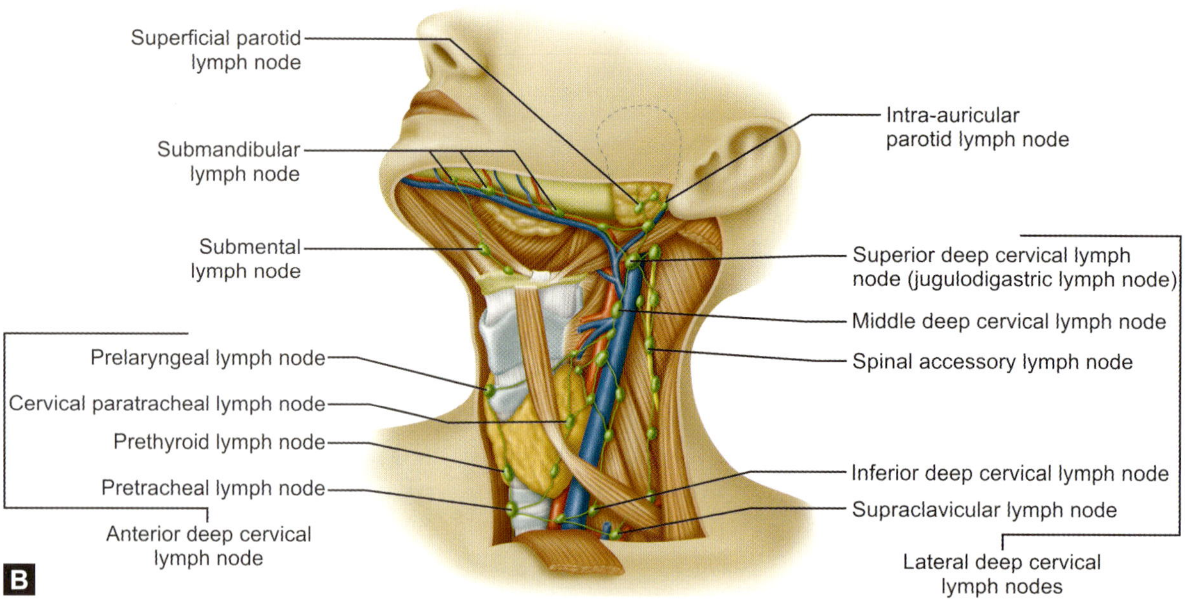

Figs. 17.1A and B: The anatomic levels of the neck (A) and major lymph node chains within each level (B).

fascial planes that separate the major structures in the anterior neck. Knowledge of the regional lymph flow within the neck allows the surgeon to accurately stage disease and guides appropriate therapy, including the selective removal of lymph nodes at highest risk for metastasis (*see* Chapter 18: Selective Neck Dissection). The lymph nodes within the neck are divided into six levels (I – VI) and six sublevels (IA, IB, IIA, IIB, VA, and VB) (Fig. 17.1A).[7] The anatomic boundaries of each level are listed in Table 17.2.

The lymph nodes within level I receive lymphatic flow from the skin over the chin and lower lip, the tip of the tongue and the floor of the mouth, and are therefore at high risk for metastasis from cancers involving these structures (Fig. 17.1B).[8,9] Similarly, level II nodes are at high risk for metastasis from cancers involving the parotid, submandibular, and submental glands, as well as the pharynx, nasal cavity, middle ear, tongue, hard and soft palate, and tonsils.[8] The nodes within level III receive flow from levels II and V, in addition to the

Table 17.2: Anatomic and radiographic boundaries of each lymph node level.

	Boundary							
	Superior		*Inferior*		*Lateral*		*Medial*	
Sublevel	Anatomic	Radiographic	Anatomic	Radiographic	Anatomic	Radiographic	Anatomic	Radiographic
I_A	Mandibular symphysis	Geniohyoid muscle	Hyoid body		Digastric muscle (anterior belly)			
I_B	Mandibular body	Mylohyoid muscle	Hyoid body		Submandibular gland (posterior edge)		Digastric muscle (anterior belly)	
II_A	Skull base	Transverse process C1	Carotid bifurcation	Hyoid bone	SAN	IJV	Submandibular gland (posterior edge)	
II_B	Skull base	Transverse process C1	Carotid bifurcation	Hyoid bone	SCM (posterior edge)		SAN	Paraspinal muscles
III	Carotid bifurcation	Hyoid bone	Omohyoid muscle	Cricoid cartilage	Cervical rootlets	SCM (posterior edge)	Sternohyoid muscle	Paraspinal muscles
IV	Omohyoid muscle	Cricoid cartilage	Clavicle	Sternoclavicular joint	Cervical rootlets	SCM (posterior edge)	Sternohyoid muscle	Paraspinal muscles
V_A	SCM and trapezius muscle		Cricoid cartilage		Trapezius muscle (anterior edge)		Cervical plexus	SCM (posterior edge)
V_B	Cricoid cartilage		Clavicle		Trapezius muscle (anterior edge)		Cervical plexus	SCM (posterior edge)
VI	Hyoid bone		Sternal manubrium (superior)		Common carotid artery			
VII	Sternal manubrium (superior edge)		Innominate artery		Innominate artery (right) Common carotid artery (left)			

(IJV: Internal jugular vein; SAN: Spinal accessory nerve; SCM: Sternocleidomastoid muscle).

retropharyngeal and pretracheal spaces, tongue base, and tonsils.[9,10] By contrast, level IV lymph nodes are rarely involved in oral cancers unless one of the more superior groups is also involved.[9,10] Instead, the level IV lymphatics receive efferent flow primarily from level III and the retropharyngeal, pretracheal, hypopharyngeal, laryngeal, and thyroid lymphatics.[9] Lymphatics in level V receive efferent flow from occipital and posterior auricular lymphatics but may become involved in tongue base, tonsillar, and oral cavity cancers if lymph flow is redirected by metastasis in higher levels.[9,10]

To achieve the aims of the MRND, the surgeon must understand and use the fascial planes separating structures in the neck from the lymphatic tissue. The fascial layers of the neck are classified into two major categories: the superficial cervical fascia and the deep cervical fascia (Fig. 17.2). The superficial fascia is a subcutaneous layer containing the muscle, cutaneous blood and lymph vessels, nerves, and a variable amount of fat (Fig. 17.2).[11]

The deep cervical fascia is classically divided into three layers: investing, pretracheal, and prevertebral. The investing, or superficial, layer of the deep cervical fascia encases the neck. When encountering the trapezius and SCMs the deep cervical fascia splits to completely invest each muscle. The pretracheal layer is located in the anterior part of the neck, extending from the hyoid to the pericardium. This layer covers the infrahyoid musculature and the thyroid, trachea, and esophagus.[12] The deep layer of the deep cervical fascia, the prevertebral layer, attaches at the posterior spinous processes and nuchal ligament, and encases the splenius, levator scapulae, and scalene muscles before crossing the midline. Notably, this fascial plane is posterior to the esophagus but anterior to the vertebral column (Fig. 17.2). Between the boundaries defined by the pretracheal and prevertebral fascia, the carotid sheath runs from the base of the skull to the base of the neck between the sternothyroid muscle and the anterior scalene muscles. Separate compartments within

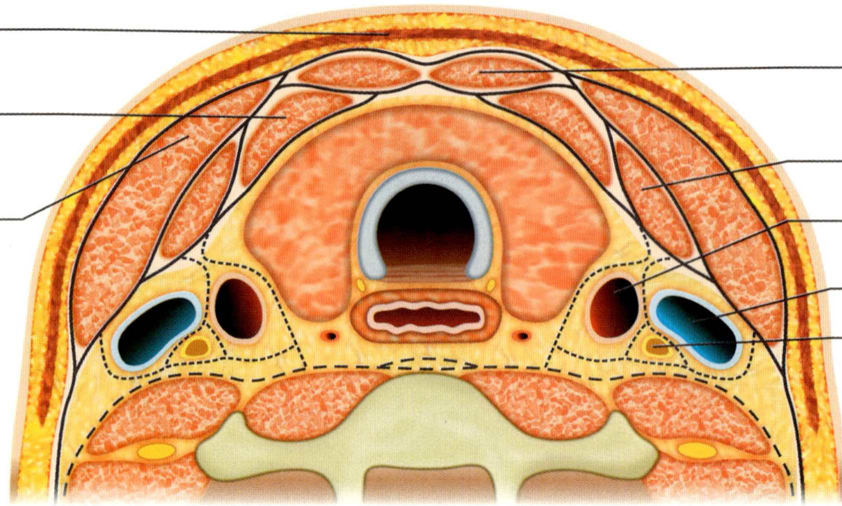

Fig. 17.2: Fascial layers of the neck at the level of C7. Dark line–superficial and pretracheal layers of the deep cervical fascia. Dashed line–prevertebral layer of the deep cervical fascia. Dotted line–carotid sheath.

this vascular bundle contain the internal jugular vein, the carotid artery, the vagus nerve, cervical lymph nodes, and sympathetic nerve fibers.[11,12]

INDICATIONS

Generally, MRND is advantageous over the radical neck dissection because the modified dissection can be performed bilaterally without significantly increasing morbidity. However, the modified dissection is best utilized when all metastatic disease is confined to lymphatic tissue. In terms of specific diseases, several authors recommend MRND for all N0 high-grade salivary gland tumors given the high propensity for such tumors to undergo subclinical lymph node metastasis.[13,14] Indeed, Nobis et al. reported that of 94 patients with salivary gland tumors, almost 40% had lymph node metastasis.[14] Similarly, ipsilateral or bilateral MRND may be indicated for oral squamous cell carcinomas (SCC).[15-18] One recent study reported that a depth of invasion ≥4 mm had a sensitivity of 83% and specificity of 57% for occult lymph node involvement, indicating that intraoperative pathology may help guide treatment.[18] Ipsilateral MRND is also indicated for SCC of the tonsils and hypopharynx, with the addition of contralateral MRND for tumors that cross the midline or have ipsilateral nodal involvement.[19,20] It should be noted that routine MRND may not be indicated for glottic laryngeal cancers because these tumors rarely involve the lymph nodes in levels I and V, so selective dissection (*see* Chapter 18) of levels II, III, and IV may be sufficient in many cases.[21,22]

For well-differentiated thyroid carcinomas current American Thyroid Association guidelines state that routine MRND is generally not indicated for small, noninvasive, clinically N0 papillary thyroid cancers and most follicular cancers.[23] However, these guidelines stipulate that compartmental en bloc dissection of level I–VI lymph nodes may improve survival for patients with lateral lymph node involvement that is detected clinically, during preoperative workup, or at the time of surgery.[23] For undifferentiated thyroid cancers, the American Thyroid Association recommends MRND for all patients with resectable disease.[24] Resectability in this case is determined by (i) the absence of distant metastatic disease and (ii) the extent of local invasion into surrounding structures such as the recurrent laryngeal, vagus, and spinal accessory nerves; the SCM; trachea; esophagus; and superior vena cava.[24]

SURGICAL TECHNIQUE

Positioning, Incision Planning, and Flap Development

The patient is placed on the operating table in the supine position with the neck extended using a shoulder roll.[25] A variety of incisions can be used for MRND; however, one of the most popular is the classical Gluck incision, or hemiapron flap, which provides excellent exposure and results in improved cosmesis (Fig. 17.3F).[11,25,26] This incision extends from the mastoid tip to the midline at the cricoid and may be extended bilaterally if a bilateral MRND is required. Alternative possibilities include extension of the Kocher incision along the posterior aspect of the sternocleidomastoid in a "hockey stick" shape (Fig. 17.3A), the Martin double-Y incision (Fig. 17.3G), the modified MacFee parallel incision (Fig. 17.3C), and the modified Schobinger incision (Fig. 17.3D). The authors recommend placing the planned incision in an existing

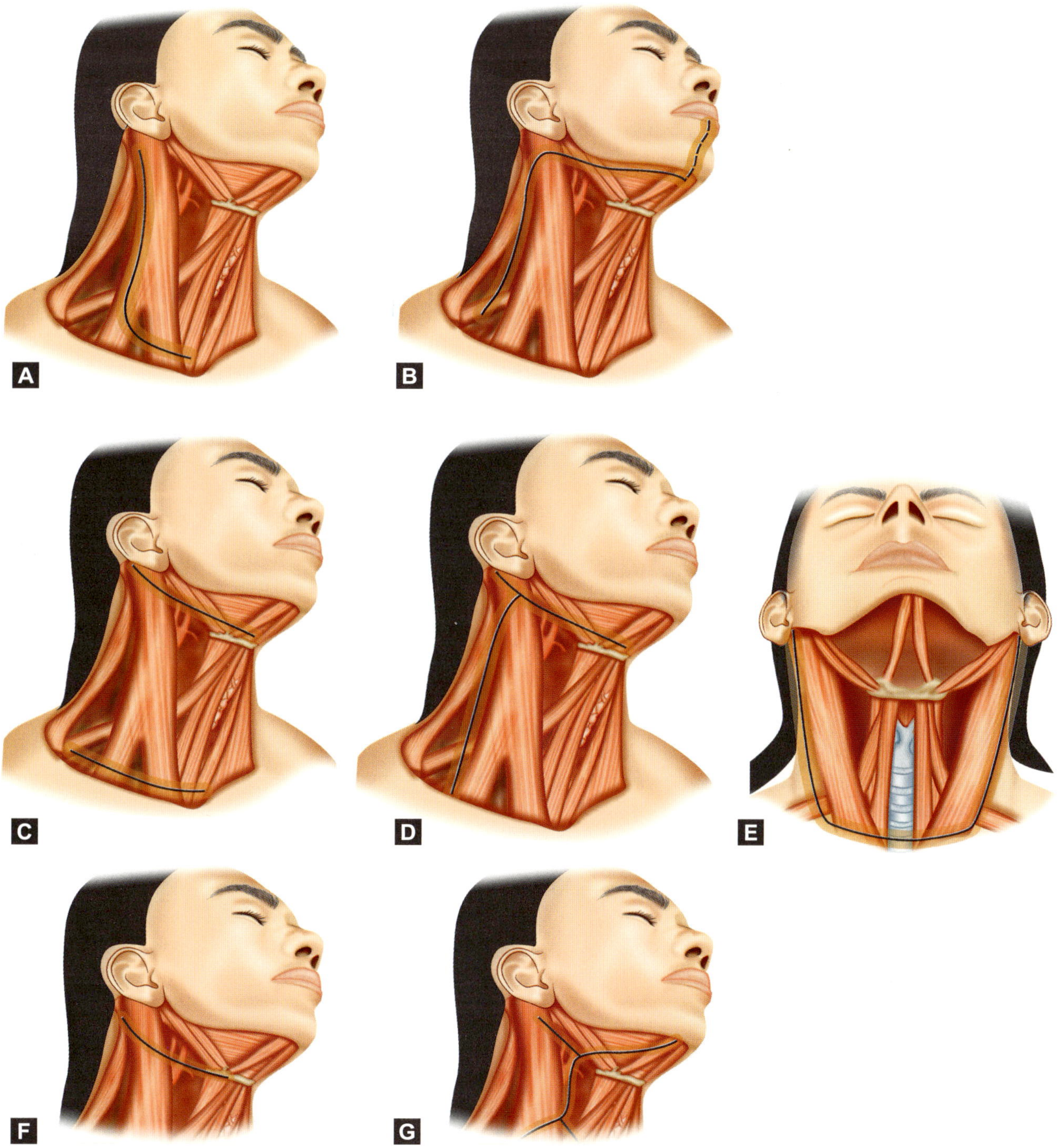
A B C D E F G

Figs. 17.3A to G: Incisions used for modified radical neck dissection: (A) Lahey (hockey stick). (B) Boomerang. (C) MacFee. (D) Modified Schobinger. (E) Apron or bilateral hockey stick. (F) Gluck. (G) Martin double-Y.

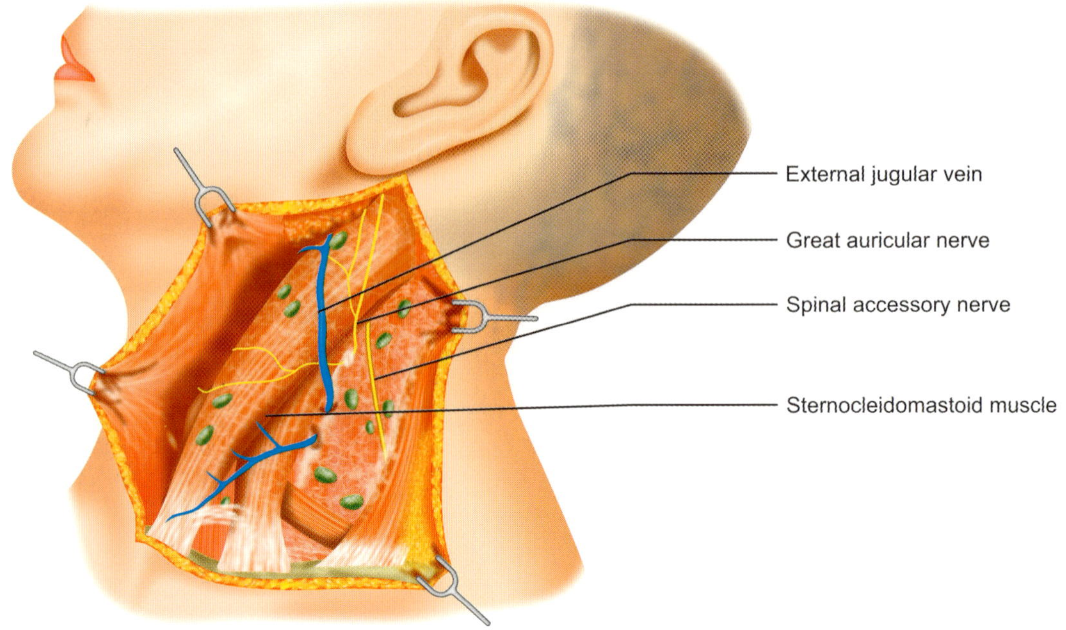

Fig. 17.4: Incision through the platysma revealing the sternocleidomastoid muscle, external jugular vein, and spinal accessory nerve.

skin crease if possible, then injecting the skin with 1% lidocaine plus 1:100,000 epinephrine. The skin incision is made with the use of a # 10- or 15-blade scalpel.

After making the incision, the skin flap is raised in a subplatysmal plane using sharp dissection with either a 15-blade or electrocautery while providing appropriate traction on the skin. At this point the SCM, external jugular vein, and great auricular nerve are identified (Fig. 17.4). The great auricular nerve innervates the skin of the earlobe and serves as an important anatomic landmark as it emerges from the posterior aspect of the sternocleidomastoid at Erb's point before coursing superiorly toward the earlobe. Dissection posterior to the platysma is performed to the level of the great auricular nerve. The subplatysmal flaps are elevated superiorly to the level of the mentum and angle of the mandible. The flaps are elevated inferiorly to the level of the clavicle and sternal notch.

Submandibular Fossa

The submandibular fossa contains the level I lymph nodes, primarily the submental and submandibular nodes, and the submandibular salivary gland. In the classical MRND the submandibular gland is preserved; however, it should be noted that many of the tumors requiring level I lymph node dissection also involve the submandibular gland, necessitating its removal. An incision in the fascia is made at the inferior border of the submandibular gland. The marginal mandibular branch of the facial nerve runs superficially in the fascia overlying the submandibular gland. The nerve may be protected by ligating the facial vein at the lower border of the submandibular gland and reflecting the ligated portion superiorly over the body of the mandible (Fig. 17.5).[11] Blunt dissection is used to identify the anterior and posterior bellies of the digastric muscle.

If the submandibular gland is to be removed, the facial artery should be ligated when dissecting the superior aspect of the gland. The mylohyoid muscle should be identified as the floor of the dissection. Next the submandibular duct and the submandibular ganglion's attachment to the lingual nerve should be ligated to free the specimen en bloc. This maneuver completes the dissection of level IB.

Moving anteriorly to remove level IA requires identifying the contralateral anterior belly of the digastric muscle. Again, the mylohyoid serves as the floor of the dissection, with the hyoid bone representing the inferior border for this level.

Dissection of the Sternocleidomastoid Muscle

The goal of the SCM dissection is to completely release the muscle from the surrounding fascia. The fascia is

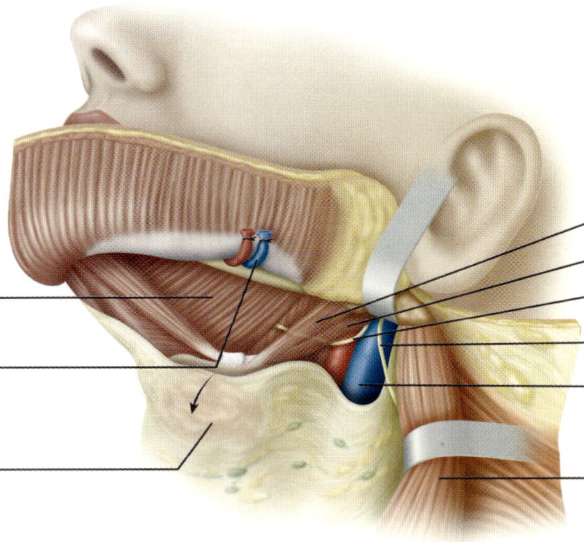

Fig. 17.5: Dissection of the submandibular fossa. The facial vein is ligated long and reflected superiorly to protect the marginal mandibular branch of the facial nerve.

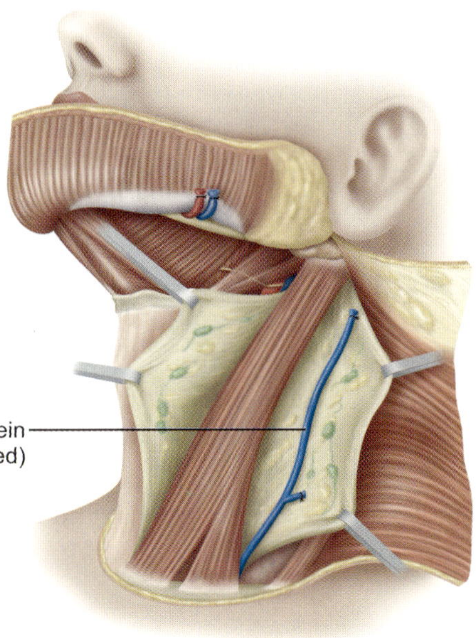

Fig. 17.6: Removal of the fascia overlying the sternocleidomastoid muscle.

incised lengthwise along the anterior border of the sternocleidomastoid using a #15-blade scalpel or electrocautery. Dissection should be carried down to level II, elevating the investing fascia on the medial aspect of the SCM towards the lateral (posterior) border of the muscle (Fig. 17.6). There are several perforating vessels along the medial edge of the muscle, which should be cauterized by an assistant as the surgeon continues the dissection. Caution should be utilized when working on the posterosuperior half of the SCM where the spinal accessory nerve pierces the muscle near the level of the transverse process of the atlas. The spinal accessory nerve exits the skull superior to the great auricular nerve and courses through the sternocleidomastoid to the trapezius on the posterolateral border of the SCM. The spinal accessory nerve can often be found about 1 cm superior and posterior to Erb's point on the posterior border of the SCM. Notably, the spinal accessory nerve divides level II into IIA and IIB. The floor of the neck in this dissection is the deep layer of the deep cervical fascia.

After the perforating vessels have been cauterized, the dissection enters an avascular plane along the posterior face of the muscle. At this point, the internal jugular vein should be visible through the fascia overlying the carotid sheath (Fig. 17.7). To completely release the muscle, the fascia covering the posterior aspect of the muscle is dissected medially and posteriorly to meet the anterior dissection.

Dissection of the Spinal Accessory Nerve

Safe identification of the spinal accessory nerve as it enters the superior sternocleidomastoid is accomplished using the aforementioned anatomic landmarks. Blunt dissection should be used to dissect tissue in the expected region of the nerve, and care should be taken to cut only

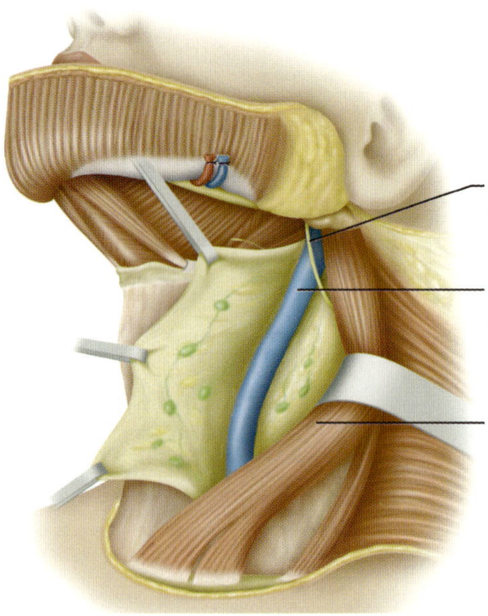

Fig. 17.7: Completion of the sternocleidomastoid muscle dissection.

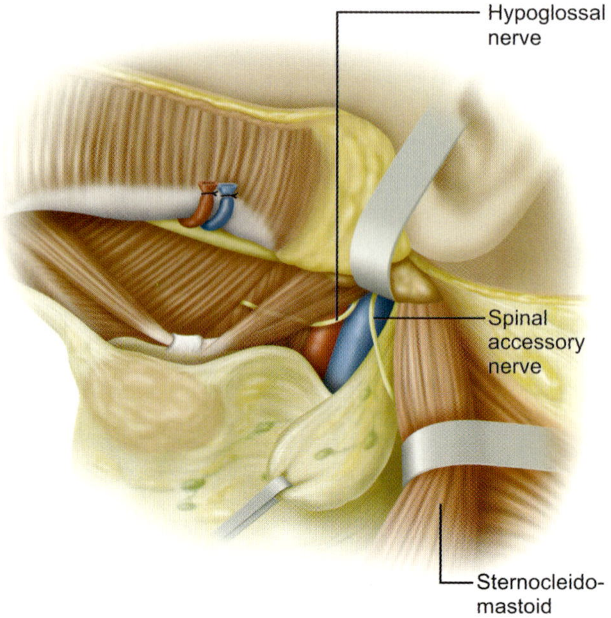

Fig. 17.8: Dissection of the submuscular triangle. The contents of level IIB are rotated under the spinal accessory nerve for removal.

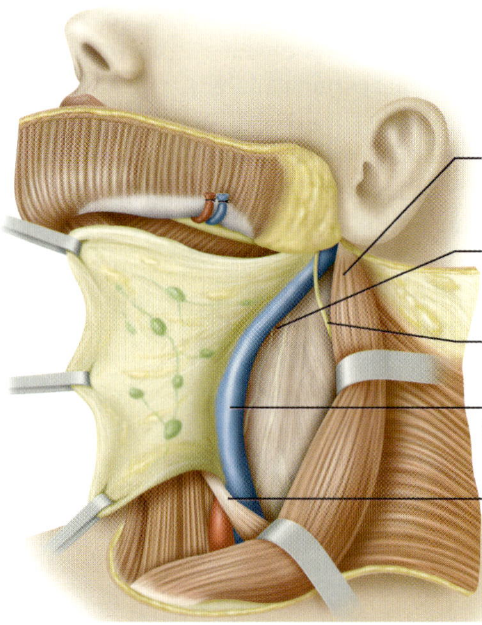

Fig. 17.9: The fascia covering the internal jugular vein is removed with anterior traction and gentle passes of the scalpel.

transparent tissue. The internal jugular vein usually lies immediately deep to the proximal spinal accessory nerve. Positive identification of the nerve can be confirmed using a nerve stimulator if necessary, resulting in movement of the shoulder.

Once the nerve is identified it is circumferentially freed from the surrounding tissues (Fig. 17.8). The fibroareolar tissue within level IIb is then dissected off of the fascia overlying the splenius capitis muscle posteriorly and the levator scapulae anteriorly. Care should be taken to avoid injuring the arterial supply in this region, namely, the occipital artery. The dissected tissue is then passed anteriorly underneath the spinal accessory nerve. Care should be taken to minimize stretching of the spinal accessory nerve, which may produce postoperative shoulder dysfunction. If disease within this region is too bulky to pass under the nerve, the specimen may be removed in two pieces.

Dissection of the Carotid Sheath

At this point, dissection continues anterior to the SCM, which is retracted posteriorly. The specimen is retracted medially while the surgeon uses a gauze pad to apply lateral traction over the deep cervical muscles. The fascia overlying the internal jugular vein is incised (Fig. 17.9). Removal of the fascia directly overlying the vein is accomplished by applying anterior traction to the fascia and gently passing a scalpel blade over the vein. Alternatively, blunt dissection with a fine hemostat and electrocautery or a harmonic shears may be used. Tributaries to the internal jugular vein including the thyroid, lingual, and facial veins should be ligated as they are encountered. After the internal jugular vein has been released from its fascia, the dissection proceeds medially to the carotid artery. Care must be taken not to injure the sympathetic trunk deep to the carotid, as this will produce a Horner syndrome. With the dissection of the fascia overlying the carotid artery, the specimen is freed from the great vessels and remains attached only to the strap muscles anteriorly (Fig. 17.10).

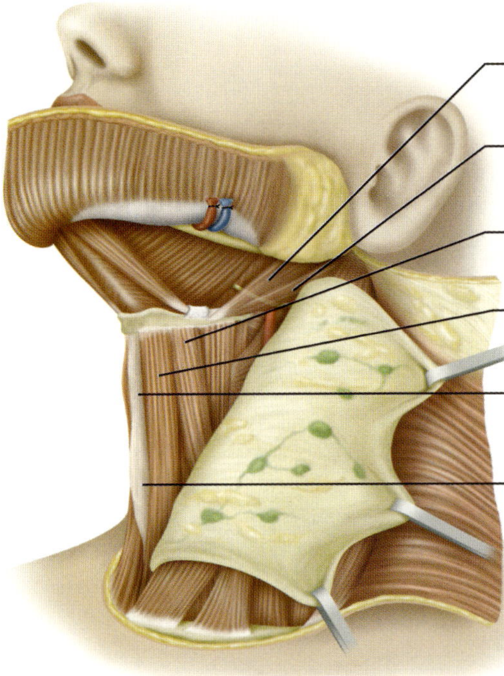

Fig. 17.10: Dissection of the anterior neck.

Posterior Triangle

At this point, attention turns to the dissection of level V lymph nodes in the posterior triangle of the neck (Fig. 17.11). To access the posterior triangle the SCM is retracted anteriorly and the accessory spinal nerve is identified as it exits the posterior border of the SCM. The dissection then proceeds medially from the anterior border of the trapezius while keeping the accessory spinal nerve in view. Superiorly, the dissection is limited by the posterior edge of the SCM and the depth should be limited to the level of the cervical plexus rootlets exiting under the posterior edge of the SCM. Contributions from the second, third, and fourth cervical nerves anastomose with the spinal accessory nerve while contributions from the third, fourth, and fifth cervical nerves form the phrenic nerve. Therefore, careful preservation of the cervical plexus is necessary for optimal functioning of the diaphragm and shoulder postoperatively. Once the carotid sheath is identified, dissection of deep cervical muscles should be stopped to avoid injury to the sympathetic trunk, which is posteromedial to the carotid sheath.

Next, the omohyoid muscle is identified and its fascia is dissected away with the contents of the posterior triangle. The omohyoid muscle may be removed if necessary, but otherwise it is retracted inferiorly. Often, the omohyoid is divided during the dissection, although it does serve as a rough guide to separate level 3 superiorly and level 4 inferiorly. The carotid sheath containing the common carotid artery, the internal jugular vein, and the vagus nerve lies immediately deep to the omohyoid muscle and must be carefully protected. The thoracic duct, which lies in the tissue immediately lateral to the jugular vein, should be ligated and sutured to prevent a chyle leak. At this point, the deep cervical fascia overlying the levator scapulae and scalene muscles is visible, and the brachial plexus may be seen between the anterior and middle scalene muscles. Keeping the dissection superficial to the deep layer of the deep cervical fascia prevents injury to the brachial plexus. The dissection proceeds medially until it reaches the level of the posterior border of the SCM. The SCM is then retracted medially and the contents of the posterior triangle may be removed en bloc (Fig. 17.12).

Wound Closure

After the complete removal of all lymphatic tissue, the wound should be inspected carefully for bleeding, then irrigated with normal saline. The presence of further bleeding or a chyle leak from the thoracic duct may be assessed by having the anesthesiologist hold a positive pressure breath (*see* Complications section). Closed suction drains are strategically placed into the wound bed and should exit the skin separately from the original incision. The wound is closed in layers with the platysma being reapproximated with absorbable sutures, the deep layers of skin closed with buried absorbable sutures, and the skin closed with staples or monofilament suture. Variations of this closure are known and acceptable. If a dressing is applied to the wound, special attention should be paid to the supraclavicular fossa because this is where most serohematomas develop.

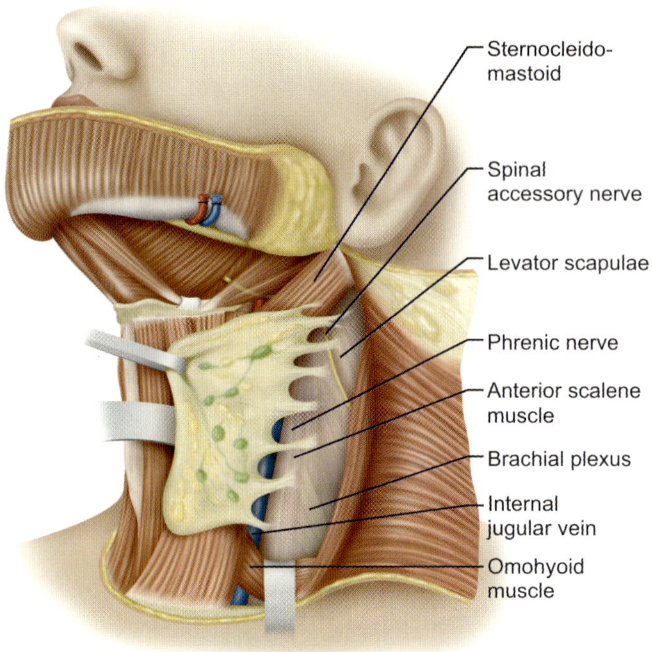

Fig. 17.11: Removal of the contents of the posterior triangle revealing the anterior scalene muscles and the brachial plexus. To protect the brachial plexus the dissection should not penetrate the prevertebral fascia.

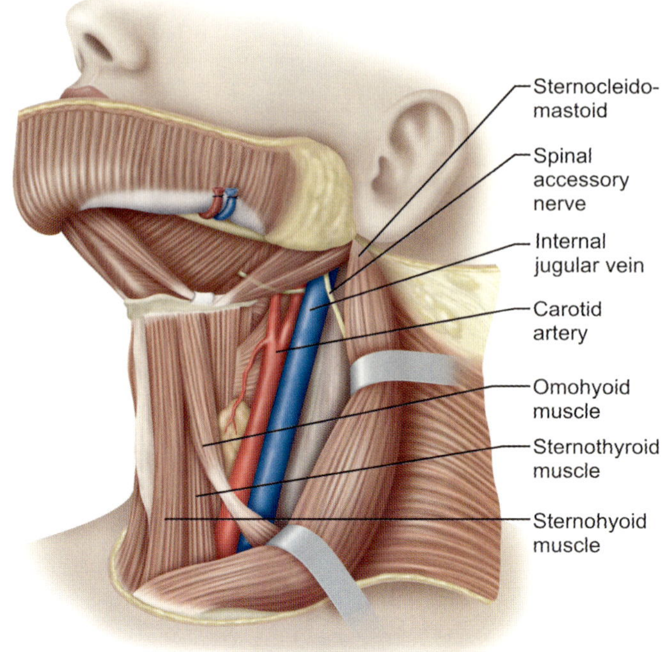

Fig. 17.12: View of the completed modified radical neck dissection.

POSTOPERATIVE CARE

A thorough postoperative nerve examination should be conducted to assess the function of the marginal mandibular branch of the facial nerve, the hypoglossal nerve, the greater auricular nerve, the spinal accessory nerve, and the brachial plexus. Transient weakness of the trapezius muscle may be noted due to disruption of the blood supply to the spinal accessory nerve or stretching of the nerve during surgery. Early intervention with physical therapy may be helpful for regaining full shoulder function. The drain(s) may be removed when the output is <30 mL per drain in a 24-hour period. General wound care should consist of cleaning the incision site twice daily with peroxide on a cotton swab tip followed by a thin layer of petroleum ointment.

COMPLICATIONS

In general, most patients tolerate MRND well and the rate of unintended complications remains relatively low; however, certain patient factors such as neoadjuvant radiation therapy may significantly increase complication rates.[9] The most common complications include injuries to nerves, vasculature, or the thoracic duct; rare complications such as increased intracranial pressure following internal jugular vein ligation have also been reported.[27] As with any surgical procedure there is risk for postoperative wound infection; however, with the use of prophylactic antibiotics the incidence of infections remains relatively low.

Neurologic Complications

The most common neurologic complication following MRND is injury to the spinal accessory nerve, which occurs in up to 27% of patients.[28] Transection of the nerve with denervation of the trapezius muscle occurs in approximately 1.7% of cases and results in "shoulder syndrome" characterized by pain, inability to fully abduct the arm, winging of the scapula, and shoulder droop.[9,29,30] However, it should be noted that significant manipulation or skeletonization of the nerve may also produce significant trapezius dysfunction and shoulder pain even if the nerve is not transected.[31-33] Accordingly, this has led some authors to argue that the lymph nodes of level IIB should not routinely be extirpated unless there is bulky metastasis in level IIA.[34-36] However, others report that there is no significant difference in spinal accessory nerve function between level IIB-dissected and level IIB-undissected patients.[33,37] We recommend that the decision to dissect level IIB be individualized and based on radiographic and physical findings and clinical judgment at the time of surgery.

If an injury to the spinal accessory nerve is observed during surgery, attempts may be made to repair the nerve using a cable graft, usually from the ipsilateral great auricular nerve.[38] Alternatively, others have used resorbable nerve guides, which have several advantages over cable grafts including the lack of donor site morbidity, a wide variety of available lengths and widths, and improved recovery of nerve function.[33,39,40] Primary repair of the nerve by suture reapproximation is not recommended as this may result in excessive tension on the nerve stumps. Patients with injury to the spinal accessory nerve should undergo physical therapy rehabilitation.

Serious complications including respiratory difficulty may result from injury to the phrenic nerve, which runs underneath the deep cervical fascia. In MRND this fascia is preserved, so the rate of phrenic nerve injuries remains low;[41] however, one should be particularly mindful when dissecting bulky disease in this region.[9] The marginal mandibular branch of the facial nerve is at risk during the dissection of level I lymph nodes. When injury to this nerve occurs, it is typically caused by retraction during surgery and results in temporary dysfunction. However, more extensive nerve damage may occur when bulky tumor is extirpated from the parotid gland. Similarly, inadvertent injury to the hypoglossal nerve may occur just anterior to the carotid artery if there is significant bleeding in the area. Other potential neurologic complications include brachial plexus injury if dissection is carried deep to the prevertebral fascia; Horner syndrome may result from injury to the cervical sympathetic trunk posterior to the carotid sheath; the vagus nerve may be injured during ligation of the internal jugular vein; and lingual nerve injury is increased during removal of primary oral cavity cancers.[9,25]

Thoracic Duct Injury

Injury to the thoracic duct on the left may occur in up to 8% of MRNDs during dissection of level IV.[42] Having the anesthesiologist hold a positive pressure breath to increase intrathoracic pressure may facilitate identification of a chyle leak, which is heralded by the appearance of milky fluid within the operative field.[9] If identified during surgery, the injury can be managed by ligation and oversewing the tissue surrounding the leaking sites with 3-0 or 4-0 nonabsorbable suture.[9,25] A muscle flap may be used to strengthen the repair and reduce the potential space in which fluid may accumulate.[25,43] Alternatively, fibrin or cyanoacrylate tissue glue may be used to effectively stop a chyle leak.[25,43]

Postoperatively, chyle leaks most commonly present with neck swelling, erythema of the skin, and increased drainage of milky fluid, which becomes more apparent once the patient begins oral nutritional intake. Any drainage of fluid with a triglyceride concentration >100 mg/dL greater than serum levels should raise suspicion for a chyle leak.[25] Low-output (<1 L/day) leaks may be managed conservatively with local pressure dressings and by reducing chyle production using a modified medium-chain triglyceride or fat-free diet or total parenteral nutrition.[43] In addition, somatostatin or octreotide may be used to reduce chyle output.[43]

In the case of high-output chyle leaks or the failure of conservative management, interventional approaches must be used. Percutaneous lymphangiography-guided cannulation with embolization of the thoracic duct is a minimally invasive interventional radiology procedure that can effectively treat chyle leak without open surgery. Alternatively, thoracoscopic ligation of the thoracic duct also provides effective treatment for high-output chyle leaks with minimal added morbidity.[44] Sometimes control requires opening the recently operated neck for exploration of the lymphatic duct. Failure to effectively identify and manage high-output chyle leaks may lead to chylothorax, a rare but potentially life-threatening complication requiring thoracentesis or chest tube placement.[25,45]

Vascular Complications

Complications involving the cervical vasculature may present either intraoperatively or postoperatively. Intraoperative vascular complications include carotid sinus sensitivity and hemorrhage. Carotid sinus sensitivity results from manipulation of the carotid body and manifests as a potentially life-threatening decrease in cardiac output with profound bradycardia.[46] In rare cases stimulation of the vasovagal reflex may also cause coronary artery vasospasm or even cardiac arrest.[47,48] Carotid sinus sensitivity may be treated with atropine intraoperatively; however, avoidance of this complication by careful and selective manipulation of the carotid bifurcation remains the best option. Subadventitial administration of small amounts (<1 mL) of 1% lidocaine may reduce the sensitivity of the carotid sinus to manipulation, although this practice is controversial.[46, 49]

Intraoperative hemorrhage is generally managed with pressure and appropriate ligation of the bleeding vessel.

The most serious bleeding can result from inadvertent injury to the internal, external, or common carotid artery. Lacerations to the common or internal carotid arteries should be repaired rapidly if the status of collateral cerebral circulation has not been determined preoperatively.[9] Importantly, the use of neoadjuvant radiotherapy may cause the formation of fibrous tissue in the neck, distorting the anatomy and making inadvertent vessel injury more likely.

Other vascular complications are associated with bilateral or, more rarely, unilateral ligation of the internal jugular vein and include increased intracranial pressure, facial edema, visual disturbance, or blindness.[27,49] Usually, the internal jugular vein remains patent after MRND. However, symptoms of internal jugular vein occlusion must be recognized early and treated with heparinization.[50] In cases where both internal jugular veins must be sacrificed, a saphenous vein graft reconstruction should be considered.

One of the most serious late vascular complications following MRND is carotid blowout. Several independent risk factors are associated with carotid blowout including body mass index <22.5 kg/m^2, primary tumor in the hypopharynx or oropharynx, an open wound in the neck, radical neck dissection, and total radiation dose to the neck of ≥ 70 Gy.[51,52] Additionally, infection may also represent a risk factor due to weakening of the arterial wall.[52] Although this complication is relatively rare, it has a mortality rate of almost 22%, and almost 15% of patients suffer neurologic sequelae after emergent management.[51] Recent literature suggests that an emergent endovascular approach may reduce mortality for carotid artery blowout when compared to traditional open ligation.[53]

Surgical Site Infections

The incidence of surgical site infections after neck dissection remains low. However, the use of a single dose of antibiotics preoperatively may lower the incidence of infection from 13.3% to 1.7%.[54] Accordingly, a single dose of antibiotics should routinely be given.

REFERENCES

1. Ferlito A, Johnson JT, Rinaldo A, et al. European surgeons were the first to perform neck dissection. Laryngoscope. 2007;117(5):797-802.
2. Martin H, Del Valle B, Ehrlich H, et al. Neck dissection. Cancer. 1951;4(3):441-99.
3. Martin H. The case for prophylactic neck dissection. Cancer. 1951;4(1):92-7.
4. Ferlito A, Robbins KT, Silver CE, et al. Classification of neck dissections: an evolving system. Auris Nasus Larynx. 2009;36(2):127-34.
5. Jesse RH, Ballantyne AJ, Larson D. Radical or modified neck dissection: a therapeutic dilemma. Am J Surg. 1978; 136(4):516-9.
6. Robbins KT, Shaha AR, Medina JE, et al. Consensus statement on the classification and terminology of neck dissection. Arch Otolaryngol—Head Neck Surg. 2008;134(5): 536-8.
7. Robbins KT, Clayman G, Levine PA, et al. Neck dissection classification update: revisions proposed by the American Head and Neck Society and the American Academy of Otolaryngology-Head and Neck Surgery. Arch Otolaryngol—Head Neck Surg. 2002;128(7):751-8.
8. Lindberg R. Distribution of cervical lymph node metastases from squamous cell carcinoma of the upper respiratory and digestive tracts. Cancer. 1972;29(6):1446-9.
9. Holmes JD. Neck dissection: nomenclature, classification, and technique. Oral Maxillofac Surg Clin North Am. 2008; 20(3):459-75.
10. Mukherji SK, Armao D, Joshi VM. Cervical nodal metastases in squamous cell carcinoma of the head and neck: what to expect. Head Neck. 2001;23(11):995-1005.
11. Gavilán J, Herranz J, Martín L. Functional neck dissection: the Latin approach. Oper Techn Otolaryngol—Head Neck Surg. 2004;15(3):168-75.
12. Moore KL, Agur AMR, Dalley AF, et al. Essential Clinical Anatomy, 5th edition. Philadelphia: Wolters Kluwer Health; 2015.
13. Kawata R, Koutetsu L, Yoshimura K, et al. Indication for elective neck dissection for N0 carcinoma of the parotid gland: a single institution's 20-year experience. Acta Otolaryngol. 2010;130(2):286-92.
14. Nobis CP, Rohleder NH, Wolff KD, et al. Head and neck salivary gland carcinomas—elective neck dissection, yes or no? J Oral Maxillofac Surg. 2014;72(1):205-10.
15. Haddadin KJ, Soutar DS, Oliver RJ, et al. Improved survival for patients with clinically T1/T2, N0 tongue tumors undergoing a prophylactic neck dissection. Head Neck. 1999;21(6):517-25.
16. Koo BS, Lim YC, Lee JS, et al. Management of contralateral N0 neck in oral cavity squamous cell carcinoma. Head Neck. 2006;28(10):896-901.
17. Lim YC, Lee JS, Koo BS, et al. Treatment of contralateral N0 neck in early squamous cell carcinoma of the oral tongue: elective neck dissection versus observation. Laryngoscope. 2006;116(3):461-5.
18. Melchers LJ, Schuuring E, van Dijk BA, et al. Tumour infiltration depth >/=4 mm is an indication for an elective neck dissection in pT1cN0 oral squamous cell carcinoma. Oral Oncol. 2012;48(4):337-42.
19. Lim YC, Lee SY, Lim JY, et al. Management of contralateral N0 neck in tonsillar squamous cell carcinoma. Laryngoscope. 2005;115(9):1672-5.
20. Koo BS, Lim YC, Lee JS, et al. Management of contralateral N0 neck in pyriform sinus carcinoma. Laryngoscope. 2006;116(7):1268-72.

21. Ferlito A, Silver CE, Rinaldo A, et al. Surgical treatment of the neck in cancer of the larynx. ORL J Otorhinolaryngol Relat Spec. 2000;62(4):217-25.
22. Amar A, Chedid HM, Franzi SA, et al. Neck dissection in squamous cell carcinoma of the larynx: indication of elective contralateral neck dissection. Braz J Otorhinolaryngol. 2012;78(2):7-10.
23. American Thyroid Association Guidelines Taskforce on Thyroid Nodules and Differentiated with Thyroid Cancer, Cooper DS, Doherty GM, et al. Revised American Thyroid Association management guidelines for patients with thyroid nodules and differentiated thyroid cancer. Thyroid. 2009;19(11):1167-214.
24. Smallridge RC, Ain KB, Asa SL, et al. American Thyroid Association guidelines for management of patients with anaplastic thyroid cancer. Thyroid. 2012;22(11):1104-39.
25. Marti J, Udelsman R. Modified radical neck dissection. In: Oertli D, Udelsman R (Eds). Surgery of the Thyroid and Parathyroid Glands. Heidelberg: Springer; 2012. pp. 223-34.
26. Gavilán J, Herranz J, DeSanto LW, Gavilán C. Functional and Selective Neck Dissection, New York: Thieme; 2002.
27. Karaman E, Saritzali G, Cansiz H. A case of increased intracranial pressure after unilateral modified radical neck dissection. Am J Otolaryngol. 2009;30(4):261-3.
28. Witt RL, Rejto L. Spinal accessory nerve monitoring in selective and modified neck dissection. Laryngoscope. 2007;117(5):776-80.
29. Prim MP, De Diego JI, Verdaguer JM, et al. Neurological complications following functional neck dissection. Eur Arch Otorhinolaryngol. 2006;263(5):473-6.
30. Nahum AM, Mullally W, Marmor L. A syndrome resulting from radical neck dissection. Arch Otolaryngol. 1961;74:424-8.
31. Saunders JR, Jr., Hirata RM, Jaques DA. Considering the spinal accessory nerve in head and neck surgery. Am J Surg. 1985;150(4):491-4.
32. Cappiello J, Piazza C, Giudice M, et al. Shoulder disability after different selective neck dissections (levels II-IV versus levels II-V): a comparative study. Laryngoscope. 2005;115(2):259-63.
33. Cappiello J, Piazza C, Nicolai P. The spinal accessory nerve in head and neck surgery. Curr Opin Otolaryngol Head Neck Surg. 2007;15(2):107-11.
34. Silverman DA, El-Hajj M, Strome S, et al. Prevalence of nodal metastases in the submuscular recess (level IIb) during selective neck dissection. Arch Otolaryngol—Head Neck Surg. 2003;129(7):724-8.
35. Paleri V, Kumar Subramaniam S, Oozeer N, et al. Dissection of the submuscular recess (sublevel IIb) in squamous cell cancer of the upper aerodigestive tract: prospective study and systematic review of the literature. Head Neck. 2008;30(2):194-200.
36. Coskun HH, Erisen L, Basut O. Selective neck dissection for clinically N0 neck in laryngeal cancer: is dissection of level IIb necessary? Otolaryngol—Head Neck Surg. 2004;131(5):655-9.
37. Koybasioglu A, Bora Tokcaer A, Inal E, et al. Accessory nerve function in lateral selective neck dissection with undissected level IIb. ORL: journal for oto-rhino-laryngology and its related specialties. 2006;68(2):88-92.
38. Weisberger EC, Kincaid J, Riteris J. Cable grafting of the spinal accessory nerve after radical neck dissection. Arch Otolaryngol—Head Neck Surg. 1998;124(4):377-80.
39. Den Dunnen WF, van der Lei B, Schakenraad JM, et al. Poly(DL-lactide-epsilon-caprolactone) nerve guides perform better than autologous nerve grafts. Microsurgery. 1996;17(7):348-57.
40. Meek MF, Den Dunnen WF, Schakenraad JM, et al. Long-term evaluation of functional nerve recovery after reconstruction with a thin-walled biodegradable poly (DL-lactide-epsilon-caprolactone) nerve guide, using walking track analysis and electrostimulation tests. Microsurgery. 1999;19(5):247-53.
41. Teymoortash A, Hoch S, Eivazi B, et al. Postoperative morbidity after different types of selective neck dissection. Laryngoscope. 2010;120(5):924-9.
42. Roh JL, Kim DH, Park CI. Prospective identification of chyle leakage in patients undergoing lateral neck dissection for metastatic thyroid cancer. Ann Surg Oncol. 2008;15(2):424-9.
43. Brennan PA, Blythe JN, Herd MK, et al. The contemporary management of chyle leak following cervical thoracic duct damage. Brit J Oral Maxillofac Surg. 2012;50(3):197-201.
44. Ilczyszyn A, Ridha H, Durrani AJ. Management of chyle leak post neck dissection: a case report and literature review. J Plast Reconstr Aesth Surg: JPRAS. 2011;64(9):e223-30.
45. Prabhu V, Passant C. Left-sided neck dissection and chylothorax: a rare complication and its management. J Laryngol Otol. 2012;126(6):648-50.
46. Babin RW, Panje WR. The incidence of vasovagal reflex activity during radical neck dissection. Laryngoscope. 1980;90(8 Pt 1):1321-3.
47. Choi SS, Lim YJ, Bahk JH, et al. Coronary artery spasm induced by carotid sinus stimulation during neck surgery. Brit J Anaesth. 2003;90(3):391-4.
48. Higuchi H, Ishii M, Nakatsuka H, et al. Sudden cardiac arrest in head and neck surgery: a case report. J Anesth. 2010;24(1):146-7.
49. Ward MJ, Faris C, Upile T, et al. Ophthalmoplegia secondary to raised intracranial pressure after unilateral neck dissection with internal jugular vein sacrifice. Head Neck. 2011;33(4):587-90.
50. Cappiello J, Piazza C, Berlucchi M, et al. Internal jugular vein patency after lateral neck dissection: a prospective study. Eur Arch Otorhinolaryngol. 2002;259(8):409-12.
51. Chen KC, Yen TT, Hsieh YL, et al. Post-irradiated carotid blowout syndrome in patients with nasopharyngeal carcinoma: a case-control study [published online ahead of print Mar 7, 2014.]. Head Neck.
52. McDonald MW, Moore MG, Johnstone PA. Risk of carotid blowout after reirradiation of the head and neck: a systematic review. Int J Radiation Oncol Biol Phys. 2012;82(3):1083-9.
53. Lu HJ, Chen KW, Chen MH, et al. Predisposing factors, management, and prognostic evaluation of acute carotid blowout syndrome. J Vasc Surg.2013;58(5):1226-35.
54. Seven H, Sayin I, Turgut S. Antibiotic prophylaxis in clean neck dissections. J Laryngol Otol. 2004;118(3):213-6.

CHAPTER 18

Selective Neck Dissection

Vijay A Patel, David Goldenberg, Neerav Goyal

INTRODUCTION

Over the last 45 years, traditional approaches to neck dissection have evolved from a radical approach where all cervical lymph nodes were removed en bloc—including locoregional structures such as the sternocleidomastoid muscle (SCM), the accessory nerve (SAN), and the internal jugular vein (IJV)—to a more selective technique where only the most at-risk lymph nodes are resected.[1] Furthermore, the work of Byers, published in 1985, introduced the concept that dissection confined only to the node levels at risk for early metastasis would produce results comparable to more extensive neck dissection.[2] The rationale for performing a selective neck dissection (SND) is based on the recognition that fascial planes separate the lymphatic structures of the neck from the nonlymphatic structures, such as muscles, vessels, and nerves. The presence of these planes facilitates removal of the lymphatics in an oncologically sound but function-preserving manner. In the past, SND was reserved for the N0 neck, but as experience and understanding of upper aerodigestive tumors has evolved, increasing numbers of reports have suggested that SND may also be useful for the clinically node positive neck under specific circumstances.[3-6]

CLASSIFICATION, PERTINENT ANATOMY, AND SURGICAL LANDMARKS BY LEVEL

Originally described by the Memorial Sloan-Kettering Group in 1981, the cervical lymph node basin classification has been further delineated in 2001 and again in 2008 by the American Head and Neck Society's Neck Dissection Committee. The classification includes seven nodal groups as well as the use of sublevels for further defining selected lymph node groups within levels I, II, and V on the basis of biologic significance.[7] The targeted lymph nodes of the neck lie superficial to the deep layer of the deep cervical fascia, which surround the scalene musculature. Figure 18.1 illustrates the different nodal groups and Table 18.1 depicts the anatomic and radiographic boundaries of each level.

Level $I_{(A/B)}$

The submental triangle corresponds to sublevel I_A, whereas the submandibular triangle corresponds to sublevel I_B. The submental triangle is the region bounded by (1) the mandibular symphysis, (2) the anterior bellies of the digastric muscle bilaterally, and (3) the hyoid bone inferiorly. The deep surface of the submental triangle is the mylohyoid muscle. The submandibular triangle is bordered by (1) the mandible superiorly, (2) the posterior belly of the digastric muscle and the stylohyoid muscle posteroinferiorly, and (3) the anterior belly of the digastric muscle anteroinferiorly. It includes the pre- and postvascular nodes that are related to the facial artery, often termed the perifacial nodes.[8]

Significant local anatomical structures include: the facial artery, the lingual artery, the submental artery, the facial vein, the hypoglossal nerve, the lingual nerve, the marginal branch of the facial nerve, and Wharton's duct (submandibular duct).

Level $II_{(A/B)}$

Level II, also known as the upper jugular region, contains two sublevels, level II_A and II_B, with the two divided by

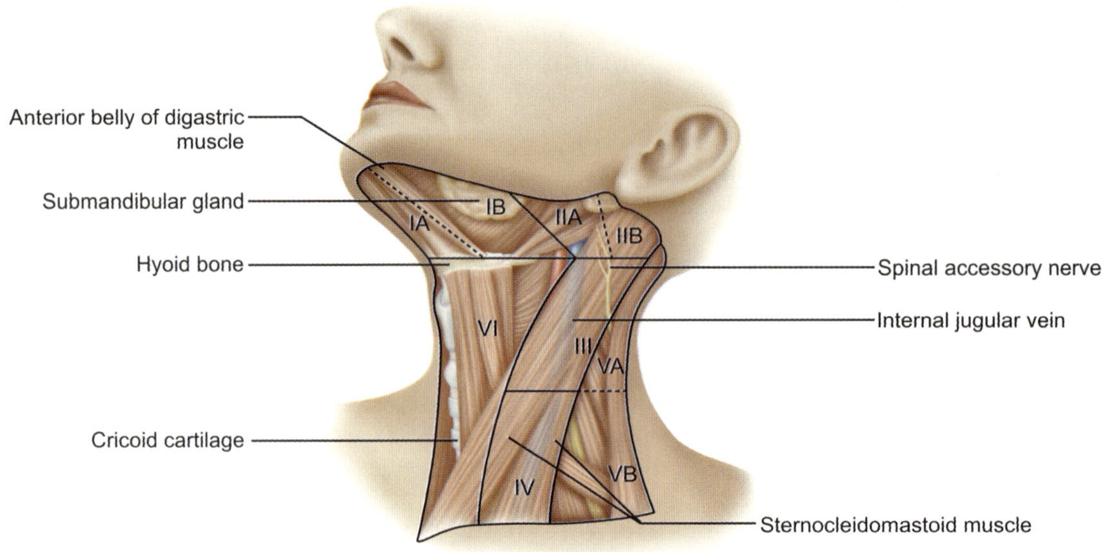

Fig. 18.1: Lymph node levels of the neck (levels I through VI).

Table 18.1: Anatomic and radiographic boundaries of each lymph node level.

	Boundary							
	Superior		*Inferior*		*Lateral*		*Medial*	
Sublevel	Anatomic	Radiographic	Anatomic	Radiographic	Anatomic	Radiographic	Anatomic	Radiographic
I_A	Mandibular symphysis	Geniohyoid muscle	Hyoid body		Digastric muscle (anterior belly)			
I_B	Mandibular body	Mylohyoid muscle	Hyoid body		Submandibular gland (posterior edge)		Digastric muscle (anterior belly)	
II_A	Skull base	Transverse process C1	Carotid bifurcation	Hyoid bone	SAN	IJV	Submandibular gland (posterior edge)	
II_B	Skull base	Transverse process C1	Carotid bifurcation	Hyoid bone	SCM (posterior edge)		SAN	Paraspinal muscles
III	Carotid bifurcation	Hyoid bone	Omohyoid muscle	Cricoid cartilage	Cervical rootlets	SCM (posterior edge)	Sternohyoid muscle	Paraspinal muscles
IV	Omohyoid muscle	Cricoid cartilage	Clavicle	Sternoclavicular joint	Cervical rootlets	SCM (posterior edge)	Sternohyoid muscle	Paraspinal muscles
V_A	SCM and trapezius muscle		Cricoid cartilage		Trapezius muscle (anterior edge)		Cervical plexus	SCM (posterior edge)
V_B	Cricoid cartilage		Clavicle		Trapezius muscle (anterior edge)		Cervical plexus	SCM (posterior edge)
VI	Hyoid bone		Sternal manubrium (superior)		Common carotid artery			
VII	Sternal manubrium (superior edge)		Innominate artery		Innominate artery (right) Common carotid artery (left)			

(IJV: Internal jugular vein; SAN: Spinal accessory nerve; SCM: Sternocleidomastoid muscle).

the course of the spinal accessory nerve (SAN). Level II_A boundaries consist of (1) the skull base superiorly, (2) the carotid bifurcation (surgically) and hyoid bone (radiographically) inferiorly, (3) the posterior belly of the digastric muscle anteriorly, (4) the vertical plane defined by the SAN posteriorly, (5) the SCM laterally, and (6) the lateral border of the sternohyoid muscle medially. Level II_B is defined (1) by the skull base superiorly, (2) the carotid bifurcation (surgically) and hyoid bone (radiographically) inferiorly, (3) the vertical plane defined by the SAN anteriorly, and (4) the posterior border of the SCM posteriorly. A subsection of level II_B, the submuscular triangle (submuscular recess), includes the most superior aspect of this zone and lies laterally to the SAN at the skull base.[9] The floor of level II is defined by the deep layer of the deep cervical fascia and the cervical rootlets. Level II contains the upper jugular lymph nodes that surround the upper third of the IJV, the SAN and the jugulodigastric node (the principal node of Kuttner), which is the most common node containing cervical metastases in oral malignancy.[9a]

Significant local anatomical structures include: branches of the external carotid artery (superior thyroid, lingual, facial, and ascending pharyngeal), the internal carotid artery, the IJV, the cervical plexus, the cervical rootlets, the common trunk of the SAN, the hypoglossal nerve, the phrenic nerve, and the vagus nerve.

Level III

Level III, also known as the middle jugular region, encompasses (1) the inferior border of level II (hyoid bone radiographically and the carotid bifurcation surgically), (2) the omohyoid muscle (surgically) and the cricoid cartilage (radiographically) inferiorly, (3) the lateral border of sternohyoid muscle anteriorly, and (4) the posterior border of the SCM posteriorly. The lateral and medial borders are identical to those of level II (the SCM laterally, the deep layer of the deep cervical fascia and the cervical rootlets medially).

Significant local anatomical structures include the common carotid artery, the IJV, the cervical rootlets, the phrenic nerve, and the vagus nerve.

Level IV

Level IV, also known as the lower jugular region, encompasses (1) the omohyoid (surgically) or the cricoid cartilage (radiographically) superiorly, (2) the clavicle inferiorly, (3) the lateral border of the sternohyoid muscle anteriorly, and (4) the posterior border of the SCM posteriorly. The medial and lateral boundaries are the same as for levels II and III (the SCM laterally, the deep layer of the deep cervical fascia and the cervical rootlets medially).

Significant local anatomical structures include the common carotid artery, the subclavian artery, the IJV, the subclavian vein, the cervical rootlets, the phrenic nerve, the vagus nerve, and the thoracic duct.

Level $V_{(A/B)}$

Level V, also known as the posterior triangle and the supraclavicular region, can be subdivided into two areas (levels V_A and V_B) by an imaginary horizontal line, extending from the inferior border of the cricoid cartilage. Level V_A is bound by (1) the intersection of the SCM and the trapezius superiorly, (2) the inferior aspect of the cricoid cartilage inferiorly, (3) the posterior border of the SCM anteriorly, (4) the anterolateral edge of the trapezius muscle posteriorly, (5) the skin and platysma laterally, and (6) the deep layer of the deep cervical fascia medially. Level V_B is defined by (1) the inferior cricoid bone superiorly, (2) the clavicle inferiorly, (3) the posterior border of the SCM anteriorly, (4) the anterolateral trapezius muscle posteriorly, (5) the skin and platysma laterally, and (6) the deep layer of the deep cervical fascia medially.

Significant local anatomical structures include the transverse cervical artery, the subclavian artery, the external jugular vein (EJV), the brachial plexus, Erb's point (punctum nervosum), the great auricular nerve, the phrenic nerve, the SAN, and the scalene muscles.

Level VI

Level VI, also known as the central compartment, encompasses (1) the hyoid bone superiorly, (2) the suprasternal notch inferiorly, and (3) the common carotid arteries laterally. This region is typically dissected only in conjunction with laryngectomy and thyroidectomy. The central compartment lymph node group is of minimal importance in primaries originating from other head and neck sites. It is made up of the lymph node bearing tissue occupying the visceral space, comprising of the paratracheal and thyroidal basins.

Significant local anatomical structures include the brachiocephalic artery (innominate artery), the cricothyroid artery, the inferior thyroid artery, the subclavian artery, the thyrocervical trunk, the vertebral artery, the anterior jugular veins, the recurrent laryngeal nerve (RLN), the vagus nerve, the cervical esophagus, the larynx, the parathyroid glands, the thyroid gland, and the trachea.

Level VII

Level VII contains the anterior superior mediastinal lymph nodes and extends from the suprasternal notch to the aortic arch inferiorly. It is bound by the superior edge of the manubrium sternum bone superiorly, the innominate artery inferiorly, and the innominate artery and left common carotid artery both medially and laterally.

Significant local anatomical structures include the innominate artery, the brachiocephalic vein, the thymus or thymic remnant, the trachea, and the upper thoracic esophagus.

Posterior Neck

The posterior neck contains two groups of lymph nodes: the suboccipital and retroauricular lymph nodes.[10,11] The suboccipital lymph nodes can be divided into three groups: the superficial occipital nodes, the deep occipital nodes, and a sole lymph node found along the splenius segment of the occipital artery. The superficial occipital nodes are located close to a cutaneous branch of the occipital artery and greater occipital nerve at the insertion of the trapezius muscle to the superior nuchal line. The deep occipital nodes are located beneath the superficial layer of the deep cervical fascia. The additional sole lymph node is found along the splenius segment of the occipital artery. The retroauricular lymph nodes can be found on or behind the mastoid process, often deep to the posterior auricular muscle. Both the suboccipital and retroauricular lymph nodes drain primarily into the level V and secondarily into level II.

Significant local anatomical structures include the occipital artery, the phrenic nerve, the levator scapulae, the splenius capitis muscle, and the trapezius muscle.

INDICATIONS AND SURGICAL TECHNIQUE OF SELECTIVE NECK DISSECTION

Relative to a classical radical neck dissection, SNDs preserve one or more nodal groups, and only remove those groups that are most likely to contain metastatic disease according to the location of the primary site.[12] Common SNDs, which will be discussed, include supraomohyoid neck dissection (SOND) (lymph node levels I–III), lateral neck dissection (LND) (lymph node levels II–IV), posterolateral neck dissection (PLND) (lymph node levels II–V, suboccipital nodes, and retroauricular nodes), and central neck dissection (CND) (lymph node levels VI–VII). Figures 18.2A to G depict the nomenclature for a variety of different incision patterns that can be used for these operations.

Supraomohyoid (Levels I–III) Neck Dissection

The use of SOND has been a controversial topic for decades; however, it is a currently accepted modality of elective treatment for patients with oral cavity cancer and either no nodal disease or low-volume nodal disease (N0–N1). The term SOND refers to removal of at-risk cervical lymph nodes contained in levels I–III.[13] The primary rationale favoring the utilization of SOND is that multiple studies have shown good prognosis for patients with clinically positive nodes at level I or II, regardless of the type of neck dissection (selective or radical) used and without jeopardizing oncologic control.[14] Furthermore, it is well appreciated that oral cavity cancer and parotid gland malignancy have a predilection for spread to levels I–III, rarely disseminating to levels IV–V.[15,16] However, relative contraindications include extensive neck disease as well as evidence of extracapsular spread either visualized radiographically and/or intraoperatively.

After induction with general anesthesia, with the patient in a supine position, we recommend using a viscoelastic polymer shoulder roll to increase neck extension as well as turning the head away from the operative side to maximize operative exposure. Both upper extremities should be appropriately tucked and cushioned. The patient is then prepped and draped in a sterile fashion. For a unilateral dissection, a "modified apron" incision is utilized to provide adequate exposure to levels I–III. If a bilateral neck dissection is necessary, a "bilateral apron" incision is utilized where the horizontal component of the unilateral "apron incision" is extended across the midline to the other side of the neck. This initial incision can be made with a knife, followed by electrocautery to begin flap elevation. The skin flaps are raised superiorly and inferiorly in the subplatysmal plane until the upper two thirds of the anterior border of the SCM, the mastoid process, the body of the mandible, and the mandibular symphysis are sufficiently exposed (Figs. 18.3A to F). This allows for preservation of both the EJV and the great auricular nerve.

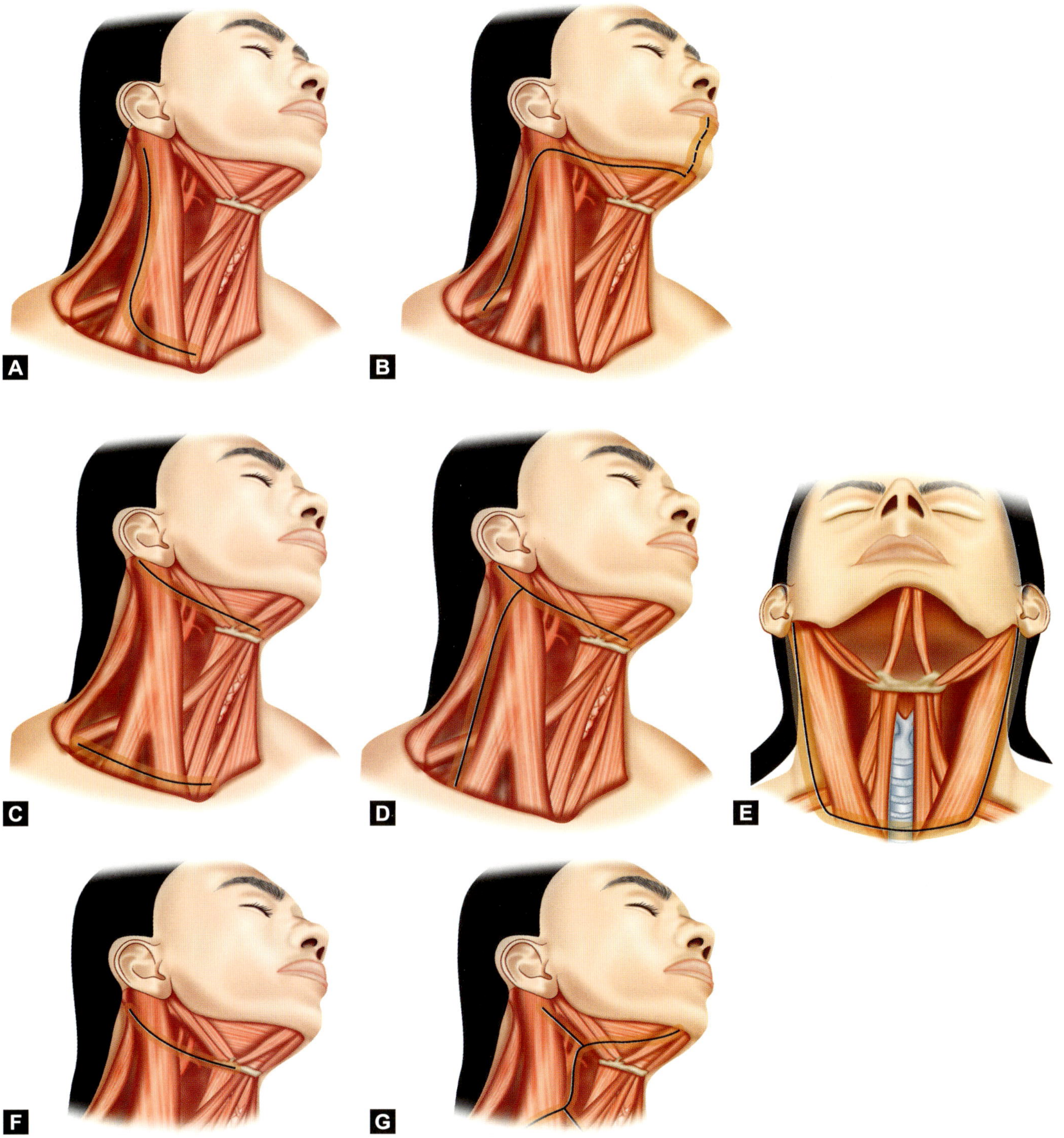

Figs. 18.2A to G: Incisions used for modified radical neck dissection: (A) Lahey (hockey stick). (B) Boomerang. (C) MacFee. (D) Modified Schobinger. (E) Apron or bilateral hockey stick. (F) Gluck. (G) Martin double-Y.

Next, the deep cervical fascia overlying the submandibular gland is incised at the inferior border of the submandibular gland and carefully raised as a separate flap to avoid injury to the mandibular branch of the facial nerve, which is often located within the superficial layer of the deep cervical fascia. To assist with retraction of this

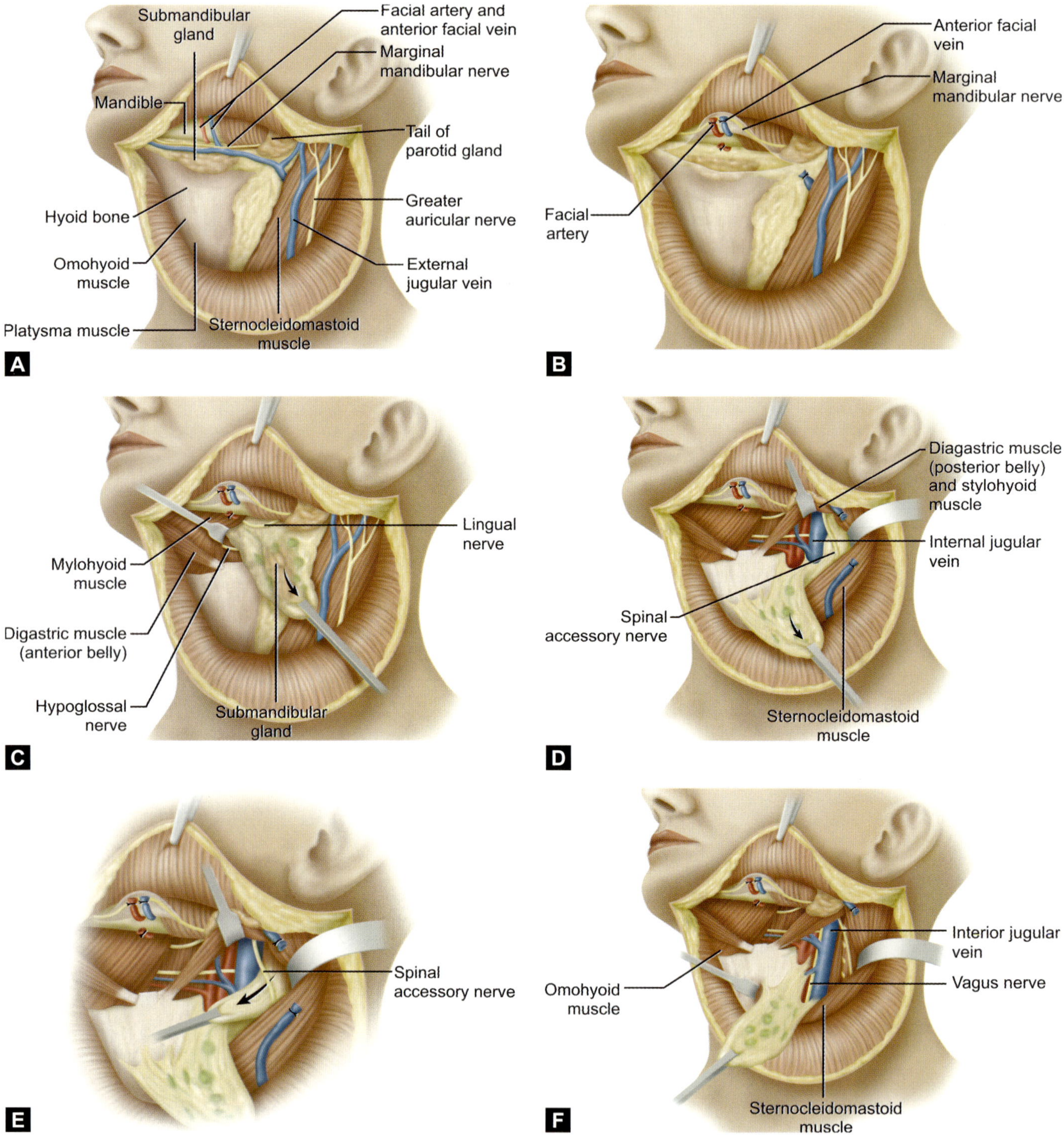

Figs. 18.3A to F: Steps to performing the supraomohyoid neck dissection. (A) The subplatysmal flaps have been raised, identifying the boundaries of the neck dissection. (B) A Hayes-Martin maneuver is shown with ligation of the facial vein and elevation of a submandibular fascial flap. The artery is also shown ligated with exposure of the inferior border of the mandible. (C) The mylohyoid muscle is identified and dissection is carried superior to the submandibular gland, exposing the lingual nerve, hypoglossal nerve, and submandibular duct. (D) The submandibular gland and duct are ligated, as well as the facial artery, allowing for the specimen to be retracted inferiorly. The spinal accessory nerve is identified, as well as the internal jugular vein. (E) Level IIb is dissected free and tucked under the nerve. (F) The rest of level II and III are elevated in a posterior to anterior direction off of the deep layer of the deep cervical fascia and cervical rootlets and off of the fascia of the internal jugular vein.

layer, often the facial vein is ligated and the ties on the facial vein are left intact and clamped to a hemostat (Hayes-Martin maneuver). Using blunt dissection along with electrocautery or ultrasonic shears, the inferior border of the submandibular gland should be well defined, along with identification of the posterior belly of the digastric muscle. The hyoid bone and the anterior belly of the contralateral digastric muscle are also skeletonized; this defines the medial boundary of dissection and the medial border of level IA. The tissue packet in level IA should be dissected off of the mylohyoid muscle, either bluntly or with electrocautery. After the tissue packet in the submental triangle has been cleared, the submandibular gland is retracted inferiorly, along with associated fat and lymph nodes with a sponge. By taking care to dissect below the submandibular fascia, the marginal mandibular nerve should be preserved. The superior border of dissection will be the inferior border of the mandible. In addition, the deep aspect of the submandibular gland should be freed, taking care not to injure the underlying venous plexus. Medially, the packet should be freed from the anterior belly of the digastric muscle, ligating any vessels and perforators encountered. The mylohyoid muscle should be identified and retracted medially. Of note, the vessel to the mylohyoid as well as the nerve to the mylohyoid will need to be addressed. Then with the gland retracted anteriorly and inferiorly, the lingual nerve, lingual artery, and submandibular duct should be easily identified. Each of these structures should be skeletonized. The afferent and efferent branches off of the lingual nerve into the submandibular gland are often visualized. The submandibular ganglion and duct is then identified, ligated, and divided, preserving the lingual nerve. The contents of the submandibular triangle are then dissected in a medial to lateral fashion. The specimen is finally swept off the posterior belly of the digastric muscle and kept pedicled to the level II neck contents. A digastric tunnel can be created, staying superficial to the digastric muscle and carrying the dissection toward the anterior border of the SCM. The hypoglossal nerve should be identified deep to the posterior belly of the digastric muscle and preserved.

Next, an incision is made in the investing (superficial) layer of the deep cervical fascia at the anterior border of the SCM, without disturbing the EJV and branches of the greater auricular nerve, which lie laterally to the SCM. The fibrofatty contents of the anterior triangle are peeled away first from the anteromedial aspect of the SCM, extending from a point close to the mastoid process above down to the level of the omohyoid muscle below, stopping when the posterior border of the muscle is reached. Vessels that are perforating through the fascia into the SCM are carefully cauterized as they are encountered. Retraction of both the SCM posteriorly and the lymph node packet anteriorly will allow for excellent visualization of the proposed plane of dissection. Next, attention should be turned to the upper third of the SCM. As the fascia is elevated off of the SCM, the SAN will come into view as it enters the muscle. It is finely dissected free of surrounding fibrofatty tissue from the level of the skull base to its point of entry into the SCM. It is also necessary to dissect along the inferior border of the posterior belly of the digastric muscle, debulk surrounding fibrofatty tissue and retract it supralaterally to provide adequate exposure of the upper carotid sheath. This triangle formed by the digastric muscle, SAN, and SCM outlines the triangular packet of tissue-bearing lymph nodes belonging to level II_B. The transverse process of the first cervical vertebrae (C1) can be palpated in this region and marks the superior border of the dissection. The IJV should be identified using blunt dissection prior to elevation of the lymph node packet as it defines its anterior border. It is important to separate this triangular packet from the underlying paraspinal muscles and to pass it under the SAN. The dissection is continued inferiorly by incising along the fibrofatty tissue corresponding with the sensory branches of the cervical plexus as the incision is carried down to the muscular floor, where it is dissected in a plane superficial to these nerves.

At this point in the procedure, it is important to carefully inspect and palpate the lower jugular chain and the posterior triangle for evidence of additional nodal disease. If found, these findings are likely due to skip metastases and the dissection would have to be extended to encompass levels IV and V.

After completion of the lateral boundary of dissection, the tissue packet is swept medially in a plane immediately above the fascia of the paraspinal muscles (the deep layer of the deep cervical fascia) and above the cervical rootlets. This maneuver allows the tissue packet to be swept over the carotid sheath and permits exposure of its structures from the level of the omohyoid muscle below to the skull base above. Sharp dissection using a scalpel is used to remove the fascia overlying the sheath while preserving the IJV. Next, the superior belly of the omohyoid muscle is skeletonized along its superior border to the level of the hyoid bone. The packet is then elevated and removed from the visceral compartment of the neck.

After the dissection is complete, the excised tissue should be marked and/or separated according to nodal level and submitted for permanent pathologic evaluation. Prior to wound closure, a closed suction drain (two if a bilateral dissection) can be placed in the surgical wound bed extending inferiorly from the digastric muscle. The platysma muscle and deep layers are carefully reapproximated with absorbable suture. The skin is closed with suture or staples. The surgeon should ensure that the drainage bulbs hold appropriate suction as well as apply gentle pressure to the incision with a towel during extubation to minimize the risk of a postoperative hematoma.

Lateral (Levels II–IV) Neck Dissection

A lateral neck dissection is indicated in the treatment of oropharyngeal, hypopharyngeal, and laryngeal cancers. In the clinically and radiographic-negative neck, LND has been shown to produce a comparable 5-year survival relative to a complete functional neck dissection with both reduced operating times and fewer short- and long-term complications.[17]

After induction with general anesthesia, with the patient in a supine position, we recommend using a visco-elastic polymer shoulder roll to increase neck extension as well as turning the head away from the operative side to maximize operative exposure. Both upper extremities should be appropriately tucked and cushioned. The patient is then prepped and draped in a sterile fashion. A single "apron" incision within a natural skin crease is used. This initial incision can be made with a knife, followed by electrocautery to begin flap elevation. The skin flaps are raised superiorly and inferiorly in the subplatysmal plane until the upper two-thirds of the anterior border of the SCM, the mastoid process, and the body of the mandible are sufficiently exposed (Figs. 18.4A to G). This allows for preservation of both the EJV and the great auricular nerve. Sharp dissection along the inferior border of the submandibular gland is then performed. Once exposed, it is retracted superiorly, and the posterior belly of the digastric muscle is exposed. The digastric muscle can be traced posteriorly toward its insertion point on the mastoid tip, delineating a "digastric tunnel." The hypoglossal nerve is then identified deep to the digastric muscle. Of note, the ranine veins are typically found superficial to the hypoglossal nerve; hence, caution should be employed during division of these vessels. Next, an incision is made in the investing (superficial) layer of the deep cervical fascia at the anterior border of the SCM, without disturbing the EJV and branches of the greater auricular nerve, which lie laterally to the SCM. The fibrofatty contents of the anterior triangle are peeled away first from the anteromedial aspect of the SCM, extending from a point close to the mastoid process above down to the level of the omohyoid muscle below, stopping when the posterior border of the muscle is reached. Vessels that are perforating through the fascia of the SCM are carefully cauterized as they are encountered. Retraction of both the SCM posteriorly and the lymph node packet anteriorly will allow for excellent visualization of the proposed plane of dissection. Next, attention should be turned to the upper third of the SCM. As the fascia is elevated off of the SCM, the SAN will come into view as it enters the muscle. It is finely dissected free of surrounding fibrofatty tissue from the level of the skull base to its point of entry into the SCM. It is also necessary to dissect along the inferior border of the posterior belly of the digastric muscle, debulk surrounding fibrofatty tissue, and retract it supralaterally to provide adequate exposure of the upper carotid sheath. The triangle formed by the digastric muscle, SAN, and SCM outlines the triangular packet of tissue-bearing lymph nodes belonging to level II_B. The transverse process of the first cervical vertebrae (C1) can be palpated in this region and marks the superior border of the dissection. Of note, the deep limit of this dissection is the fascia ("muscular carpet") overlying the splenius capitis muscle posteriorly and the levator scapulae muscle anteriorly.[18] The IJV should be identified using blunt dissection prior to elevation of this packet as it defines the anterior border of the packet. It is important to separate this triangular packet from the underlying paraspinal muscles and to pass it under the SAN to join Level IIA. The dissection is continued inferiorly by incising along the fibrofatty tissue corresponding with the sensory branches of the cervical plexus as the incision is carried down to the muscular floor, where corresponding fibrofatty tissue is dissected in a plane superficial to these nerves (brachial plexus and phrenic nerve).

After completion of the lateral boundary of dissection, the tissue packet is swept medially in a plane immediately above the fascia of the paraspinal muscles (the deep layer of the deep cervical fascia) and above the cervical rootlets. This maneuver allows the tissue packet to be swept over the carotid sheath and permits exposure of its structures from the level of the omohyoid muscle below to the skull base above. Sharp dissection using a scalpel is used to remove the fascia overlying the sheath while preserving the IJV. Branches of the IJV (thyroid and facial branches) are ligated (ties or clips) as they are identified along the course of the vessel. The specimen is then dissected away from the sternohyoid muscles inferiorly, the hypoglossal nerve, branches of the IJV, and the external carotid artery superiorly. Care is taken not to injure the thoracic duct as one approaches the fibrofatty tissue adjacent to the IJV.[18]

The lymph node tissue packet is completely dissected away from the visceral compartment of the neck and removed. The excised tissue should be marked and/or separated according to nodal level and submitted for permanent pathologic evaluation. A closed suction drain is inserted (two if a bilateral dissection) through a separate incision and secured to the skin. The platysma muscle and deep layers are carefully reapproximated using 3-4 Vicryl sutures. The skin is closed with 4–5 Prolene sutures or staples. The incision is appropriately cleaned with a moist sponge, and topical antibiotic ointment is applied. The surgeon should ensure that the drainage bulbs can hold appropriate suction as well as apply gentle pressure to the incision with a towel to minimize the risk of a hematoma during extubation.

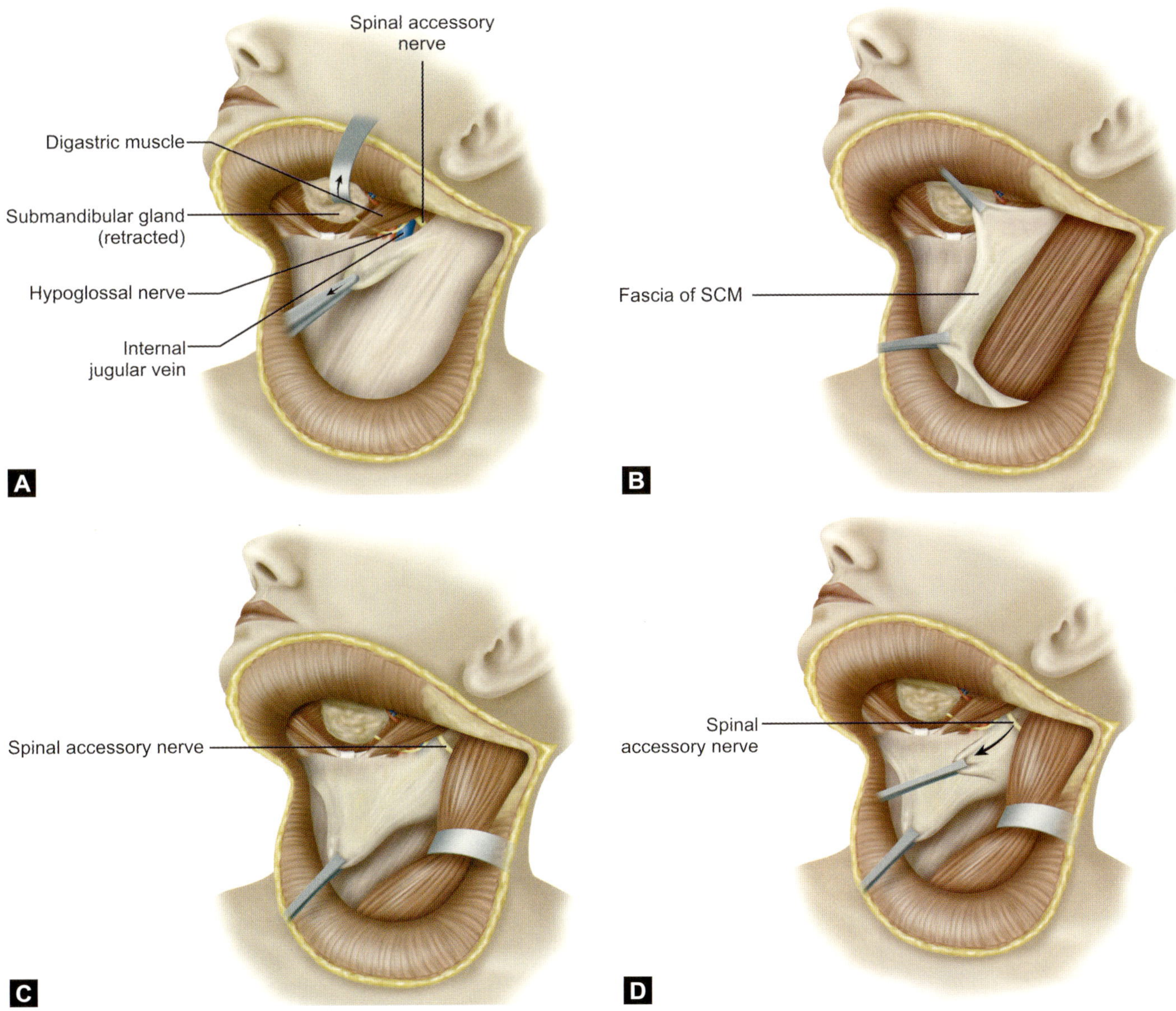

Figs. 18.4A to D: Steps to performing the lateral neck dissection. (A) The subplatysmal flaps have been raised, identifying the boundaries of the neck dissection. The hypoglossal nerve is traced backwards, where the IJV is identified. (B) Anterior retraction of the SCM fascia. (C) Identification of the SAN, entering the SCM. (D) Passage of level IIB lymphatic contents deep to SAN.

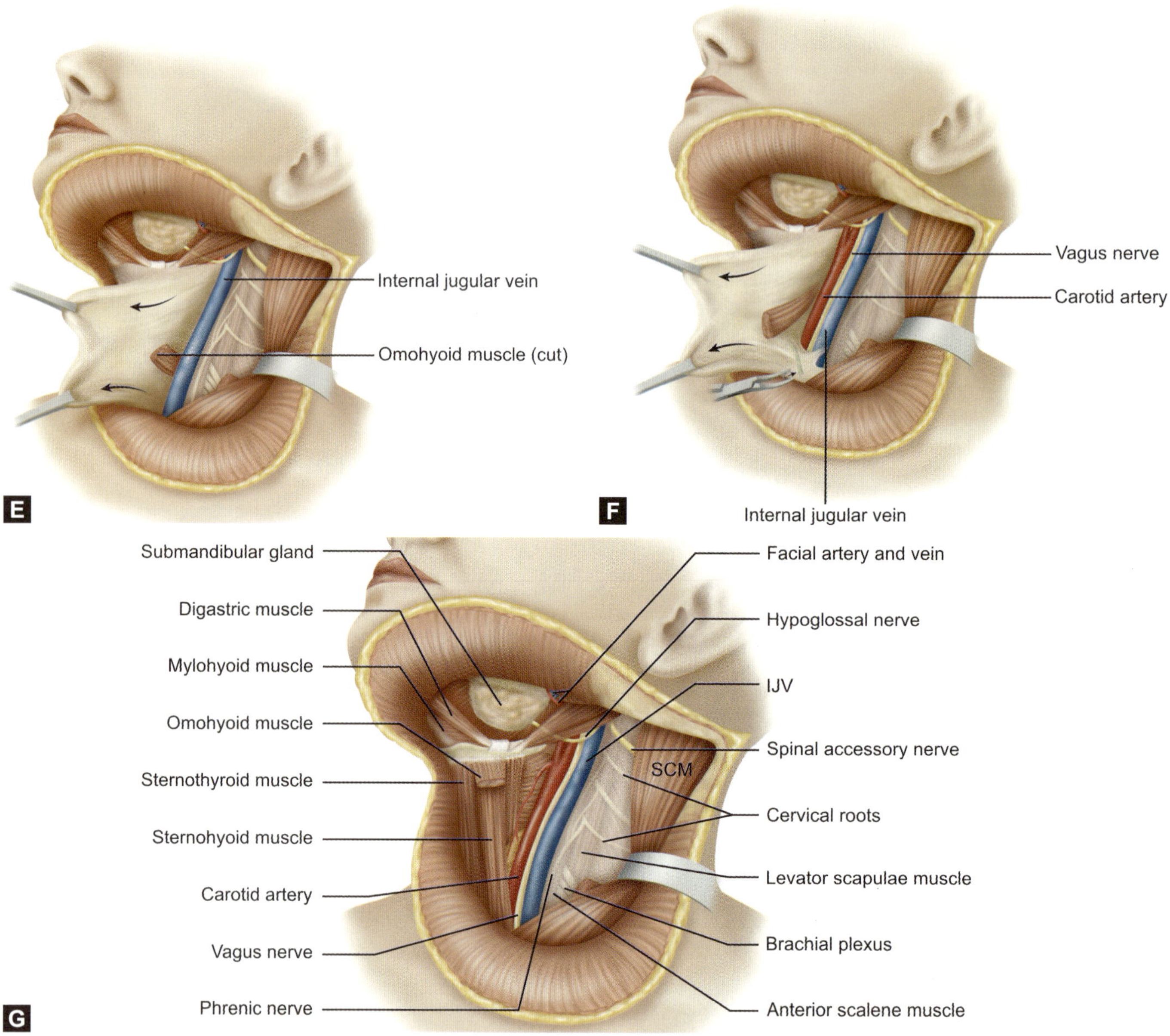

Figs. 18.4E to G: (E) Fine dissection across the IJV. (F) Continued fine dissection across the carotid sheath. (G) Fully dissected visceral compartment of the neck.

Posterolateral (Levels II–V, Suboccipital, and Retroauricular) Neck Dissection

A posterolateral neck dissection is indicated in the treatment of melanomas, squamous cell carcinomas, or other skin tumors with metastatic potential located in the posterior neck and/or scalp due to their complex lymphatic drainage patterns in these areas.[10,19] A line drawn in a coronal plane at the level of the external auditory canal is often used to differentiate anteriorly versus posteriorly draining tumors (Fig. 18.5).[20]

After induction with general anesthesia, the patient is placed in the supine position, with a viscoelastic polymer shoulder roll placed under the ipsilateral shoulder as well as turning the head away from the operative side to maximize operative exposure. Both upper extremities should be appropriately tucked and cushioned and the operating table should be rotated 180°. If a bilateral dissection is required, the patient is positioned in a prone position,

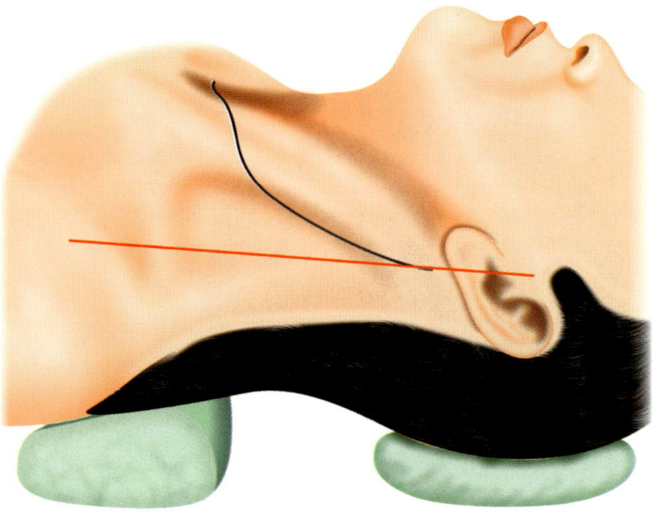

Fig. 18.5: Operative positioning—a line drawn in a coronal plane at the level of the external auditory canal is often used to differentiate anteriorly versus posteriorly draining tumors.

with the neck positioned in slight flexion.[10] The patient is then prepped locally with a povidone-iodine solution and draped in a sterile fashion while maintaining sterile exposure of the posterior neck. For a unilateral dissection, a "hockey stick" or "S" incision is designed starting in a natural skin crease along the midline of the anterior neck, which travels horizontally and extends superiorly towards the mastoid tip. This incision is then extended horizontally and posteriorly along the inferior nuchal line towards the occiput. The initial incision, planned by a marker pen, can be made with a knife, followed by electrocautery to begin flap elevation (Figs. 18.6A to D).[11]

The skin flaps are raised superiorly and inferiorly in the subplatysmal plane until the upper two-thirds of the anterior border of the SCM, the mastoid process, the body of the mandible, and the mandibular symphysis are sufficiently exposed. This allows for preservation of both the EJV and the great auricular nerve. In this case, dissection should continue posteriorly until the trapezius muscle is identified and dissected off the occiput to C3-C4 with subsequent removal of any underlying node-bearing tissue. This defines the extent of the dissection posteriorly. Raising the posterior flap requires both avoidance of including the superficial suboccipital lymph nodes deep to the flap as well as avoidance of raising a thin flap, which can cause necrosis and/or "button holding" of the skin. While the nodal dissection can occur in a variety of progressions, we will describe first dissecting level V, then the suboccipital and retroauricular nodes, and finally levels II–IV, allowing for the entire nodal packet to be removed in an en bloc fashion.

The nodal dissection first begins in the posterior triangle by first identifying the SAN. The SAN should be carefully traced and dissected to its insertion point on the trapezius muscle, while carefully avoiding inadvertent injury to the nerve or other branches of the cervical plexus.

Next, attention is turned to dissection of the suboccipital and retroauricular nodes. The suboccipital nodes can be found along the occipital artery, deep to the trapezius muscle, and superficial to the splenius capitis muscle. At this point, the dissection proceeds inferiorly towards the deep neck musculature. First, the superficial occipital nodes can be dissected off the underlying splenius capitis muscle. Branches of the occipital artery with any nodal tissue may also be ligated and removed as they are encountered along the splenius capitis muscle. Next, the retroauricular nodes are dissected away from the mastoid and the SCM. Similarly, any nodal tissue found superior to the omohyoid muscle is removed. To expose the tranverse cervical artery and vein, the omohyoid muscle is divided. These vessels are subsequently ligated, allowing access to level VB. Both the phrenic nerve and the brachial plexus can now be identified and preserved along their anatomic position within the floor of the neck. With identification of these structures, the remaining nodal tissue packet can now be safely dissected off the scalene musculature. The SCM can now be skeletonized and preserved, serving as the lateral dissection boundary. The IJV is also skeletonized using a scalpel, serving as the anterior and superior boundaries of the dissection. At this point, the nodal tissue packet can either be divided and sent off for permanent pathology or swept deep to the SCM and maintained pedicled to the submuscular recess contents, which will be subsequently dissected.[20]

Attention is then directed to the anterior dissection for levels II–IV. Refer to the "Lateral Neck Dissection" section for additional details with regards to surgical technique.

Two closed suction drains are placed in the surgical wound bed, one anterior to the IJV and one in level V, which are secured to the skin using a separate incision. The platysma muscle and deep layers are carefully reapproximated using 3-4 Vicryl sutures. The skin is closed with 4-5 Prolene sutures or staples. The incision is appropriately cleaned with a moist sponge, and topical antibiotic ointment is applied. The surgeon should ensure that the drainage bulbs can hold appropriate suction as well as apply gentle pressure to the incision with a towel to minimize the risk of a hematoma during extubation.

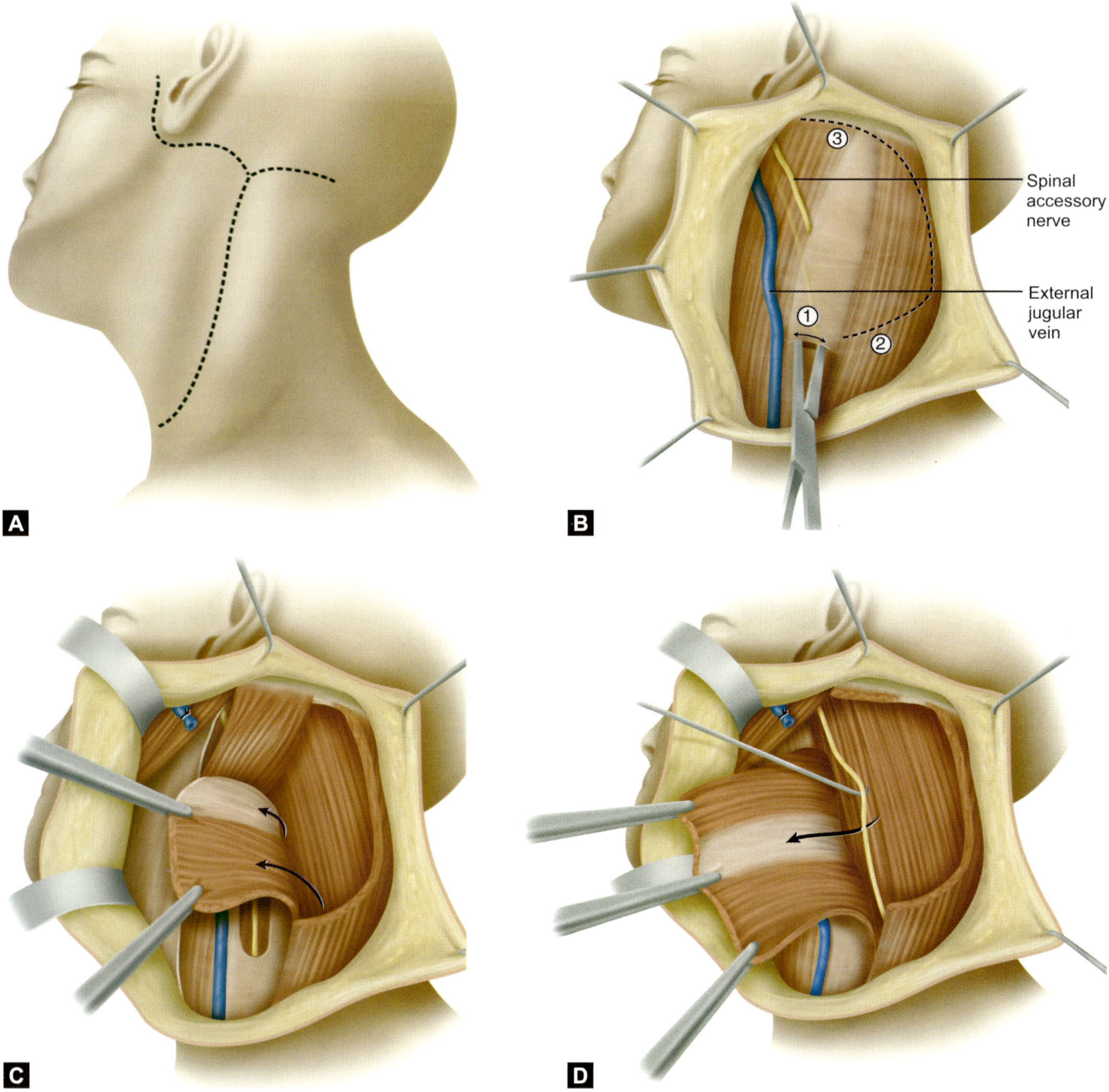

Figs. 18.6A to D: Steps to performing a posterolateral neck dissection. (A) Planned incision (hockey stick or S). (B) Elevation of platysma muscle. (C) Elevation of the trapezius flap and en bloc resection of lymphatic tissue. (D) Fully dissected visceral compartment of the neck.

Central Neck Dissection (Levels VI–VII)

Indications for a CND include high-grade thyroid carcinoma as well as advanced neck disease (laryngeal, esophageal, and tracheal cancer). Therapeutic neck dissections in thyroid cancer are recommended for patients with documented metastatic disease based on imaging and/or cytologic evaluation by fine-needle aspiration of involved lymph nodes. The rationale for a standardized compartment-oriented central neck dissection is that it may decrease the risk of recurrent thyroid cancer within the central neck.[21,22]

After induction with general anesthesia, the patient is placed in the supine position and a viscoelastic polymer shoulder roll is placed to increase neck extension and maximize surgical exposure. Both upper extremities should be appropriately tucked and cushioned on the patient's side. The use of a nerve-monitoring system may be a helpful adjunct to test the electrophysiologic integrity of the RLN before commencing dissection on the contralateral side or in reoperative cases where scar tissue makes identification difficult. The patient is then prepped locally with a povidone–iodine solution and draped in a sterile fashion. A standard Kocher thyroidectomy incision within a natural skin crease provides sufficient exposure for dissection. The initial incision, planned with a marking pen, can be made with a knife, followed by electrocautery to begin flap elevation. Skin flaps are raised superiorly to the thyroid notch and inferiorly to the sternal notch, respectively. The fascial plane between the sternohyoid and sternothyroid muscles is divided in order to maximize lateral retraction. For reoperative cases, due to the degree of fibrosis, the strap muscles can be divided horizontally, or resected to maximize lateral exposure (Figs. 18.7A to C). The prelaryngeal lymph node, located anterior to the cricothyroid membrane, is usually encountered at the level of the thyroid pyramidal lobe and isthmus. The carotid artery is identified on either side and is skeletonized from the level of the thyroid cartilage down to the clavicle. The paratracheal lymph nodes are then separated from the carotid sheath, and the dissection line is extended inferiorly to the level of the innominate artery.

Given that the superior boundary of the central neck compartment is the hyoid bone, lymph nodes are not usually found above the junction of the inferior thyroid artery and the RLN as it enters the cricothyroid membrane. Radiographic imaging and/or direct visualization intra-operatively is usually helpful in determining if this region requires dissection.

Dissection for the right and left central neck compartment differ slightly due to the anatomical course of the RLN. Since the right RLN travels around the subclavian artery, lymph nodes are present both anterior and posterior to the right RLN, dividing the right paratracheal lymph nodes into two compartments. Using a fine-tipped instrument, careful dissection of lymph-bearing tissue is completed along the course of the RLN both anteriorly and posteriorly to the level of the clavicle. The posterior compartment lymph nodes are then mobilized anteriorly and transposed under the nerve using a nerve hook. The lymphatic tissue inferior to the inferior thyroid artery and deep to the RLN is then mobilized off the prevertebral fascia and esophagus. This dissection should be carried down to the level of the innominate artery to incorporate the superior mediastinal lymph nodes with the paratracheal lymph nodes. In addition, especially in larger patients, the upper pleural membrane is sometimes visible posterior to the lymphatic tissue, warranting careful dissection in this area to avoid an iatrogenic pneumothorax.

In contrast, the left RLN travels around the aortic arch and travels along the tracheoesophageal groove. Unlike the right side, there typically is a paucity of lymph nodes deep to the left RLN, which can be dissected once the paratracheal nodes are separated from the carotid sheath as described earlier. Dissection of the left superior mediastinal lymph nodes should be carried out in a similar fashion as described above for the right superior mediastinal lymph nodes. The excised tissue should be marked and/or separated according to nodal level and submitted for permanent pathologic evaluation. The deep layers are carefully reapproximated using 3-4 Vicryl sutures. The skin is closed with 4–5 Prolene sutures or staples. The incision is appropriately cleaned with a moist sponge, and topical antibiotic ointment is applied. The surgeon should ensure that the drainage bulbs can hold appropriate suction as well as apply gentle pressure to the incision with a towel to minimize the risk of a hematoma during extubation.

COMPLICATIONS

Hematoma

Postoperative hematoma usually occurs within the first 24 hours and may result in a life-threatening situation. The hemorrhage may originate from sutured incisional wounds, a mucosal surface in the mouth, pharynx or larynx, and/or major vessels inadequately ligated intra-operatively. It is important to appreciate that bleeding into upper aerodigestive tract may compromise the patency of the airway, either by direct obstruction or as a result of aspiration of blood into the respiratory tract. The potential for a hematoma is highest at extubation, where patients may experience extensive coughing and increased intra-thoracic pressures. Hence, gentle pressure at the incision site with a towel is recommended as primary means of prevention during extubation and emergence from anesthesia. Surgical exploration for evacuation of clots and control of the bleeding vessel are best accomplished in the operating room.[10,17] Conservative management includes regularly "milking" drains as well as pressure dressings.

Chylous Fistula

Postoperative chyle leaks can occur through thoracic duct injury as well as arterial and venous bleeding due to inadequate vessel ligation intraoperatively. A simple Valsalva maneuver prior to wound closure can confirm vessel patency as well as any potential compromised sources. Otherwise, conservative management includes closed wound drainage, pressure dressings, somatostatin and a low-fat diet. However, large chyle leaks

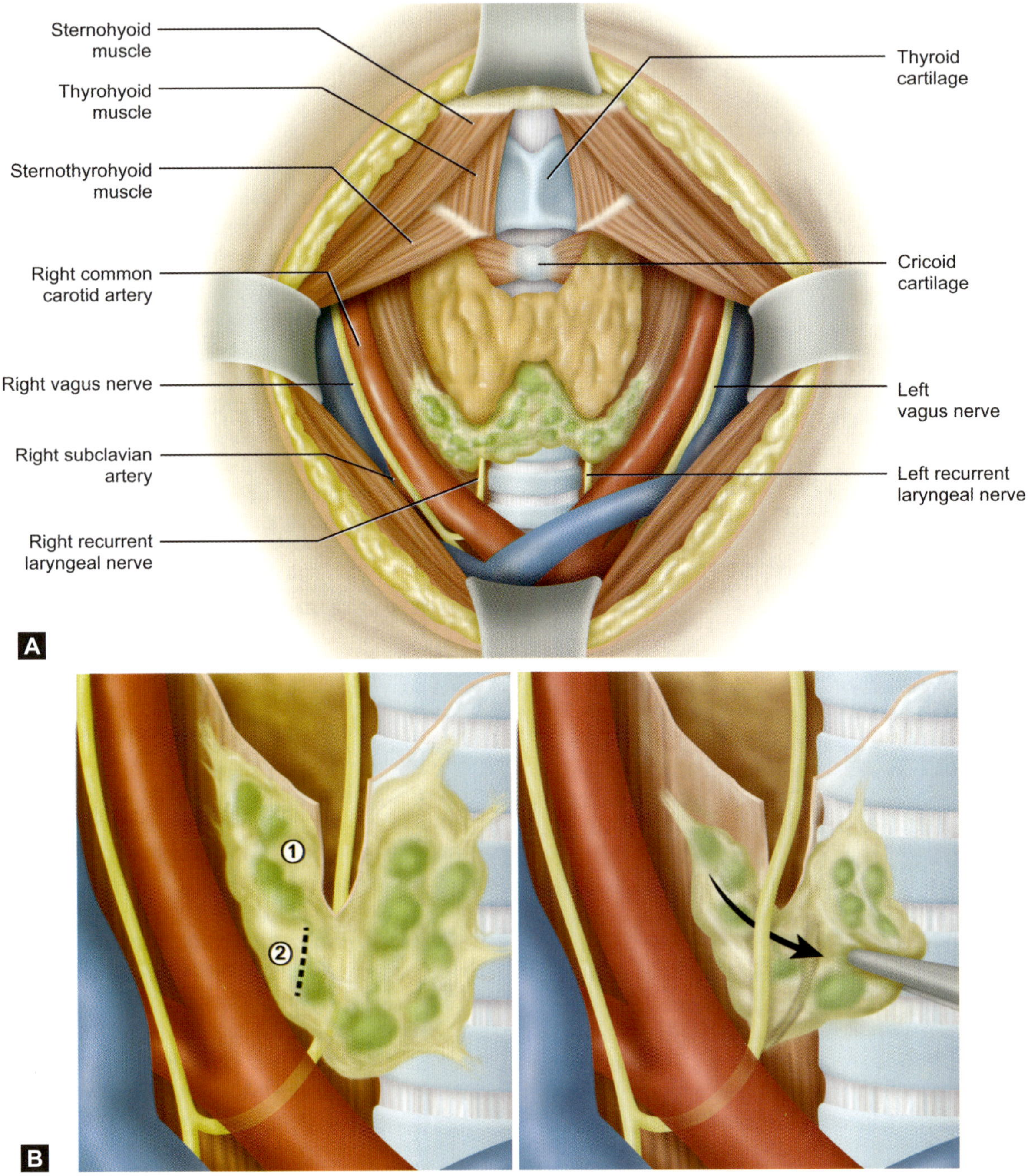

Figs. 18.7A and B: Steps to performing a central neck dissection. (A) Central compartment anatomy. (B) Dissection of central neck compartment along the right RLN, exposing the paratracheal lymph nodes. After carefully freeing the posterior lymphatics, they are transposed under the RLN and swept anteriorly.

CHAPTER

19

Thyroidectomy

Neerav Goyal, Darrin V Bann, David Goldenberg

INTRODUCTION

The thyroid, so named for being "shield shaped", is one of the larger endocrine glands and plays a key role in regulating metabolism by secreting tri-iodothyronine (T_3) and thyroxine (T_4). The gland is composed of both follicular and parafollicular (or "C cells") cells. This chapter will focus on the surgical treatment of pathology arising from these cells.

ANATOMY AND EMBRYOLOGY

The thyroid is a butterfly-shaped organ that normally weighs between 15 and 25 g, although the weight and size of the gland may vary considerably. It is composed of two lobes that lie on either side of the trachea and the isthmus, which overlies the anterior trachea, and joins the lobes. Each lobe measures approximately 4 cm in length and 2 cm in width in the normal patient.[1] Female patients generally have heavier and larger thyroid glands, which further enlarge during pregnancy.

The follicular cells of the thyroid are derived from a median diverticulum of the pharyngeal floor—the foramen cecum—between the 3rd and 4th weeks. The foramen cecum develops caudal to the first pharyngeal arch and rostral to the second pharyngeal pouch and grows inferiorly and posteriorly as a tubular duct called the thyroglossal duct. By the 7th week, the thyroid gland descends anterior and inferior to the hyoid bone, thyroid cartilage and cricoid cartilage to rest anterior to the trachea. Between the 7th and 10th weeks the thyroglossal duct degenerates, although the inferior-most aspect of this structure may persist in up to 50% of patients as the pyramidal lobe of the isthmus. During development, the ultimobranchial bodies from the fifth pharyngeal pouches are enveloped by the thyroid lobe and develop into the parafollicular cells. Figure 19.1 demonstrates the embryology and formation of the thyroid gland.[2-4]

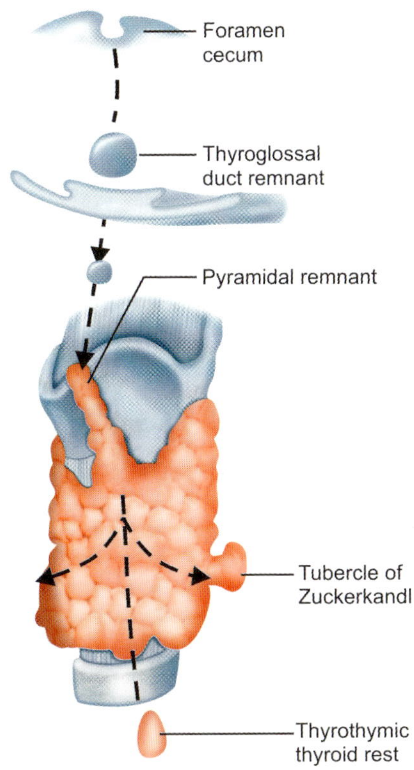

Fig. 19.1: Embryology and formation of the thyroid gland. The thyroid develops caudal to the first pharyngeal arch and rostral to the second pharyngeal pouch, growing inferiorly and posteriorly as a tubular duct called the thyroglossal duct. By the 7th week, the thyroid gland descends anterior and inferior to the hyoid bone, thyroid cartilage, and cricoid cartilages to rest anterior to the trachea.

The thyroid gland lies in the middle layer of the deep cervical fascia and is attached to the thyroid and cricoid cartilages via an anterior suspensory ligament and to the

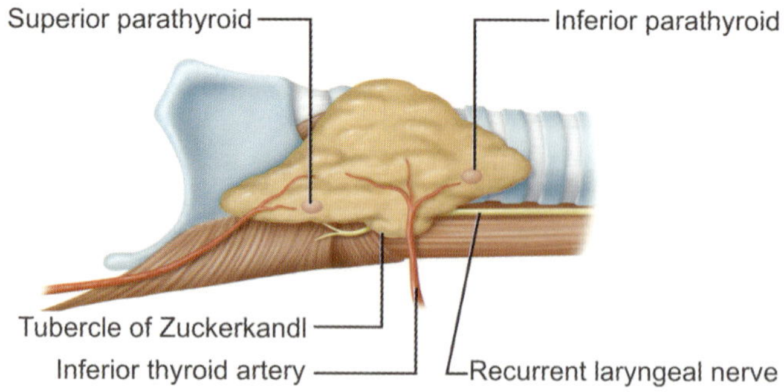

Fig. 19.2: The tubercle of Zuckerkandl marks the posterolateral aspect of the thyroid lobe and is most often found lateral to the recurrent laryngeal nerve. The tubercle can be found in 80% of thyroids and when found can lead directly to the recurrent laryngeal nerve, as 93% of the nerves are found medial to this tubercle. Most often, the nerve is found in a groove between the tubercle and the lobe of the thyroid gland.

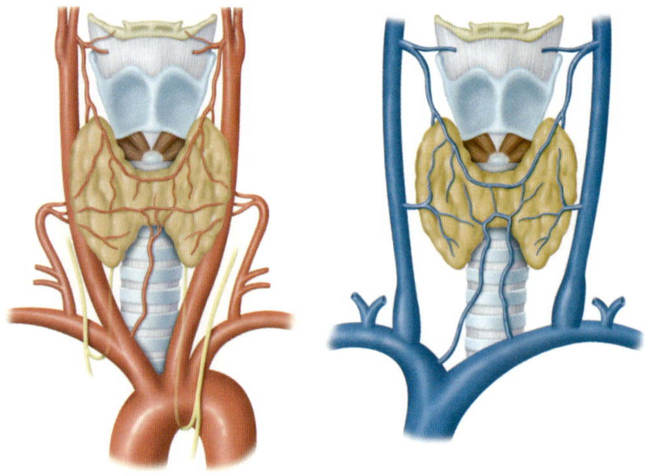

Fig. 19.3: The vascular supply and venous drainage of the thyroid gland.

first and second tracheal rings and the cricoid cartilage via a posterior suspensory ligament (Berry's ligament).[5] The thyroid lies anterior to the pretracheal fascia and trachea and posterior to the sternohyoid and sternothyroid muscles. There is often a slight outgrowth of thyroid tissue at the posterolateral aspect of each thyroid lobe referred to as the tubercule of Zuckerkandl (Fig. 19.2).[3,6]

The gland is innervated by sympathetic fibers from the superior, middle, and inferior cervical ganglia and parasympathetic fibers from the vagus nerve.[2,4] The vascular supply to the thyroid consists of the superior and inferior thyroid arteries, which are derived from the external carotid artery and the thyrocervical trunk, respectively (Fig. 19.3). In 2–12% of patients, the thyroidea ima artery supplies the thyroid through the inferior border of the isthmus. This artery may arise from the innominate artery, subclavian artery, right common carotid artery, the internal mammary artery, or may branch directly from the aortic arch (Fig. 19.3). Vascular outflow from the thyroid is provided by the superior, middle, and inferior thyroid veins, which drain into either the internal jugular or innominate veins (Fig. 19.3). Typical lymphatic drainage is to the prelaryngeal, pretracheal, paratracheal, and supraclavicular nodes (Fig. 19.4).[3,4]

In discussing the anatomy of the thyroid, it is also crucial to discuss the anatomy of the recurrent laryngeal nerve (RLN), as the nerve runs in close proximity to the gland and is an important structure to identify and preserve during surgery. Embryologically, the nerve is associated with the sixth branchial arch, and branches off of the vagus nerve to innervate the muscles of the larynx. As the larynx ascends during fetal development, the sixth aortic arch persists on the left as the ductus arteriosus and right sixth aortic arch degenerates. As such, the RLN on the left loops around the aorta. On the right, however, the nerve recurs around the subclavian artery, which is derived from the fourth branchial arch. With aberrant vascular formation, such as an aberrant right subclavian artery, it is possible for the right RLN nerve to be nonrecurrent, which occurs in 0.5–1% of the population.[3]

The left RLN tends to be more closely approximated to the trachea within the tracheoesophageal groove as compared to the right nerve. In addition, the right nerve travels in a more anterior plane and tends to have a thicker fascia overlying it. In half the population, the nerve is found within the tracheoesophageal groove, and in the remaining population it may lie slightly anterior or posterior to the groove.[3] The RLNs tend to be intimately related to Berry's ligament, and also tend to lie just medial to the tubercle of Zuckerkandl.[3,5,6] The nerves are also closely related to the inferior thyroid artery, although they can lie either superficial or deep to the artery (Fig. 19.5).[24-26]

The external branch of the superior laryngeal nerve innervates the cricothyroid muscle. On either side of the trachea, it follows closely with the superior laryngeal artery and vein and courses near the superior pole of each thyroid lobe. The distance between the nerve and the superior pole of the thyroid is variable, although between 23% and 42% of identified nerves are located at least 1 cm superior to the superior pole. In the remaining instances, the superior laryngeal nerve is < 1 cm cranial to the superior pole, with 14-54% of nerves found deep to the superior pole of the thyroid.[7]

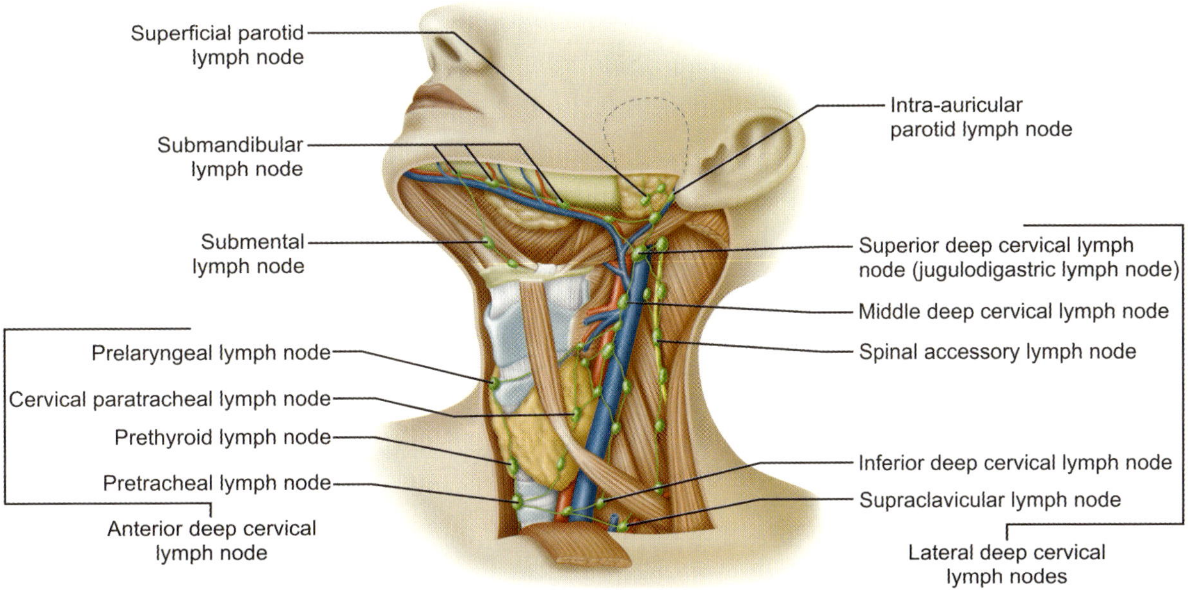

Fig. 19.4: Lymphatic drainage of the thyroid gland.

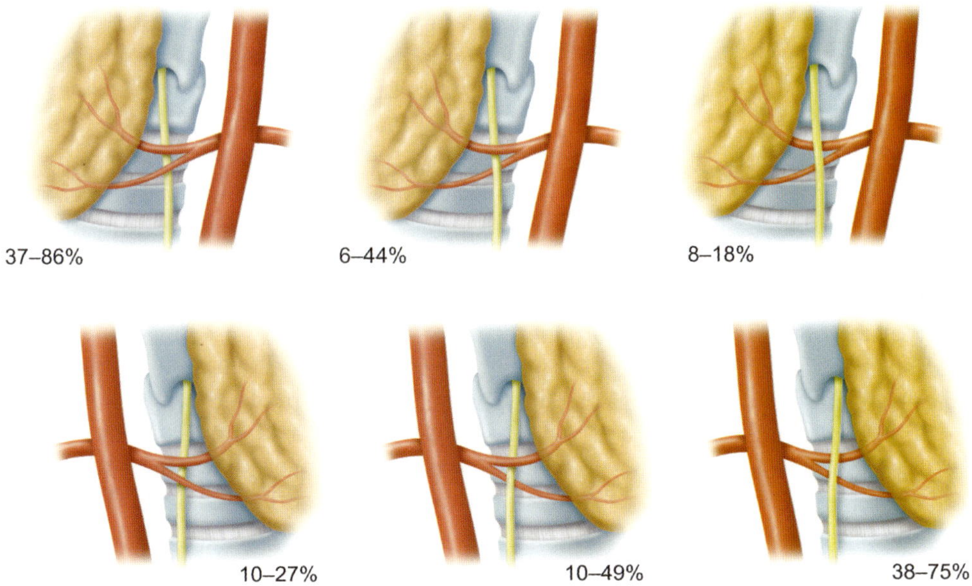

Fig. 19.5: Relationship variants between the recurrent laryngeal nerve and inferior thyroid artery.

INDICATIONS AND CONTRAINDICATIONS FOR SURGERY

Indications for thyroid surgery include thyroid cancer, hyperthyroidism (Graves disease), thyroid masses (or nodules), and goiters. Although the diagnosis and evaluation of thyroid cancer is beyond the scope of this chapter, thyroid cancer is most often diagnosed by fine-needle aspiration biopsy of a thyroid nodule identified on examination or by imaging. A total thyroidectomy is indicated in patients with medullary thyroid cancer and for most papillary thyroid cancers. Current research suggests performing a hemithyroidectomy for patients with a single focus of papillary microcarcinomas (in a thyroid nodule <10 mm in size).[8,9] For patients with follicular or Hürthle cell lesions on fine-needle aspiration, a hemithyroidectomy is indicated with the possibility of a completion thyroidectomy if the pathology of the operative specimen indicates malignancy. Fifteen to thirty percent of fine-needle aspiration biopsy specimens fall into the "indeterminate" category. In this category there are three subgroups: (1) atypical, (2) follicular neoplasm, and (3) suspicious for cancer. Various molecular diagnostic procedures are now being used to clarify whether the indeterminate category represents malignant or benign disease and to determine whether a thyroidectomy is appropriate therapy.

For patients with hyperthyroidism refractory to medical treatment, a subtotal or total thyroidectomy is a viable option, rendering the patient iatrogenically hypothyroid after surgery. However, uncontrolled hyperthyroidism is a relative contraindication to surgery due to the risk of developing intraoperative or postoperative thyroid storm.

Patients who present with symptoms of dysphagia, dyspnea, shortness of breath, and/or hoarseness thought to be secondary to compression from a large goiter are also candidates for removal of the goiter via thyroid lobectomy or total thyroidectomy. Often, dysphagia to solids is the earliest presenting symptom. Occasionally, patients will present with solely aesthetic concerns regarding a large goiter without overt compressive symptoms.

SURGICAL TECHNIQUE

The technique described below is performed under general anesthesia and refers to the capsular dissection of a thyroid lobe, which can be mirrored for a total thyroidectomy. A variety of instrumentation is available to perform the blunt and sharp dissection described in this procedure, including sharp dissection with suture ligation of vessels, electric cautery, and ultrasonic scalpels.

Prior to making the incision, it is important to extend the neck to maximize access to the thyroid. This can be achieved by placing a roll underneath the scapula. For the initial incision, the authors typically plan a traditional collar incision (Fig. 19.6), which is created in a curvilinear fashion across the midline within a skin crease approximately two finger breadths (2 cm) above the superior edge of the clavicle and sternal notch. A variety of incision lengths are described in the literature; however, in the authors' experience a length between 6 and 8 cm allows for adequate exposure while minimizing stretch injury to the surrounding skin. In addition, some researchers suggest that the use of smaller cervical incisions for thyroidectomy does not result in significant improvements in patient satisfaction.[10-12]

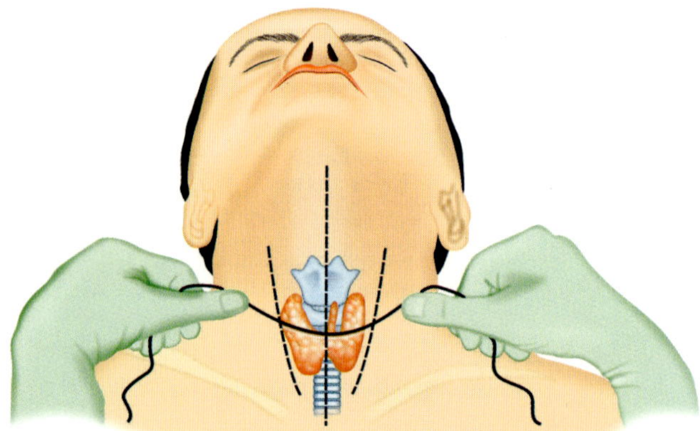

Fig. 19.6: Kocher incision.

After marking the planned skin incision and injecting local anesthetic, the skin is incised with a #15 blade through the epidermis and dermis. Dissection proceeds through the subcutaneous fat to identify the platysma, which is often partially dehiscent in the midline. The platysma is incised in a transverse plane, and subplatysmal flaps are raised superiorly and inferiorly, allowing for adequate exposure from the cricoid to the sternal notch. Care is taken not to disrupt the anterior jugular veins, although these veins may be ligated should increased exposure become necessary. After raising the subplatysmal flaps, the authors use a self-retaining retractor, such as a Mahorner thyroid retractor or a Gelpi retractor, which is placed in the subplatysmal plane and allows for maximal exposure.

The cervical linea alba is the decussation of the fascia between the paired sternothyroid and sternohyoid muscles (Fig. 19.7). Dissection is carried through this line, separating the strap muscles laterally, down to the thyroid capsule. To reduce bleeding, the authors will often use bipolar cautery to ligate any larger veins evident on the thyroid capsule.

Once the thyroid capsule is exposed, the authors proceed in a systematic fashion by first identifying the lateral border of the thyroid, then identifying and taking down the attachments at the superior pole, elevating the thyroid lobe medially, identifying the RLN, and then removing the specimen (in the case of a hemithyroidectomy).

Dissection toward the lateral border of the thyroid is carried out using a combination of blunt dissection and electrocautery or an ultrasonic scalpel. Any large veins are addressed as they are encountered to reduce the risk of bleeding during the operation. Usually, the carotid artery

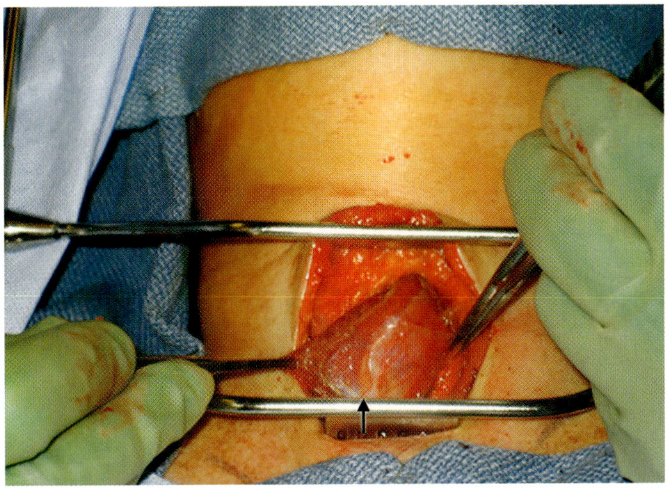

Fig. 19.7: The cervical linea alba (arrow).

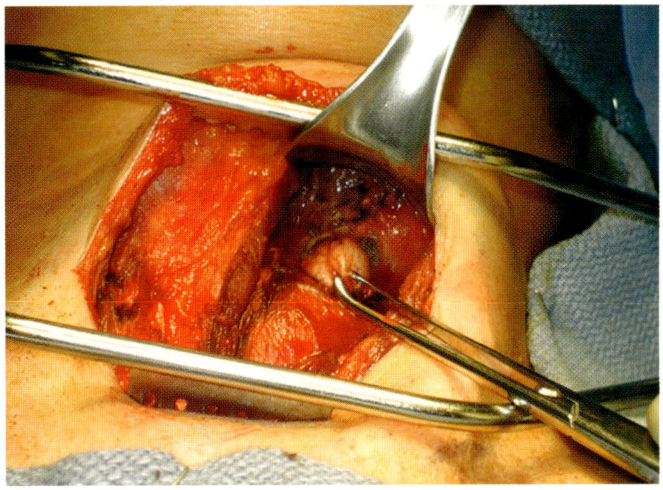

Fig. 19.8: Intraoperative photograph showing an upward and lateral retraction of the strap muscles and a downward and medial retraction of the superior pole of the thyroid, allowing for easy visualization of the superior thyroid artery.

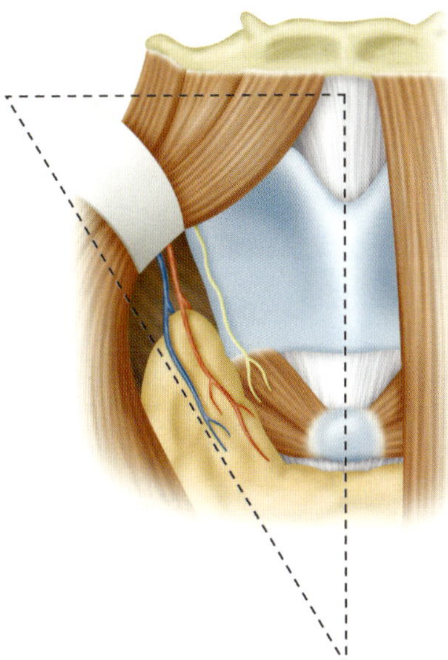

Fig. 19.9: Joll's triangle is formed by the midline of the trachea medially, the strap musculature superiorly and laterally, and the superior pole and pedicle of the thyroid lobe inferiorly and laterally. The floor is defined by the cricothyroid muscle.

is identified just adjacent and lateral to the lateral edge of the thyroid lobe. With larger or more nodular lobes, it is often helpful to transect the sternothyroid and sternohyoid muscles to provide additional exposure. The authors often use the ultrasonic scalpel to divide the muscles, which are reapproximated at the end of the procedure.

After identifying the lateral border of the sternothyroid muscle, a retractor is placed underneath the muscle near its superior attachment. With a superior vector of retraction, the superior pole of the thyroid lobe is easily visualized. To assist with the dissection, the authors will retract the thyroid lobe inferiorly with the use of an Allis clamp (Fig.19.8). The pole is then freed from its medial and lateral facial attachments. Joll's triangle, defined by the tracheal midline, the strap muscles and the superior pole and pedicle of the thyroid, is a useful landmark to identify the external branch of the superior laryngeal nerve (Fig. 19.9). The superior thyroid artery and vein are then dissected out and isolated before being ligated, either with a suture or with the ultrasonic scalpel. Care is taken to preserve the superior laryngeal nerve. The superior parathyroid can be identified adjacent and often superior to the superior pole.

Next, a second Allis clamp is placed on the inferolateral aspect of the thyroid lobe and the thyroid lobe is retracted medially. Often, the middle thyroid vein is encountered during this maneuver and can be safely ligated. Using blunt dissection, the posterior aspect of the thyroid lobe is elevated. The inferior thyroid vein can be visualized near the inferior pole of the gland. The inferior parathyroid gland is frequently identified superficial to the inferior thyroid vein.

The next step is to identify the RLN. A variety of landmarks have been described in the literature to identify the nerve (Table 19.1). The recurrent laryngeal nerve forms one side of Beahrs triangle with the common carotid and inferior thyroid artery forming the other two sides (Fig. 19.10). Simon's triangle refers to an imaginary triangle

Table 19.1: Landmarks for identifying the recurrent laryngeal nerve (RLN).

- The tubercle of Zuckerkandl—most often, the nerve is found medial and deep to the tubercle (*see* Fig. 19.2)
- Berry's ligament can be used for identification, since the nerves are found in close proximity to the ligament (warning—various anatomic relationships between the two structures)
- Simon's triangle: triangle bordered by the common carotid artery, the inferior thyroid artery, and the esophagus
- The inferior thyroid artery can also be used as a landmark for the RLN, with its close association with the pathway of the nerve. (Warning—variations exist, branches of the inferior thyroid artery may be anterior or posterior to the nerve, or the nerve can run in between the branches of the artery) (*see* Fig. 19.5)
- Beahrs triangle—RLN forms the third side of a triangle formed by the common carotid artery and the inferior thyroid artery low in the tracheoesophageal groove (Fig. 19.10)
- Relation to the cricothyroid joint: the RLN enters the larynx anteromedial to the cricothyroid joint

bordered by the common carotid artery, the inferior thyroid artery, and the esophagus.[27] The RLN runs within Simon's triangle toward the larynx.[3,13] Other landmarks include the tracheoesophageal groove, the ligament of Berry, and the tubercle of Zuckerkandl.[3,5,6] The RLN generally courses between the tubercle and the trachea. The authors use a combination of these landmarks, usually by first identifying the inferior thyroid artery and the tracheoesophageal groove, followed by elevating the tubercle of Zuckerkandl. Using this combination of landmarks allows increased accuracy in identifying the RLN, given variations in vascular and nervous anatomy within the population. After the nerve has been identified, it can be traced toward its insertion into the larynx. This ensures that the RLN remains protected and uninjured while removing the thyroid lobe.

Lastly, the ligament of Berry is divided close to its attachment to the thyroid capsule. After dividing the ligament, the lobe is only attached inferiorly and by the pretracheal fascia. If a hemithyroidectomy is being performed the inferior thyroid artery can be ligated, ensuring that the blood supply to the parathyroid glands

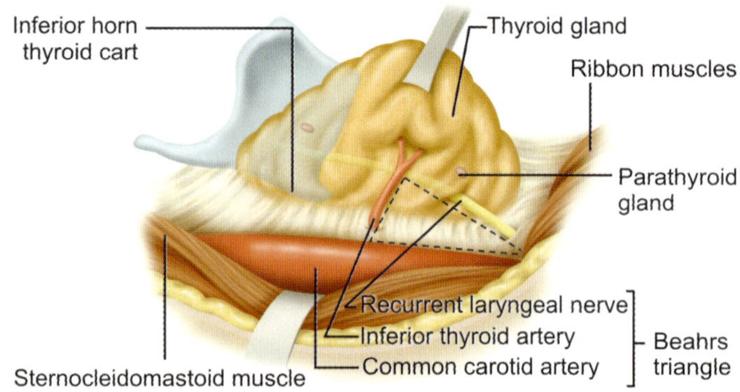

Fig. 19.10: The recurrent laryngeal nerve forms one side of Beahrs triangle with the common carotid and inferior thyroid artery forming the other two sides.

remains intact. The dissection can then proceed along the isthmus and the trachea, dividing the thyroid and removing the specimen from the wound. If a total thyroidectomy is indicated, the authors usually leave the isthmus attached, repeat the procedure for the contralateral lobe and subsequently dissect the entire specimen en bloc.

After removing the specimen, the authors will grossly inspect the specimen to ensure there was no iatrogenic amputation of a parathyroid gland. Should this occur, autoimplantation of the parathyroid can be performed into the sternocleidomastoid muscle. The explanted parathyroid gland is divided sharply into 15–20 pieces, which are implanted into a pocket made in the sternocleidomastoid. The implantation site is then marked with staples or nonabsorbable suture.

Minimally Invasive Approaches

Since the description of the capsular dissection by Halsted and Evans,[14] there have been a variety of modifications to the technique. One of the major areas of development has been to decrease the size of the neck incision. Initial techniques to reduce incision size involved the use of carbon dioxide insufflation in the neck, similar to abdominal laparoscopic procedures.[15,16] These techniques allow for a small incision (usually 15 mm in length) placed either at the sternal notch[16] or at the medial border of the sternocleidomastoid[17] for the larger trochar and specimen retrieval, with the use of additional trochars for instrumentation. Operative times vary, with average reported times between 98 and 220 minutes.[16,17] However, the insufflation technique has produced complications including hypercarbia and significant subcutaneous emphysema.[18]

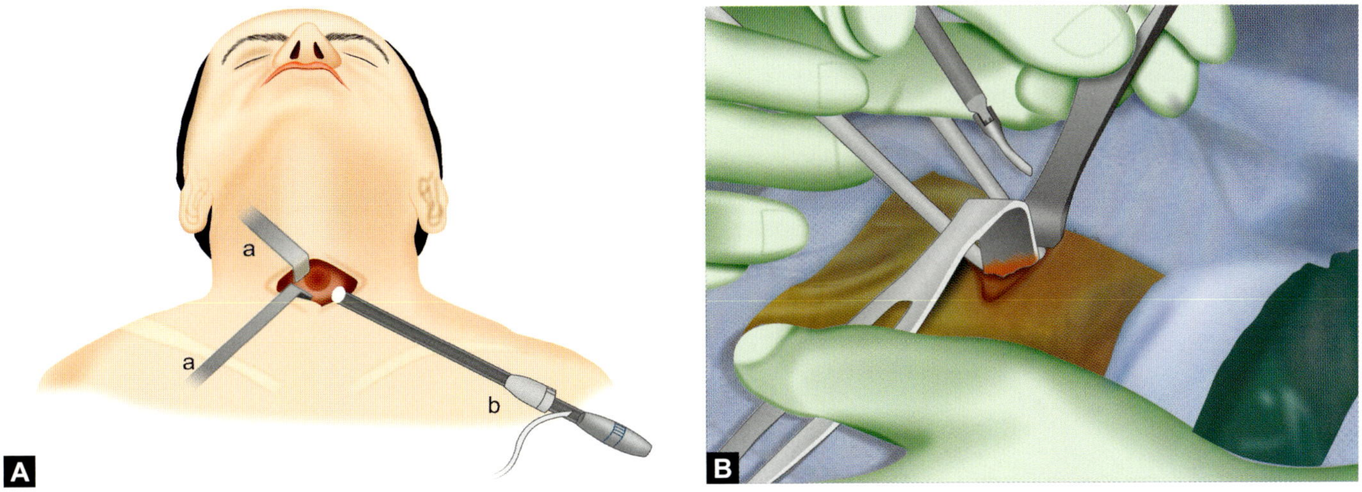

Figs. 19.11A and B: (A) Illustration of an endoscopic approach to the superior pole using retractors (a) and an endoscope (b). (B) Another illustration demonstrating lateral dissection with a combination of retractors, endoscope and an ultrasonic scalpel.

Miccoli et al. describe a minimally invasive video-assisted thyroidectomy approach, which uses a smaller cervical incision without insufflation.[19] In this technique, Miccoli and colleagues utilize an incision between 15 and 30 mm in length in a slightly superior location to a traditional collar incision. In addition, the patient's neck is less extended as compared to a conventional thyroidectomy. The thyroid capsule is approached in a similar fashion to a conventional thyroidectomy. After exposing the thyroid capsule, a 30° endoscope and specialized retractors and dissectors are used to identify and skeletonize the vessels of the superior pole. Figures 19.11A amd B display a schematic of how the instruments are oriented for the procedure. The ultrasonic scalpel is used to ligate these vessels, and the thryoidectomy proceeds with identification of the RLN and the parathyroids. Of note, the procedure requires a primary surgeon and two assistants, with one holding the retractors and the other maneuvering the endoscope. A multi-institutional study demonstrated a slightly longer operative time for the video-assisted approach compared to a conventional thyroidectomy as well as the increased costs of instrumentation and additional assistants. The study also describes criteria for appropriate patient selection for the procedure, including[19]:

- Thyroid nodule < 3.5 cm
- Absence of thyroiditis
- Thyroid volume < 15 mL
- Cytologic and clinical evidence of benign disease, follicular tumor, or low-risk papillary thyroid cancer.

Terris et al. describe a modification to the minimally invasive approach described by Miccoli et al. Their approach similarly requires a more superior incision compared to conventional thyroidectomy. With the Terris technique, a larger incision approximately 4-6 cm in length is used and the superior aspects of the strap muscles are transected to provide access to the superior poles of the thyroid lobes. However, similar to the Miccoli technique, endoscopes are used to assist with visualization and dissection.[20]

Substernal Goiter

The substernal goiter presents a significant challenge due to the size and location of the goiter. In the authors' experience, maximal exposure is necessary to ensure removal of the goiter, which can be facilitated by optimal extension of the neck. Often, these thyroid glands tend to be more vascular in nature, and therefore meticulous attention must be paid to hemostasis. Transecting the sternothyroid and sternohyoid muscles can greatly increase the exposure of the goiter. After identifying the lateral border and freeing the superior pole, dissection should be carried along the posterior aspect of the capsule to identify the RLN and parathyroid glands. Of note, the RLN can occasionally be displaced by a goiter, even such that the nerve is superficial to the goiter, as shown in Figure 19.12.[21-23] Once these borders have been freed, the inferior pole of the thyroid can usually be elevated into the surgical bed using digital dissection along the thyroid capsule (Fig. 19.13). Since the goiters originate in the neck, they do not usually have a mediastinal blood supply. Substernal goiters rarely require a sternotomy for removal.

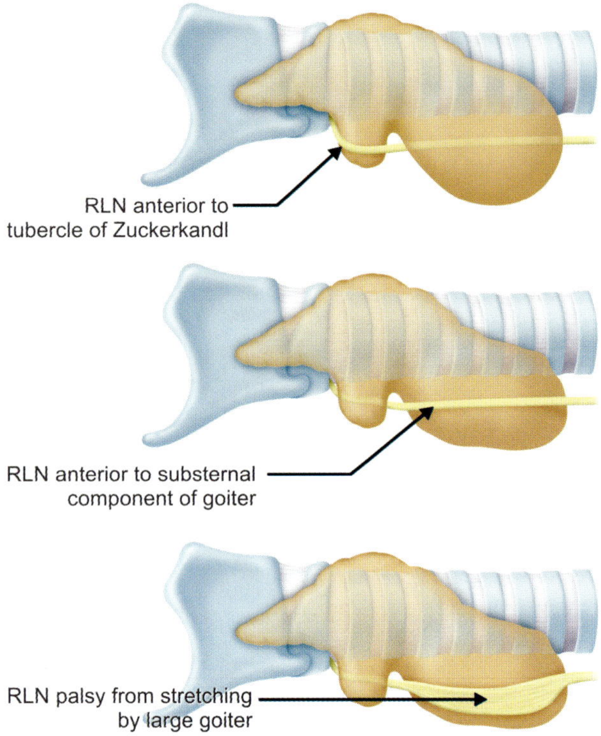

Fig. 19.12: Typically a goiter will lie superficial to the recurrent laryngeal nerve (RLN). Specific anatomic anomalies should be considered where (from top to bottom) the RLN lies anterior to the tubercle of Zuckerkandl and deep to the goiter, the RLN lies anterior to the substernal component of the goiter, and the RLN is stretched by the goiter.

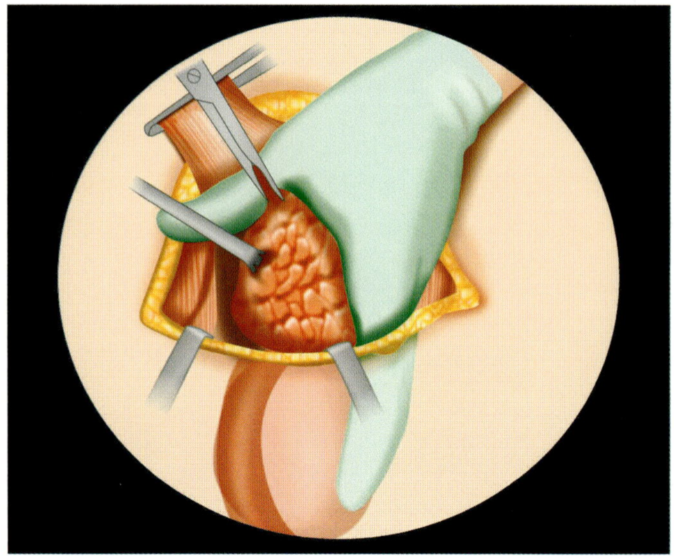

Fig. 19.13: Finger dissection can be used to bluntly dissect around goiters and help elevate them from below the sternum into the neck.

COMPLICATIONS

Recurrent Laryngeal Nerve Injury

Recurrent laryngeal nerve paralysis is a known and specific complication of thyroid surgery. RLN paralysis rates vary because many studies do not include postoperative laryngeal examination, which is essential to accurately determine postoperative RLN paralysis rates. The incidence of RLN paralysis increases with bilateral surgery, revision surgery, surgery for malignancy, surgery for postoperative substernal goiter, and in patients brought back to surgery for postoperative bleeding. Prevention is key in preventing RLN paralysis: the RLN should be clearly identified and dissected along its entire course at thyroidectomy, and identification should be made both visually and through neural electric stimulation. Such stimulation is safe and allows the surgeon to identify a neurapraxic nerve injury and potentially postpone contralateral thyroid surgery.[28]

In cases of unilateral vocal cord paralysis, corrective procedures may be delayed for 6 months to a year to allow time for improvement in a reversible injury, unless the nerve was known to be transected during surgery; bilateral paralyses may necessitate a tracheotomy.

Superior Laryngeal Nerve Injury

Injury to the external branch of the superior laryngeal nerve occurs in 0–25% of thyroidectomies. The superior laryngeal nerve is highly vulnerable during ligation of superior pedicle of thyroid gland. Trauma to the nerve results in an inability to lengthen a vocal fold and subsequent inability to create a high-pitched sound; this may particularly devastating for singers. On laryngoscopy, posterior glottic rotation toward the paretic side and bowing of the vocal fold on the weak side may be noted.

Hypoparathyroidism

Hypoparathyroidism may result from trauma to the parathyroid glands, devascularization of the glands, or avulsion of the glands during surgery. Temporary hypoparathyroidism, defined as < 6 months duration, occurs in 17–40% of patients after total thyroidectomy. Permanent hypoparathyroidism after total thyroidectomy occurs in up to 10% of patients. Hypoparathyroidism may be asymptomatic or may result in perioral and digital paresthesias. Progressive neuromuscular irritability results in spontaneous carpopedal spasm, abdominal cramps, laryngeal stridor, mental status changes, QT prolongation on the electrocardiogram, and ultimately tetanic contractions.

Evaluation of parathyroid function is performed by ionized calcium (or total calcium and albumin) levels perioperatively or by measuring PTH postoperatively; a normal level accurately predicts normocalcemia.

Postoperative Bleeding

The incidence of bleeding after thyroid surgery is low (0.3–1%), but an unrecognized or rapidly expanding hematoma can cause airway compromise and asphyxiation. No evidence suggests that the usage of drains prevents the formation of a hematoma or seroma. A drain, if placed, is not a substitute for intraoperative hemostasis. Postoperative bleeding may present with neck swelling, neck pain, or signs and symptoms of airway obstruction (e.g. dyspnea, stridor, hypoxia). Any patient presenting with these symptoms after thyroidectomy should be immediately examined for evidence of hematoma. If a neck hematoma is causing airway compromise, open the surgical incision at the bedside to release the collection of blood and immediately transfer the patient to the operating room.

In the case of a hematoma without impending airway obstruction, transfer the patient to the operating room as soon as is practical. Remain with the patient and be prepared to assist with airway management as direct visualization of the glottis may be difficult in these cases.

Infection

Currently, postoperative infection occurs in < 1–2% of all thyroid surgery cases.

Seroma

Postoperative surgical site seromas may be followed clinically and allowed to resorb if small and asymptomatic. Large seromas may be aspirated under sterile conditions.

CONCLUSION

The thyroid gland is derived from the foramen cecum and is positioned anterior to the trachea and inferior to the thyroid and cricoid cartilages. For both benign and malignant disease processes, either a thyroid lobectomy or total thyroidectomy may be indicated. When performing a thyroidectomy, care must be taken to identify and protect the recurrent laryngeal nerve, which innervates the muscles of the larynx. Fortunately, a variety of landmarks can be used to assist with the identification and preservation of the nerve (Table 19.1). One of the most serious complications from the procedure is injury to the recurrent laryngeal nerve, resulting in hoarseness (if unilateral) or airway obstruction (if bilateral). Additionally, although the incidence of postoperative bleeding is low, a rapidly expanding hematoma can cause significant airway obstruction. Therefore, any patient presenting with neck pain, swelling, or symptoms of airway obstruction after thyroidectomy must be evaluated immediately. With good exposure and knowledge of anatomy, a thyroidectomy can be performed safely with a low risk of complications.

REFERENCES

1. Mohebati A, Shaha AR. Anatomy of thyroid and parathyroid glands and neurovascular relations. Clin Anat N Y N. 2012;25(1):19-31.
2. Gray H, Standring S. Gray's Anatomy: The Anatomical Basis of Clinical Practice. Edinburgh: Churchill Livingstone Elsevier; 2008.
3. Fancy T, Gallagher D, 3rd, Hornig JD. Surgical anatomy of the thyroid and parathyroid glands. Otolaryngol Clin North Am. 2010;43(2):221-7, vii.
4. Bliss RD, Gauger PG, Delbridge LW. Surgeon's approach to the thyroid gland: surgical anatomy and the importance of technique. World J Surg. 2000;24(8):891-7.
5. Leow CK, Webb AJ. The lateral thyroid ligament of Berry. Int Surg. 1998;83(1):75-8.
6. Yun J-S, Lee YS, Jung JJ, et al. The Zuckerkandl's tubercle: a useful anatomical landmark for detecting both the recurrent laryngeal nerve and the superior parathyroid during thyroid surgery. Endocr J. 2008;55(5):925-30.
7. Kochilas X, Bibas A, Xenellis J, et al. Surgical anatomy of the external branch of the superior laryngeal nerve and its clinical significance in head and neck surgery. Clin Anat NYN. 2008;21(2):99-105.
8. Wu AW, Wang MB, Nguyen CT. Surgical practice patterns in the treatment of papillary thyroid microcarcinoma. Arch Otolaryngol Head Neck Surg. 2010;136(12):1182-90.
9. Gershinsky M, Barnett-Griness O, Stein N, et al. Total versus hemithyroidectomy for microscopic papillary thyroid cancer. J Endocrinol Invest. 2012;35(5):464-8.
10. Linos D, Economopoulos KP, Kiriakopoulos A, et al. Scar perceptions after thyroid and parathyroid surgery: comparison of minimal and conventional approaches. Surgery. 2013;153(3):400-7.
11. O'Connell DA, Diamond C, Seikaly H, et al. Objective and subjective scar aesthetics in minimal access vs conventional access parathyroidectomy and thyroidectomy surgical procedures: a paired cohort study. Arch Otolaryngol Head Neck Surg. 2008;134(1):85-93.

12. Toll EC, Loizou P, Davis CR, et al. Scars and satisfaction: do smaller scars improve patient-reported outcome? Eur Arch Oto-Rhino-Laryngol. 2012;269(1):309-13.
13. Khatri VP. Operative Surgery Manual. Philadelphia, PA: Saunders; 2003. p. 332.
14. Halsted WS, Evans HM. I. The parathyroid glandules. Their blood supply and their preservation in operation upon the thyroid gland. Ann Surg. 1907;46(4):489-506.
15. Hüscher CS, Chiodini S, Napolitano C, et al. Endoscopic right thyroid lobectomy. Surg Endosc. 1997;11(8):877.
16. Gagner M, Inabnet WB, 3rd. Endoscopic thyroidectomy for solitary thyroid nodules. Thyroid Off J Am Thyroid Assoc. 2001;11(2):161-3.
17. Henry J-F. Minimally invasive surgery of the thyroid and parathyroid glands. Br J Surg. 2006;93(1):1-2.
18. Linos D. Minimally invasive thyroidectomy: a comprehensive appraisal of existing techniques. Surgery. 2011;150(1): 17-24.
19. Miccoli P, Berti P, Conte M, et al. Minimally invasive surgery for thyroid small nodules: preliminary report. J Endocrinol Invest. 1999;22(11):849-51.
20. Terris DJ, Bonnett A, Gourin CG, et al. Minimally invasive thyroidectomy using the Sofferman technique. Laryngoscope. 2005;115(6):1104-8.
21. Fritts L, Thompson NW. The surgical treatment of substernal goiter. Oper Tech Otolaryngol-Head Neck Surg. 1994; 5(3):179-88.
22. Maruotti RA, Zannini P, Viani MP, et al. Surgical treatment of substernal goiters. Int Surg. 1991;76(1):12-7.
23. Gurleyik E. Two cases of enlarged Zuckerkandl's tubercle of the thyroid displacing the recurrent laryngeal nerve laterally. Case Rep Med. 2011;2011:303861.
24. Campos BA, Henriques PR. Relationship between the recurrent laryngeal nerve and the inferior thyroid artery: a study in corpses. Rev Hosp Clínicas. 2000;55(6):195–200.
25. Kulekci M, Batioglu-Karaaltin A, Saatci O, Uzun I. Relationship between the branches of the recurrent laryngeal nerve and the inferior thyroid artery. Ann Otol Rhinol Laryngol. 2012;121(10):650–6.
26. Tang W-J, Sun S-Q, Wang X-L, et al. An applied anatomical study on the recurrent laryngeal nerve and inferior thyroid artery. Surg Radiol Anat. 2012;34(4):325–32.
27. Simon MM. RLN in thyroid surgery: triangle for its recognition and protection. Am J Surg. 1943;60:212-22.
28. Goldenberg D, Randolph G. Thyroid and parathyroid glands. In: Lee KJ (Ed.). Essential Otolaryngology Head and Neck Surgery, 10th ed. New York: McGraw-Hill; 2011.

CHAPTER

20

Parathyroid Surgery

Darrin V Bann, Neerav Goyal, David Goldenberg

The parathyroid glands exhibit variation in anatomical location and number,[1-3] so successful parathyroid surgery requires an intimate knowledge of parathyroid anatomy, as well as an understanding of the typical and atypical locations of the parathyroid glands. In this light, preoperative studies are focused on identifying the location of abnormal parathyroid tissue (in the case of primary hyperparathyroidism), while the procedure itself is best thought of as a systematic exploration of the anterior neck with a focus on distinguishing parathyroid tissue from the surrounding fat and lymphatics. The goal of this chapter is therefore not to discuss the merits and drawbacks of various approaches to parathyroid surgery, but rather to provide a broad overview of the surgical management of parathyroid disease.

ANATOMY AND EMBRYOLOGY

The parathyroid glands are two sets of small (approximately 6 × 3.5 × 1.5 mm), paired, yellow-brown glands typically located near the thyroid. Embryologically, the superior parathyroid glands are derived from the fourth pharyngeal pouch. The superior parathyroid glands typically exhibit less anatomic variation than the inferior glands, and 80% of superior parathyroid glands are found at the cricothyroid junction, approximately 1 cm superior to where the recurrent laryngeal nerve crosses the inferior thyroid artery. However, it should be noted that in approximately 1% of the population, normal superior parathyroid glands may be located in the paraesophageal or retroesophageal space, allowing these glands to descend into the anterior or posterior mediastinum (Fig. 20.1).[4-6]

The inferior parathyroid glands and the thymus are derived from the third pharyngeal pouch and exhibit more anatomical variation than the superior parathyroid glands. During development the inferior glands migrate caudally with the thymus until they reach their final position, which in 50% of patients is within 1 cm lateral, inferior, or posterior to the inferior pole of the thyroid.[7] Alternatively, the inferior parathyroids may fail to descend and instead remain near the carotid bifurcation, or may descend into the mediastinum with the thymus (Fig. 20.1). Most commonly, ectopic inferior parathyroid glands may be found within the thyrothymic ligament or within the superior thymus gland. Vascular supply to both the superior

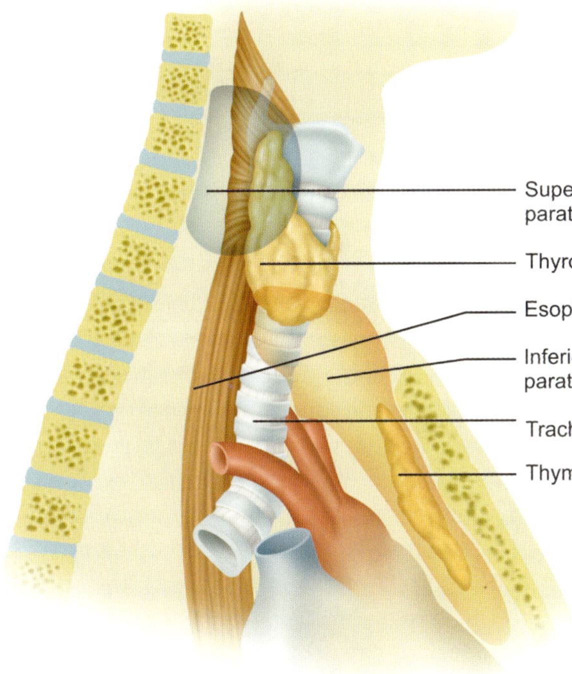

Fig. 20.1: Migration patterns of the parathyroid glands. Shaded areas on the sagittal sections indicate the most likely location for the superior and inferior parathyroid glands.

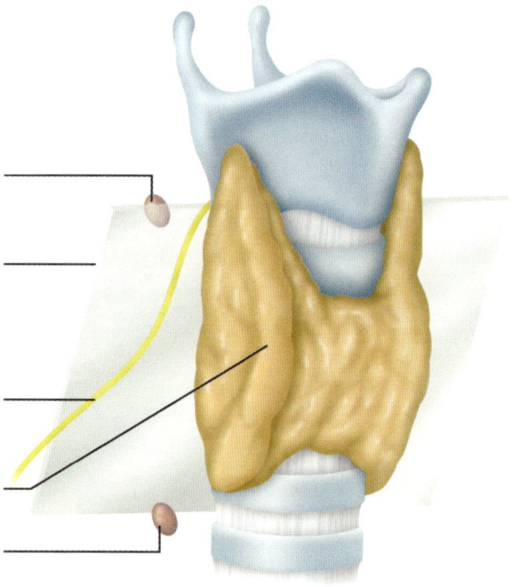

Fig. 20.2: The locations of the superior and inferior parathyroid glands relative to a coronal plane drawn along the course of the recurrent laryngeal nerve. The superior glands are usually dorsal to the plane, while the inferior glands are usually ventral to the plane.

Table 20.1: Symptoms of chronic hypercalcemia.

- Nephrolithiasis
- Polyuria-polydipsia
- Bone pain, cysts, demineralization, and fracture
- Arthritis
- Gout
- Band keratitis, palpebral fissure calcium deposition
- Abdominal pain
- Duodenal and peptic ulcers
- Constipation
- Pancreatitis
- Memory changes
- Confusion
- Depression
- Malaise
- Fatigue

and inferior parathyroid glands occurs by way of a small hilar vessel derived from the inferior thyroid artery in the majority of the cases (76-86%). Some patients will have a superior parathyroid artery from the superior thyroid artery.[8]

Although identification of the recurrent laryngeal nerve is not always mandated during parathyroid surgery, the nerve itself may serve as an important landmark in identifying parathyroid glands. After looping under the subclavian artery (left) or the aorta (right), the left and right recurrent laryngeal nerves track superiorly in the tracheoesophageal groove posterior to the thyroid gland. If a coronal plane is drawn along the path of the recurrent laryngeal nerve, the superior parathyroid glands will be dorsal or posterior to this plane while the inferior parathyroid glands will be anterior to the plane (Fig. 20.2). However, it should be noted that if dissection proceeds into the retroesophageal space the recurrent laryngeal nerve should be identified and protected to prevent injury.

INDICATIONS FOR PARATHYROIDECTOMY

The primary function of the parathyroid glands is to regulate calcium homeostasis by releasing parathyroid hormone (PTH) in response to low levels of ionized calcium. Primary hyperparathyroidism occurs in 1/500 females and 1/2,000 males and may be sporadic, familial, or associated with multiple endocrine neoplasia (MEN) type I or MEN IIa. Parathyroid adenomas account for 80–90% of cases of primary hyperparathyroidism. Most parathyroid adenomas are spontaneous and affect only one gland, although 2–10% of patients may have two-gland (double) adenomas.[9-11] Hyperplasia of all four glands occurs in 5–15% of cases and may be sporadic or associated with MEN I or MEN IIa. In cases where serum calcium and PTH are significantly elevated parathyroid carcinoma may be considered, although this condition remains relatively rare, occurring in only 1–2% of the population.

The classical albeit "passé" presentation of hyperparathyroidism can be remembered by the phrase "stones, bones, groans, and psychiatric overtones" representing the nephrolithiasis (stones), bone pain (bones), abdominal pain (groans), and memory changes (psychiatric overtones) frequently encountered with chronic hypercalcemia (Table 20.1). However, at the present time, most cases of hyperparathyroidism are detected through routine laboratory testing while the patient is still relatively asymptomatic. Although primary hyperparathyroidism is an important cause of hypercalcemia that can be addressed through surgery, the differential diagnosis of hyperparathyroidism includes many other causes of hypercalcemia not amenable to surgery (Table 20.2).

Table 20.2: Differential diagnosis of chronic hypercalcemia.

Parathyroidectomy indicated	*Parathyroidectomy not indicated*
• Parathyroid adenoma	• Benign familial hypercalciuric hypercalcemia (BFHH)
• Parathyroid carcinoma	• Secondary hyperparathyroidism
• Parathyroid hyperplasia	• Pseudohyperparathyroidism
	• Sarcoidosis
	• Granulomatous disease
	• Milk-alkali syndrome
	• Malignancy (breast, lung, multiple myeloma)
	• Pheochromocytoma
	• Vitamin D intoxication
	• Lithium
	• Thiazide diuretic use
	• Hyperthyroidism
	• Adrenal insufficiency
	• Paget disease

Notably, the autosomal dominant disorder benign familial hypocalciuric hypercalcemia (BFHH) is associated with high calcium and PTH levels similar to primary hyperparathyroidism. Benign familial hypocalciuric hypercalcemia is caused by excessive renal Ca^{2+} reabsorption, resulting in increased serum calcium with low-urinary calcium. Surgery is not indicated for BFHH, and therefore, this disorder must be distinguished from hyperparathyroidism before surgery is considered.

Diagnosis of primary hyperparathyroidism fundamentally rests on an elevated serum Ca^{2+} with a normal or elevated PTH level. However, secondary hyperparathyroidism due to kidney disease should be ruled out by measuring 1,25-dihydroxyvitamin D3 levels. Additionally, BFHH may be ruled out by performing a 24-hour urine Ca^{2+} to creatinine ratio. A 24-hour urine Ca^{2+} to creatinine clearance ratio of <0.01 is indicative of BFHH. From the 2002 National Institute of Health guidelines on managing asymptomatic primary hyperparathyroidism, parathyroidectomy is indicated for patients with a diagnosis of primary hyperparathyroidism and serum Ca^{2+} >1.0 mg/dL above the upper limit of normal; patients with hypercalciuria >400 mg/dL or renal stones; creatinine clearance <30% of predicted for age; bone density T-score of <2.5 at any site; patients <50 years old; and any patient requesting surgery or for whom surveillance and follow-up are difficult or impossible.[5] In 2008, these guidelines were updated to exclude the requirement for hypercalciuria and the creatinine clearence criteria was changed to being <60 mL/min.

PREOPERATIVE LOCALIZATION STUDIES

The goal of preoperative imaging in the context of guided or focused parathyroid surgery for hyperparathyroidism is to locate the abnormal gland, thereby sparing the patient a bilateral neck exploration. A common modality for preoperative parathyroid imaging is sestamibi scanning, which uses technetium-99m-methoxyisobutyl isonitrile (Tc^{99}MIBI) to visualize abnormal glands (Fig. 20.3A). Tc^{99}MIBI is initially taken up by the thyroid and parathyroid glands;[12] however, the marker is cleared from the thyroid after 1–3 hours but is retained by adenomatous parathyroid glands, allowing the affected gland to be visualized by imaging at 15 minutes and 2.5 hours postinjection of Tc^{99}MIBI.[13] The sensitivity for sestamibi scanning ranges from 70% to 100% and can be increased by 2% to 3% by adding single proton emission computed tomography (SPECT), which also provides three-dimensional information regarding gland localization (Figs. 20.3B and C).[14] By contrast, contrast CT scanning alone has 40% specificity and 86% sensitivity for identifying ectopic parathyroid glands.[15,16] The sensitivity is improved to 88% by 4D-CT scanning, which images changes in contrast perfusion over time (Fig. 20.3D).[17] Drawbacks to sestamibi and CT-mediated imaging include the need for specialized equipment, the time required for these studies, high cost, the need for the professional expertise of both radiologists and the surgeon, and added radiation exposure to the patient.

As an alternative to nuclear imaging studies, ultrasound (US) may be used to visualize parathyroid glands. Parathyroid adenomas usually appear as well-circumscribed, ovoid, solid masses that are homogenously hypoechoic relative to the surrounding tissue (Fig. 20.3E). The sensitivity of US is highly operator dependent but in experienced hands may reach 70–100%, although the sensitivity decreases to 47–84% in the setting of concurrent thyroid disease.[14] Newer methods including

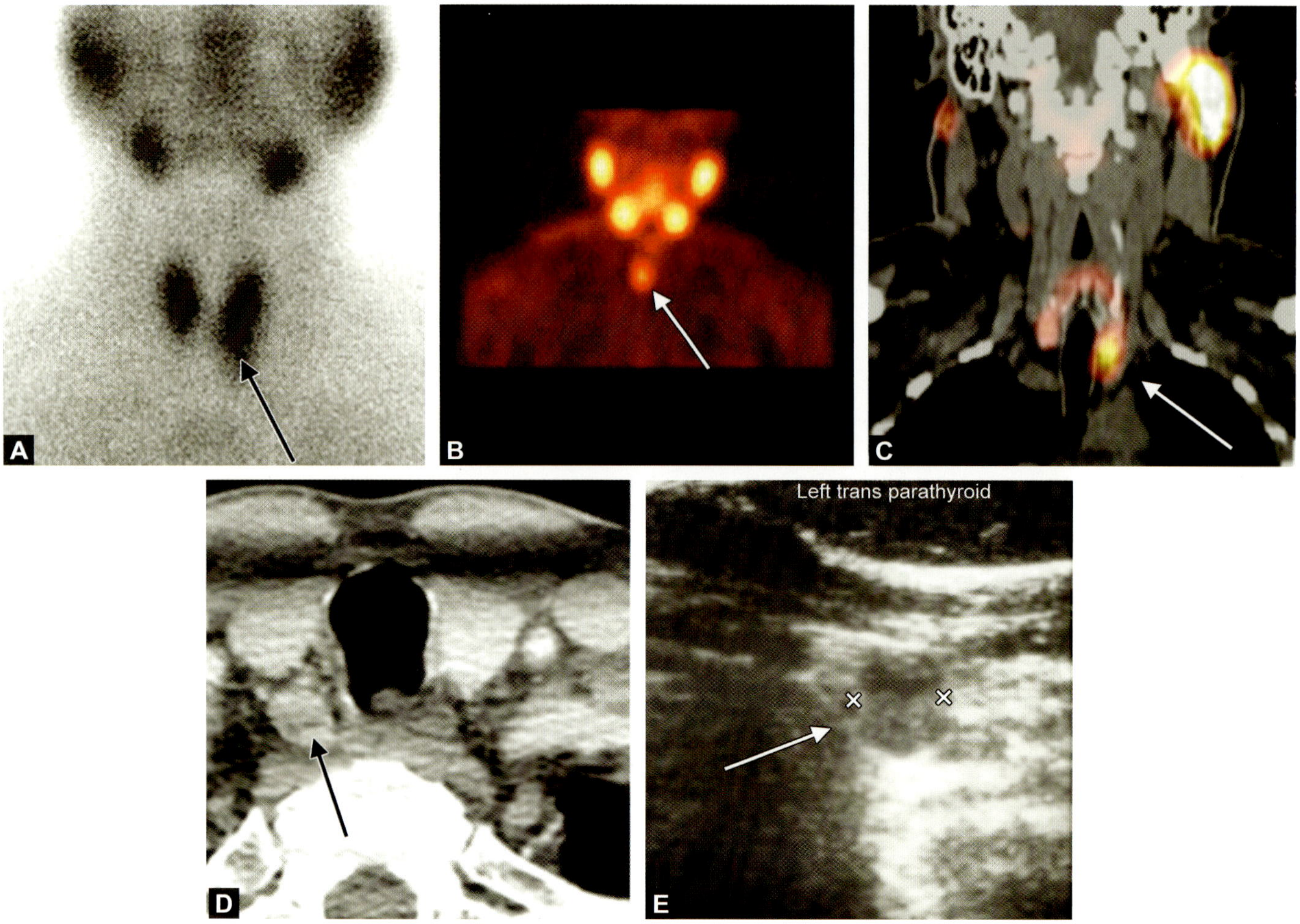

Figs. 20.3A to E: Imaging modalities for preoperative localization studies. (A) Sestamibi. (B) Single positron emission computed tomography (SPECT). (C) SPECT/CT. (D) 4D-CT. (E) Ultrasound. Arrows indicate the location of adenomatous parathyroid glands.

high-resolution US and contrast-enhanced US may approach or surpass the sensitivity of sestamibi scans.[18-20] Ultrasound studies may be performed in the office, are relatively inexpensive, and provide rapid and dynamic imaging by the surgeon. However, the sensitivity of the study is subject to interoperator variability. Also, US can be a suboptimal modality for identifying ectopic parathyroid glands, particularly when the glands are located in the mediastinum or within the thyroid.[15]

Recent cost–benefit analysis suggests that sestamibi-SPECT and US with or without 4D-CT scanning are the most cost-effective modalities for parathyroid imaging.[22] However, among patients for whom US- or CT-based imaging is suboptimal, MRI may also be used to identify abnormal parathyroid glands. The parathyroids are normally isointense with the surrounding muscle on T1-weighted imaging; however, hyperfunctional glands show gadolinium contrast enhancement on T1 scans. Additionally, all parathyroid glands are hyperintense relative to the surrounding tissue in T2-weighted imaging. The sensitivity of MRI ranges from 69% to 88%, which is generally lower than SPECT-CT or US-mediated imaging.[14]

OPERATIVE TECHNIQUES

General considerations of parathyroid surgery include the use of a systematic approach to exploration of the neck to locate and identify parathyroid glands and the maintenance of excellent hemostasis so that the field is not bloodstained, which makes it difficult to identify parathyroid glands amidst the surrounding fat. The use of loupe magnification and intraoperative monitoring of the recurrent laryngeal nerve can be considered for parathyroid surgery.

Parathyroid Exploration

A Kocher incision is made two fingerbreadths (~2 cm) above the suprasternal notch and carried through the platysma (Fig. 20.4). At this point, the superior flap may be dissected superiorly toward the notch of the thyroid cartilage, while the inferior flap is dissected toward the suprasternal notch, exposing the midline strap muscles. Two approaches may be used to dissect through the strap muscles: a midline approach, which requires more dissection and is therefore more time-consuming but provides a more familiar view of the relevant anatomy (Figs. 20.5A and B); and a lateral approach (Figs. 20.6A and B). In the midline approach the midline raphe of the strap muscles is identified and separated from the thyroid notch to the suprasternal notch, which allows the sternocleidomastoid, sternohyoid, sternothyroid, and omohyoid muscles to be retracted laterally. The muscles on the side to be explored first are lifted away from the thyroid capsule. Care must be taken to maintain hemostasis while dissecting through the highly vascular plane between the sternothyroid muscle and the thyroid capsule. If needed, the sternothyroid muscle may be divided to gain additional exposure. The middle thyroid vein is then identified, ligated, and divided, and the ipsilateral thyroid lobe is rotated anteromedially using Babcock or Allis clamps placed under direct visualization (*see* Figs. 20.5A and B). Division of the superior or inferior thyroid arteries is not usually necessary, but may be considered if additional exposure is required.

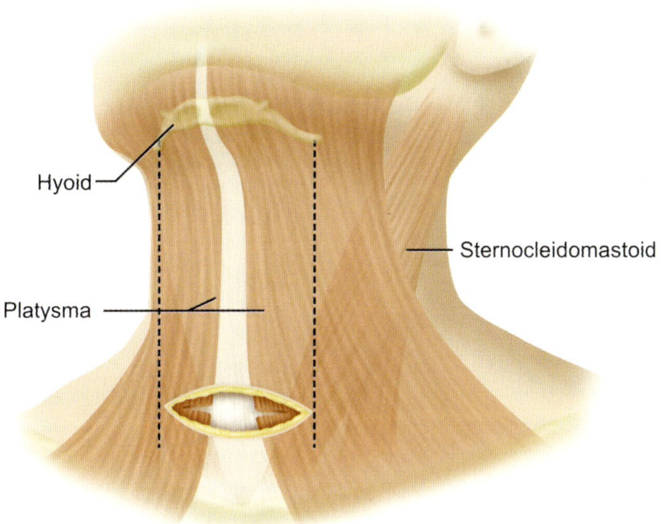

Fig. 20.4: Midline incision for parathyroid exploration. A Kocher incision is created approximately 2 cm above the sternal notch and carried through the platysma. The hyoid bone may serve as a guide for the length of the incision.

For the lateral approach, the fascia along the medial border of the sternocleidomastoid is divided between the carotid sheath and the lateral border of the strap muscles (Figs. 20.6A and B). The middle thyroid veins are identified, ligated, and divided along the thyroid capsule, and Babcock clamps are used to grasp the thyroid with the overlying strap muscles as a unit, which is then rotated anteromedially to expose the parathyroid glands. It should be noted that the more limited exposure from this approach makes it difficult to access low-lying parathyroid glands and the superior mediastinum.

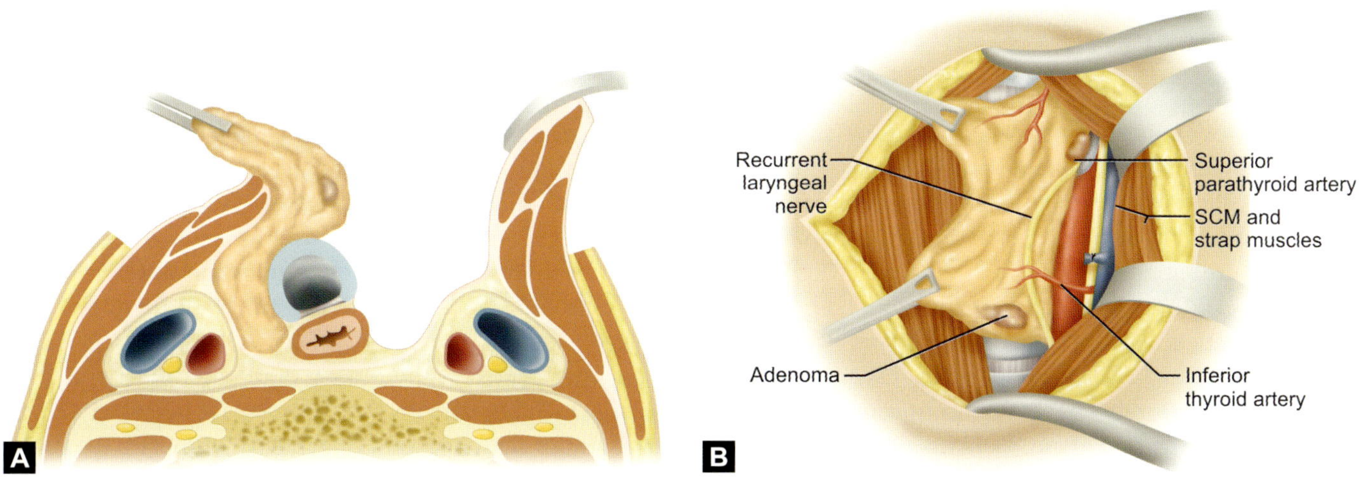

Figs. 20.5A and B: Medial approach to parathyroid exploration. An axial view (A) and surgeon's view (B) showing the division of the strap muscles along the median raphe with lateral retraction of the sternocleidomastoid, omohyoid, sternohyoid, and sternothyroid muscles to access the parathyroid glands.

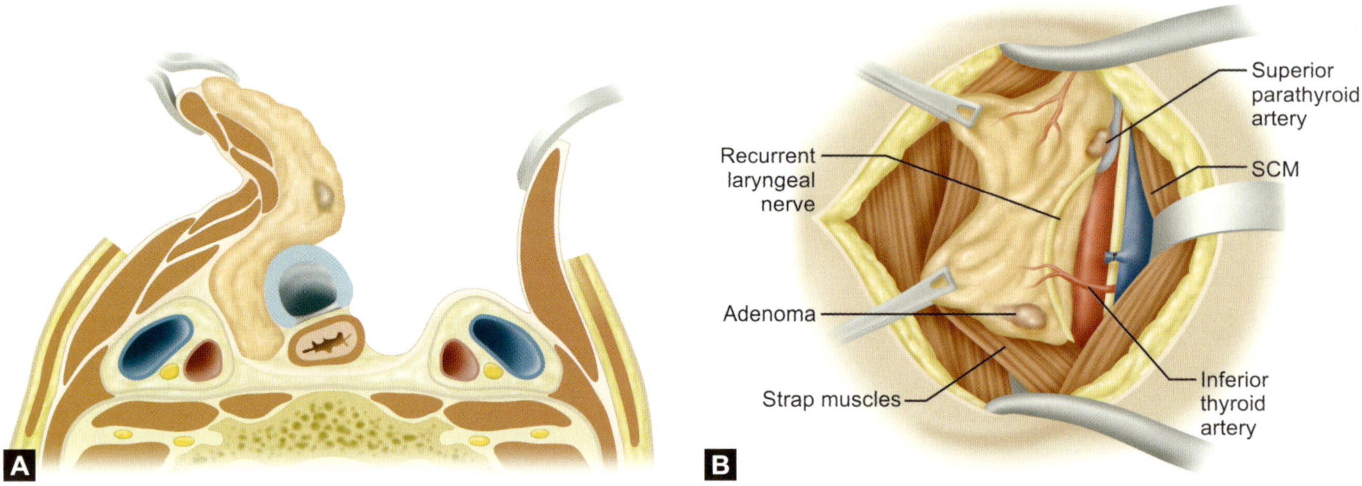

Figs. 20.6A and B: Lateral approach to the parathyroid glands. (A) Axial and (B) surgeon's view showing the fascial incision along the medial border of the sternocleidomastoid muscle with anteromedial retraction of the thyroid and overlying strap muscles.

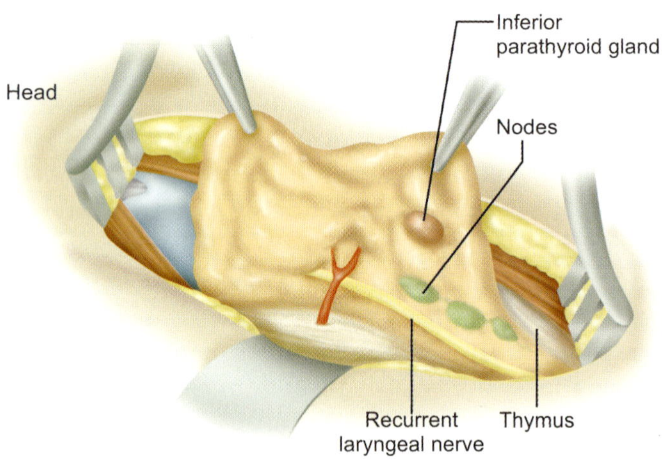

Fig. 20.7: The inferior parathyroid glands are commonly found along the thyroid capsule anterior and medial to the crossing of the recurrent laryngeal nerve and the inferior thyroid artery.

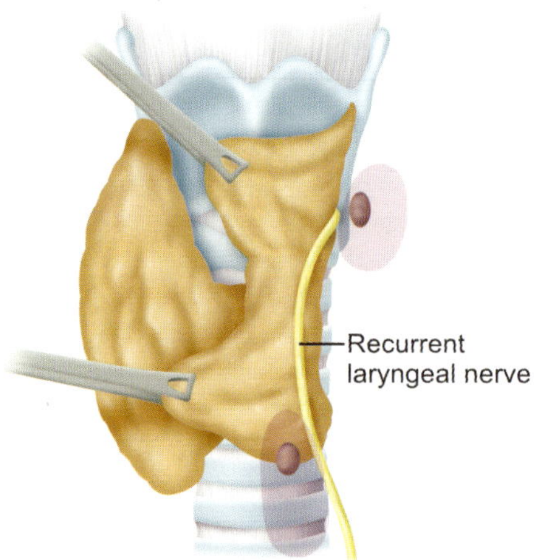

Fig. 20.8: Relationship of the superior (shading) and inferior (shading) parathyroid glands to the recurrent laryngeal nerve.

The fibroareolar tissue surrounding the thyroid gland may be dissected using Kocher or peanut dissectors. This technique allows the glands to be visualized with minimal bloodstaining, thereby permitting the identification of normal and abnormal glands. Care should be taken to remain close to the thyroid capsule to allow for identification of glands embedded within the fibrous tissue surrounding the thyroid (Fig. 20.7). Additional exposure may be gained by dissecting the pretracheal fascia connecting the carotid sheath and the thyroid gland, yielding access to the paraesophageal and retroesophageal spaces. While identification of the recurrent laryngeal nerve is not uniformly necessary for every parathyroid surgery, any dissection within the paraesophageal or retroesophageal spaces merits identification and protection of the recurrent laryngeal nerve.

Usually, the inferior parathyroid glands are sought first. These glands tend to be larger and have a more anterior location than the superior parathyroid glands. Although the anatomical location of the inferior parathyroid glands tends to be more variable, they are most commonly found along the posterior thyroid capsule anterior and slightly medial to the crossing of the recurrent laryngeal nerve and the inferior thyroid artery (Fig. 20.8). While adenomatous glands may be readily apparent on dissection, care should be taken not to remove the adenomatous gland before the other ipsilateral gland has been identified because removal

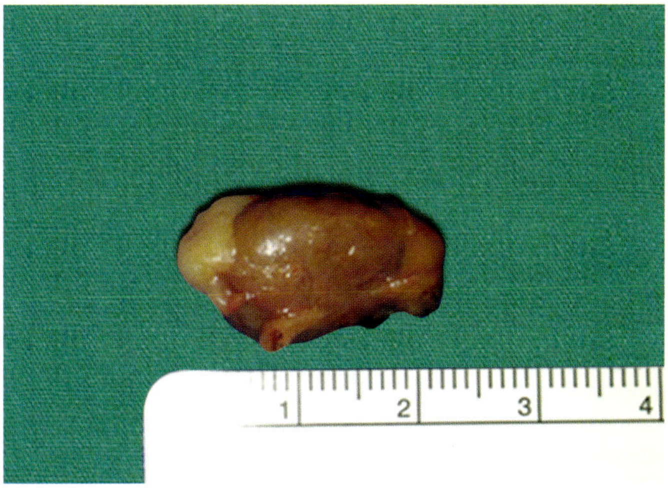

Fig. 20.9: Parathyroid adenoma. Note the fat cap on the left and the ocher coloration of the parathyroid gland.

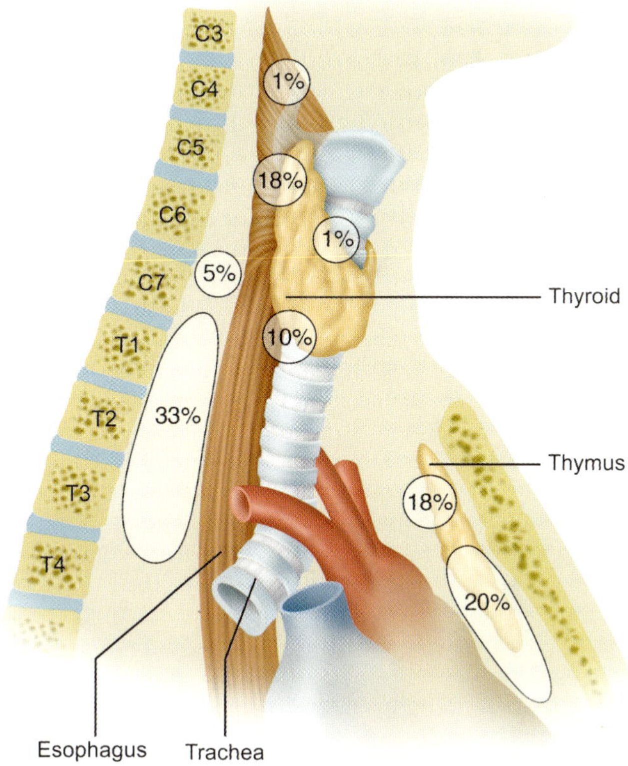

Fig. 20.10: Common locations of ectopic parathyroid glands.

of the adenoma may distort anatomical relationships and the normal gland may be small in size due to suppression by the adenoma.

Parathyroid glands have several physical features that aid in their identification amidst the surrounding fat. Primarily, parathyroid tissue is darker and browner (caramel color) compared to yellow fat or white thymus tissue (Fig. 20.9). Parathyroid glands also have a distinct vascular pedicle, best visualized under loupe magnification, which is most often derived from the inferior thyroid artery. Accordingly, tracing the branches of the inferior thyroid artery may aid in the identification of parathyroid glands. Finally, if tissue is removed, parathyroid tissue tends to sink when placed in saline, whereas fat tends to float.[1] Abnormal glands may frequently be palpated before they are visualized. Palpation along the paraesophageal space just dorsal to the recurrent laryngeal nerve and the inferior thyroid artery may therefore reveal glands that can subsequently be exposed by further dissection. Similarly, glands may be palpated on the posterior aspect of the thyroid capsule underneath the pretracheal fascia.

Once a parathyroid gland has been identified, dissection should be initiated at the outermost tip of the gland with the goal of preserving the vascular supply until the decision is made to remove the gland. Abnormal glands should be sampled for pathology and ipsilateral normal glands may also be sampled for pathologic analysis. If the paired gland is normal or suppressed, the surgeon may decide whether or not to proceed with contralateral neck dissection or to limit the operation to a unilateral procedure. Any glands that are unintentionally devascularized or avulsed should be verified by pathology and placed in ice-cold saline until they can be minced and reimplanted.

If a gland suspected to be an adenoma cannot be identified or if all glands cannot be located in the case of hyperplasia, a thorough dissection should be carried out to identify ectopic glands. The most common locations for ectopic parathyroid glands include the retroesophageal or retrotracheal spaces, the anterior mediastinum, the carotid sheath, and the hyoid bone or the angle of the mandible. Rarely, intrathyroid glands may also be found (Fig. 20.10). All areas accessible through a cervical excision should be explored including the retroesophageal space and the carotid sheath (Figs. 20.11A and B). Additionally, thymus tissue should be removed from the superior mediastinum and inspected (Fig. 20.11C). Failure to locate all glands after these steps may require a thyroid lobectomy to identify parathyroid glands within the thyroid (Fig. 20.11D); however, removal of normal thyroid tissue should only be considered as a last resort. It should be noted that only 0.2% of all parathyroid glands (2% of ectopic parathyroid glands) are located within the thyroid.[4]

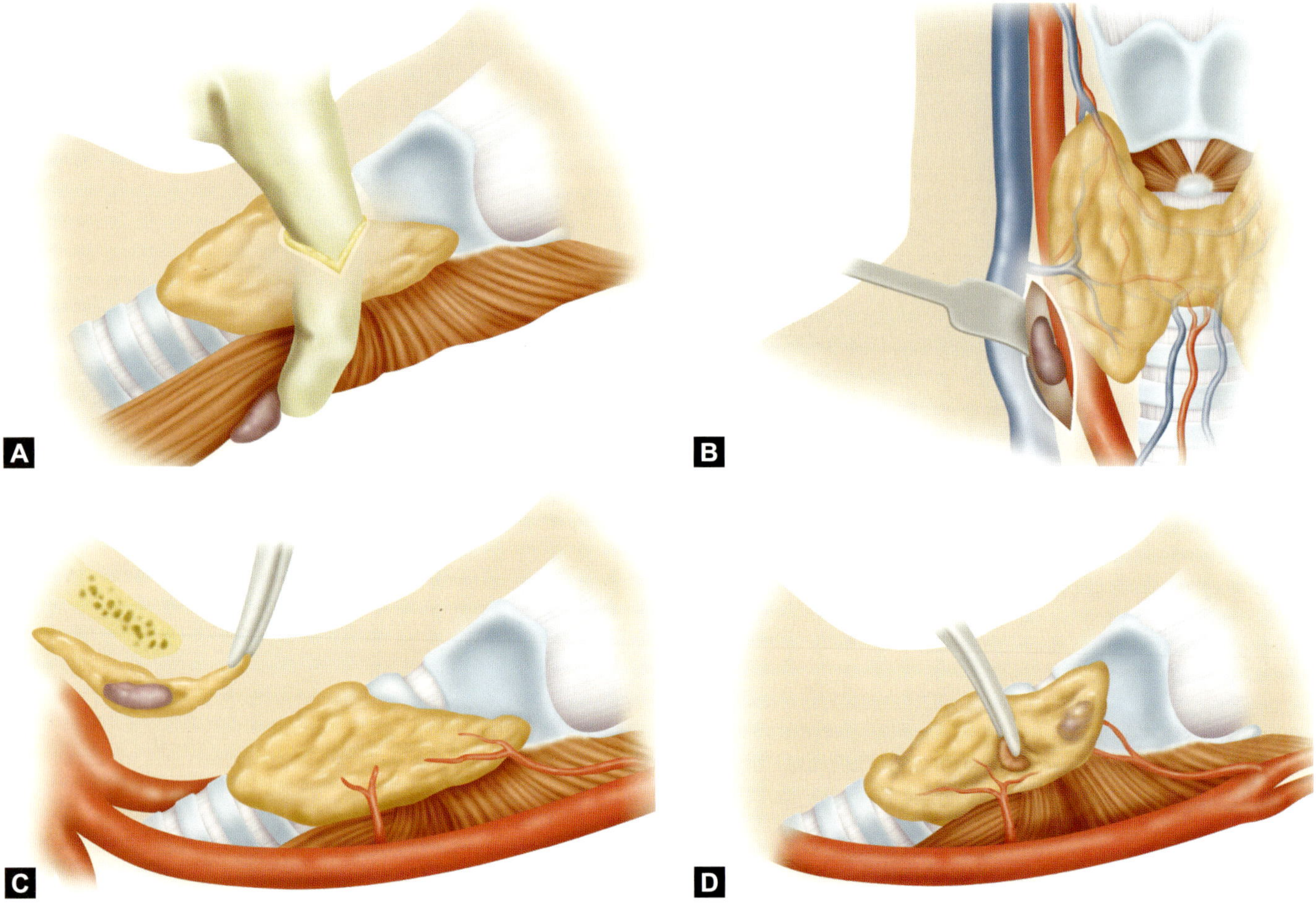

Figs. 20.11A to D: Identification of ectopic thyroid glands. All areas accessible through a cervical incision should be thoroughly searched until the ectopic gland(s) have been identified including palpation of the retroesophageal space (A), inspection of the carotid sheath (B), removal of the thymus from the anterior mediastinum (C), and assessing for intrathyroid parathyroid glands (D).

In the case of four-gland hyperplasia, three and a half glands may be removed (subtotal parathyroidectomy) or all four glands may be removed with approximately half of one gland selected for reimplantation (total parathyroidectomy with auto-reimplantation). The selected gland should be sharply minced into 15–20 pieces (Fig. 20.12A), which can then be implanted into small pockets created in the sternocleidomastoid muscle. The implantation site should be marked with surgical clips or nonabsorbable suture to facilitate future identification should the reimplanted gland become adenomatous. Alternatively, the gland may be reimplanted into the brachioradialis muscle, which requires less-invasive procedures to remove the gland should a parathyroid adenoma develop (Fig. 20.12B).[22]

Minimally Invasive Parathyroidectomy

Advances in imaging combined with a desire from surgeons and the public for less invasive procedures have led to the increased use of minimally invasive techniques for parathyroid surgery. Advantages of these approaches include decreased recovery time, shortened operative time, fewer complications, and improved cosmetic outcome. Minimally invasive guided parathyroid surgery requires that patients first undergo an imaging localization procedure as previously described. Only patients with preoperative imaging studies indicating a single adenoma are candidates for guided surgery.

The incisions used for minimally invasive parathyroidectomy range in length from 15 to 40 mm and are placed 20–40 mm above the sternal notch, preferably in a skin crease overlying the suspected adenoma. Midline and lateral approaches to the parathyroid have been described. The midline approach has been used for glands that are superficial (i.e. at the same depth of the thyroid) and inferior to the thyroid, while the lateral approach may be more appropriate for glands that are posterior to the thyroid lobe or deep to the carotid artery.[23]

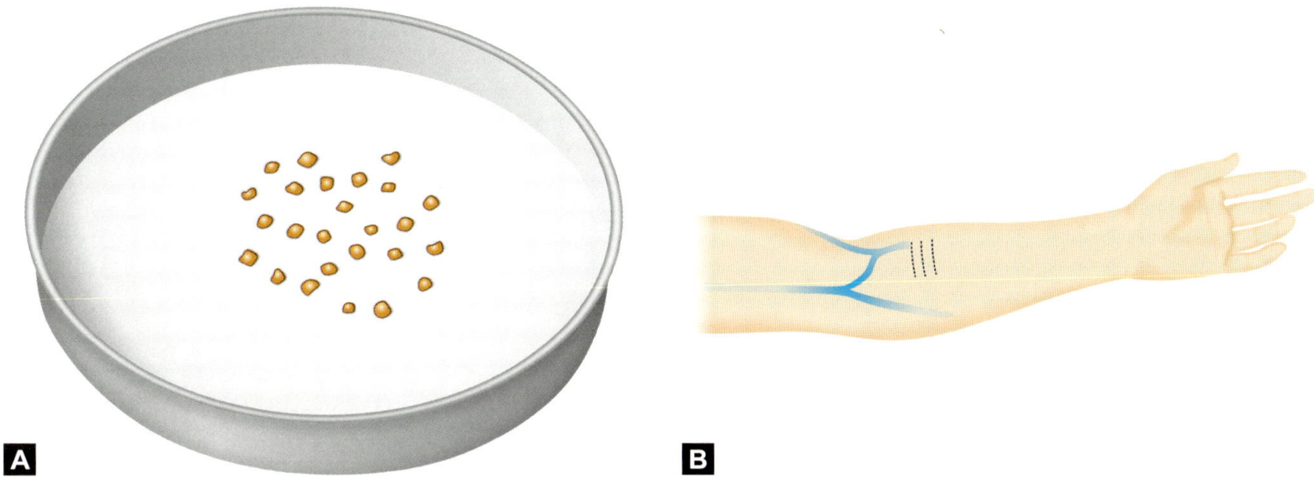

Figs. 20.12A and B: Autotransplantation of parathyroid tissue. One half of a removed gland may be cut into 1-mm cubes (A) and reimplanted into small pockets created in the sternocleidomastoid muscle or in the brachioradialis muscle (B).

For the midline approach, a 15–25 mm horizontal incision is made across the midline at the level of the suspected adenoma (Fig. 20.13A). The subplatysmal planes are then circumferentially elevated from the thyroid cartilage to the sternal notch and a small quantity of subcutaneous fat is removed to create an operative space above the strap muscles (Fig. 20.13B). A self-retaining retractor may be used to help increase exposure. The sternothyroid muscles are then separated along the midline using electrocautery or an ultrasonic scalpel to expose the fascia overlying the thyroid gland (Fig. 20.13C). At this point, blunt dissection is performed in the tissue surrounding the suspected adenoma. Once the adenoma is identified, it is freed from the surrounding fascia with blunt dissection and a bipolar cautery or ultrasonic scalpel is used to ligate the vascular supply to the gland and remove the specimen (Fig. 20.13D).

The initial reports describing the lateral approach placed a 20-mm incision directly over the affected gland;[25] however, others have used a slightly more midline incision.[23] In this approach, access to the parathyroid is gained by dissecting between the anterior border of the sternocleidomastoid muscle and the lateral border of the strap muscles. The sternocleidomastoid is then retracted laterally, and dissection is carried posteriorly in a plane medial to the carotid sheath and lateral to the thyroid lobule to the depth of the prevertebral fascia. The surgeon may then dissect medially in a plane posterior to the thyroid to expose the parathyroid adenoma. Once the adenoma is identified, the vasculature is ligated and the gland is removed similarly to the anterior approach.

Minimally Invasive Radioguided Parathyroidectomy

To help identify the abnormal gland a handheld gamma detection device (gamma probe) may be used intraoperatively in conjunction with Tc-99m sestamibi scanning. This technique allows the localization and removal of the adenoma to be combined in a "single-day" protocol. In this scenario, the patient is injected with a 20 mCi (740 MBq) dose of Tc-99m sestamibi on the day of surgery.[25] Based on the results of the imaging, an ink mark is placed on the skin over the diseased gland and the patient is optimally brought to the operating room within hours of Tc-99m sestamibi injection. A gamma probe is calibrated and three readings of the patient's background radiation level are recorded by pointing the probe at the patient's leg. The location of the skin marking is then confirmed using the gamma probe to conduct 10-second counts through the skin overlying the affected gland.

Using either a midline or lateral approach, the gamma probe is used to help localize the "hot" parathyroid adenoma within the surgical wound. After removal of the suspected adenoma three 10-second gamma readings are taken from the specimen and the surgical bed. Complete removal of the adenoma is confirmed if the gamma readings from the specimen are at least 20% of the readings obtained from the surgical bed (the "20% rule").[26,27] Intraoperative PTH levels may also be obtained to confirm the removal of the affected gland as described below.

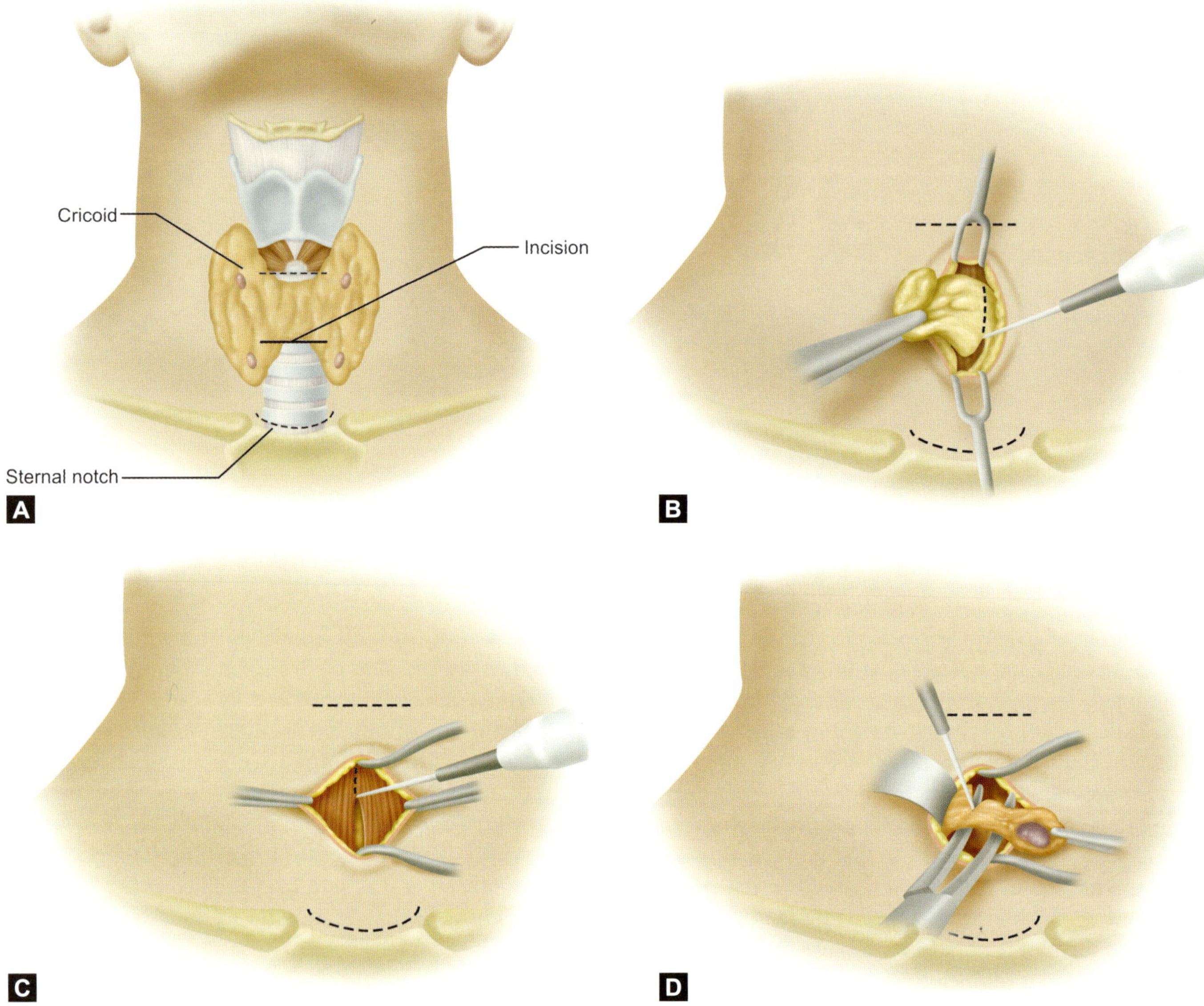

Figs. 20.13A to D: Minimally invasive parathyroidectomy. (A) Following preoperative imaging studies, midline incisions are created at the level of the adenomatous gland. (B) A small amount of subcutaneous fat is removed to create an operative space above the strap muscles, and (C) the strap muscles are divided along the midline and the thyroid gland is medialized. (D) The abnormal gland is identified and excised.

Ultrasound-Guided Parathyroidectomy

As an alternative to radiotracer imaging on the day of surgery, some reports describe the use of intraoperative ultrasound to help identify and confirm the removal of parathyroid adenomas. With this technique, once the thyroid bed has been exposed the ultrasound probe is used to assist with the approach to the localized gland.[27,28] Although published reports of this technique only include relatively small numbers of patients, 100% success rates have been reported, indicating that intraoperative ultrasound may be valuable for the identification of parathyroid adenomas.

Video-Assisted Parathyroidectomy

Recently, video-assisted endoscopic techniques have also been used for surgical management of hyperparathyroidism. These techniques access diseased glands through small incisions in the upper chest wall or the cervical region.[29-31] Additionally, the use of surgical robots has permitted a transaxillary approach to parathyroidectomy.[32] Benefits of endoscopic parathyroid surgery include excellent cosmetic outcome, reduced patient discomfort, and fewer problems with cervical motion following the procedure. However, it should be noted that the extended intraoperative time associated with endoscopic or robot-assisted procedures and the potential for conversion to an open procedure may negate some of the potential benefits.[30,33] Candidate patients for these procedures must undergo preoperative imaging and must have single-gland disease without significant thyroid enlargement or nodularity.[30,34] Furthermore, patients receiving endoscopic parathyroid surgery should undergo intraoperative PTH monitoring to confirm the successful removal of the abnormal gland.[30] However, in appropriately selected patients endoscopic parathyroidectomy has a 98% success rate.[30]

Intraoperative PTH Monitoring

The half-life of PTH is 2–5 minutes, permitting intraoperative monitoring of PTH levels to confirm the removal of abnormal glands. This technique may be used to prove that affected parathyroid tissue has been removed during bilateral neck explorations; however, it is most beneficial during minimally invasive procedures because an appropriate reduction in PTH after removal of the abnormal gland obviates the need for bilateral exploration. PTH levels are measured from peripheral blood when the abnormal gland is identified (baseline) and 10 minutes after all suspected hyperfunctional glands have been removed. A post-excisional PTH level that is normal or near-normal and is at least 50% lower than baseline is highly predictive of the successful removal of all abnormal tissue.[36] Importantly, a decrease in the PTH level of <50% may indicate that abnormal parathyroid tissue is still present and may necessitate a bilateral neck exploration.

POSTOPERATIVE CARE AND COMPLICATIONS OF PARATHYROIDECTOMY

Hypocalcemia

After successful parathyroidectomy serum calcium levels usually drop, reaching a nadir 48–96 hours after surgery.[37] The drop in serum calcium levels may result in symptoms of hypocalcemia or tetany in some patients despite normal serum calcium levels. Additionally, postoperative hypocalcemia may result in "bone hunger" in some patients with severe depletion of skeletal calcium. Serum calcium levels should be monitored at least once during the first 24 hours after surgery, and normocalcemia and normal PTH levels at 6 months postsurgery indicate that the procedure was successful.

For experienced surgeons 5% of patients with primary hyperparathyroidism have persistent postoperative hypercalcemia.[38] However, the rate of postoperative hypercalcemia ranges from 10% to 15% in patients with parathyroid hyperplasia, secondary hyperparathyroidism, or some forms of inherited hyperparathyroidism including MEN I.[38] The reasons for surgical failure include inability to find the adenomatous gland, failure to locate or identify a second adenomatous gland, failure to recognize four-gland hyperplasia, failure to locate or identify a supernumerary gland, regrowth of an adenoma from unresected parathyroid tissue following removal of an adenomatous gland, unrecognized parathyroid carcinoma, or incorrect diagnosis. Permanent hypoparathyroidism may also occur after parathyroidectomy and is seen in approximately 5% of patients with single-gland adenoma. However, up to 10–30% of patients with four-gland hyperplasia may experience permanent hypoparathyroidism.

Recurrent Laryngeal Nerve Injury

Recurrent laryngeal nerve injury is an uncommon complication of parathyroidectomy, occurring in 0.2–2% of patients.[38-40] Furthermore, bilateral recurrent laryngeal nerve injury during initial parathyoridectomy is estimated to occur only in 1/5,000 patients, which has led some authors argue against the routine use of recurrent laryngeal nerve monitoring during routine parathyroidectomy.[38] However, recent studies have indicated that parathyroid adenomas, particularly of the right superior gland, are frequently located within 2.5 to 3.9 mm of the RLN, placing the nerve at risk of injury during parathyroidectomy.[40] Even though Untch et al.[40] reported no recurrent laryngeal nerve injuries in their study, other evidence indicates that visual identification of the recurrent laryngeal nerve during parathyroid exploration may reduce the incidence of permanent recurrent laryngeal nerve paresis.[41] Accordingly, during dissections involving the paraesophageal space or retroesophageal space the RLN should be identified; however, confirmation of the recurrent laryngeal nerve by using neural electric stimulation may reflect the personal preference of the surgeon.

REFERENCES

1. Cohen J. Parathyroid exploration. Oper Tech Otolaryngol Head Neck Surg. 2003;14(2):109-17.
2. Akerstrom G, Malmaeus J, Bergstrom R. Surgical anatomy of human parathyroid glands. Surgery. 1984;95(1):14-21.
3. Numano M, et al. Surgical significance of supernumerary parathyroid glands in renal hyperparathyroidism. World J Surg. 1998;22(10):1098-102; discussion 1103.
4. Lappas D, et al. Location, number and morphology of parathyroid glands: results from a large anatomical series. Anatomic Sci Int. 2012;87(3):160-64.
5. Bilezikian JP, Khan AA, Potts JT. Guidelines for the Management of Asymptomatic Primary Hyperparathyroidism: Summary Statement from the Third International Workshop. J Clin Endocrinol Metab. 2009 Feb;94(2):335–9.
6. Summers GW. Parathyroid update: a review of 220 cases. Ear Nose Throat J. 1996;75(7):434-9.
7. Fancy T, Gallagher D 3rd, Hornig JD. Surgical anatomy of the thyroid and parathyroid glands. Otolaryngol Clin North Am. 2010;43(2):221-7, vii.
8. Alveryd A. Parathyroid glands in thyroid surgery. I. Anatomy of parathyroid glands. II. Postoperative hypoparathyroidism—identification and autotransplantation of parathyroid glands. Acta Chir Scand. 1968;389:1-120.
9. Harness JK, et al. Multiple adenomas of the parathyroids: do they exist? Arch Surg. 1979;114(4):468-74.
10. Attie JN, Bock G, Auguste LJ. Multiple parathyroid adenomas: report of thirty-three cases. Surgery. 1990;108(6):1014-9; discussion 1019-20.
11. Tezelman S, et al. Double parathyroid adenomas. Clinical and biochemical characteristics before and after parathyroidectomy. Ann Surg. 1993;218(3):300-307; discussion 307-9.
12. Coakley AJ, et al. 99Tcm sestamibi—a new agent for parathyroid imaging. Nucl Med Commun. 1989;10(11):791-4.
13. Mariani G, et al. Preoperative localization and radioguided parathyroid surgery. J Nucl Med. 2003;44(9):1443-58.
14. Mohebati A, Shaha AR. Imaging techniques in parathyroid surgery for primary hyperparathyroidism. Am J Otolaryngol. 2012;33(4):457-68.
15. Gross ND, et al. The diagnostic utility of computed tomography for preoperative localization in surgery for hyperparathyroidism. Laryngoscope. 2004;114(2):227-31.
16. Ishibashi M, et al. Localization of ectopic parathyroid glands using technetium-99m sestamibi imaging: comparison with magnetic resonance and computed tomographic imaging. Eur J Nucl Med. 1997;24(2):197-201.
17. Rodgers SE, et al. Improved preoperative planning for directed parathyroidectomy with 4-dimensional computed tomography. Surgery. 2006;140(6):932-40; discussion 940-41.
18. Haber RS, Kim CK, Inabnet WB. Ultrasonography for preoperative localization of enlarged parathyroid glands in primary hyperparathyroidism: comparison with (99m) technetium sestamibi scintigraphy. Clin Endocrinol. 2002; 57(2):241-9.
19. Agha A, et al. The role of contrast-enhanced ultrasonography (CEUS) in comparison with 99mTechnetium-sestamibi scintigraphy for localization diagnostic of primary hyperparathyroidism. Clin Hemorheol Microcirc. 2014; 58(4):515-20.
20. Agha A, et al. Highly efficient localization of pathological glands in primary hyperparathyroidism using contrast-enhanced ultrasonography (CEUS) in comparison with conventional ultrasonography. J Clin Endocrinol Metab. 2013;98(5):2019-25.
21. Schneider R, et al. Frequency of ectopic and supernumerary intrathymic parathyroid glands in patients with renal hyperparathyroidism: analysis of 461 patients undergoing initial parathyroidectomy with bilateral cervical thymectomy. World J Surg. 2011;35(6):1260-65.
22. Lo CY. Parathyroid autotransplantation during thyroidectomy. ANZ J Surg. 2002;72(12):902-7.
23. Shindo ML, Rosenthal JM, Lee T. Minimally invasive parathyroidectomy using local anesthesia with intravenous sedation and targeted approaches. Otolaryngol Head Neck Surg. 2008;138(3):381-7.
24. Agarwal G, et al. Minimally invasive parathyroidectomy using the 'focused' lateral approach. I. Results of the first 100 consecutive cases. ANZ J Surg. 2002;72(2):100-104.
25. Rubello D, et al. Minimally invasive (99m)Tc-sestamibi radioguided surgery of parathyroid adenomas. Panminerva Med. 2005;47(2):99-107.
26. Murphy C, Norman J. The 20% rule: a simple, instantaneous radioactivity measurement defines cure and allows elimination of frozen sections and hormone assays during parathyroidectomy. Surgery. 1999;126(6):1023-8; discussion 1028-9.
27. Quillo AR, et al. Minimally invasive parathyroid surgery, the Norman 20% rule: is it valid? Am Surg. 2011;77(4): 484-7.
28. Kell MR, et al. Minimally invasive parathyroidectomy with operative ultrasound localization of the adenoma. Surg Endosc. 2004;18(7):1097-8.
29. Ashcroft AJ, et al. Intra-operative ultrasound localisation of a parathyroid adenoma. Ann R Coll Surg Engl. 2011; 93(2):172.
30. Prades JM, et al. Endoscopic surgery of the parathyroid glands: methods and principles. Eur Ann Otorhinolaryngol Head Neck Dis. 2013;130(3):157-60.
31. Fouquet T, et al. Totally endoscopic lateral parathyroidectomy: prospective evaluation of 200 patients. ESES 2010 Vienna presentation. Langenbecks Arch Surg. 2010;395(7): 935-40.
32. Kang J, et al. Trans-areola single-site endoscopic parathyroidectomy: report of one case. Surg Innov. 2013;20(6): 16-20.
33. Landry CS, et al. Robot assisted transaxillary surgery (RATS) for the removal of thyroid and parathyroid glands. Surgery. 2011;149(4):549-55.
34. Landry CS, et al. Robot-assisted transaxillary thyroid surgery in the United States: is it comparable to open thyroid lobectomy? Ann Surg Oncol. 2012;19(4):1269-74.

35. Mihai R, et al. Surgical strategy for sporadic primary hyperparathyroidism an evidence-based approach to surgical strategy, patient selection, surgical access, and reoperations. Langenbecks Arch Surg. 2009;394(5):785-98.
36. Richards ML, et al. An optimal algorithm for intraoperative parathyroid hormone monitoring. Arch Surg. 2011; 146(3):280-85.
37. Mittendorf EA, Merlino JI, McHenry CR. Post-parathyroidectomy hypocalcemia: incidence, risk factors, and management. Am Surg. 2004;70(2):114-19; discussion 119-20.
38. Carty SE. Prevention and management of complications in parathyroid surgery. Otolaryngol Clin North Am. 2004; 37(4):897-907, xi.
39. Allendorf J, et al. 1112 consecutive bilateral neck explorations for primary hyperparathyroidism. World J Surg. 2007;31(11):2075-80.
40. Untch BR, et al. Tumor proximity to the recurrent laryngeal nerve in patients with primary hyperparathyroidism undergoing parathyroidectomy. Ann Surg Oncol. 2012; 19(12):3823-6.
41. Steurer M, et al. Advantages of recurrent laryngeal nerve identification in thyroidectomy and parathyroidectomy and the importance of preoperative and postoperative laryngoscopic examination in more than 1000 nerves at risk. Laryngoscope. 2002;112(1):124-33.
42. Thompson NW, Eckhauser FE, Harness JK. The anatomy of primary hyperparathyroidism. Surgery. 1982;92(5):814-21.

Section 6

Salivary and Parapharyngeal Space Tumors

Section Editor: ***Jason G Newman***

Chapters

CHAPTER

21

Parotidectomy

Steven M Sperry, Jason G Newman

INTRODUCTION

The parotidectomy procedure that we know today, involving tumor extirpation along with removal of the surrounding gland while preserving the branches of the facial nerve, has been performed for over 100 years for benign and malignant processes of the salivary gland. A total parotidectomy with nerve preservation was described in 1907 by Carwardine, and further advocates of the procedure were Bailey[1] and Kidd.[2] However, it was not until the 1960s that the approach of parotidectomy with nerve dissection was more generally accepted as a way to protect the integrity of the facial nerve. The historical alternatives included local excision without nerve identification, incision and biopsy, and enucleation; these alternative procedures have historically led to high tumor recurrence rates and complication rates, and are considered inferior to the current standard of care of facial nerve identification and preservation with tumor extirpation including a margin of normal salivary tissue. Most surgeons today perform a partial parotidectomy procedure, removing just the portion of the gland surrounding the tumor, as opposed to the entire lobe of parotid gland superficial or deep to the facial nerve. There are currently advocates of extracapsular dissection of benign parotid tumors, with even closer margins of resection just outside the tumor capsule. This chapter, however, focuses on describing the more common partial parotidectomy procedure practiced today.

Parotid lesions can be benign or malignant, and non-neoplastic or neoplastic. As 80% of parotid tumors are benign, the procedure is most frequently performed for benign indications; however, the question of malignancy and the possibility of altering the extent of surgery based on surgical findings makes for complex intraoperative decision making. Fine-needle aspiration has been utilized to aid in the preoperative diagnosis of salivary tumors, and is fairly accurate in differentiating between benign and malignant lesions. The parotidectomy procedure is still indicated for suspected benign and malignant tumors for definitive diagnosis and surgical treatment. Intraoperative frozen section may be utilized to confirm the diagnosis and guide the extent of surgery, and has been shown to be reliable for decision making.[3]

ANATOMY[4]

The parotid is the largest of the paired major salivary glands. Each gland is located at the upper boundary of level II of the neck, superficial to the sternocleidomastoid muscle (SCM), posterior belly of the digastric, and masseter muscle. The platysma and superficial cervical fascia are continuous with the superficial musculoaponeurotic system (SMAS) fascia of the face, and the parotid lies deep to and separate from this layer of fascia (Figs. 21.1 and 21.2). The gland is invested by a fascia of the superficial layer of the deep cervical fascia (which similarly also invests the other major salivary glands), termed the parotid-masseteric fascia. This fascia superiorly is firmly attached to the zygomatic process, and inferiorly it condenses into the SCM muscle fascia. On the deep medial surface of the parotid the fascia condenses at the stylomandibular ligament. Superior to this ligament, the investing fascia is often weak and discontinuous, which allows the passage of glandular tissue through a tunnel-like space superior to the stylomandibular ligament into the parapharyngeal space (forming a so-called dumbbell tumor).

Gland Structure

The parotid gland is an excretory gland composed of epithelial cells and salivary tissue. The deep cervical fascia

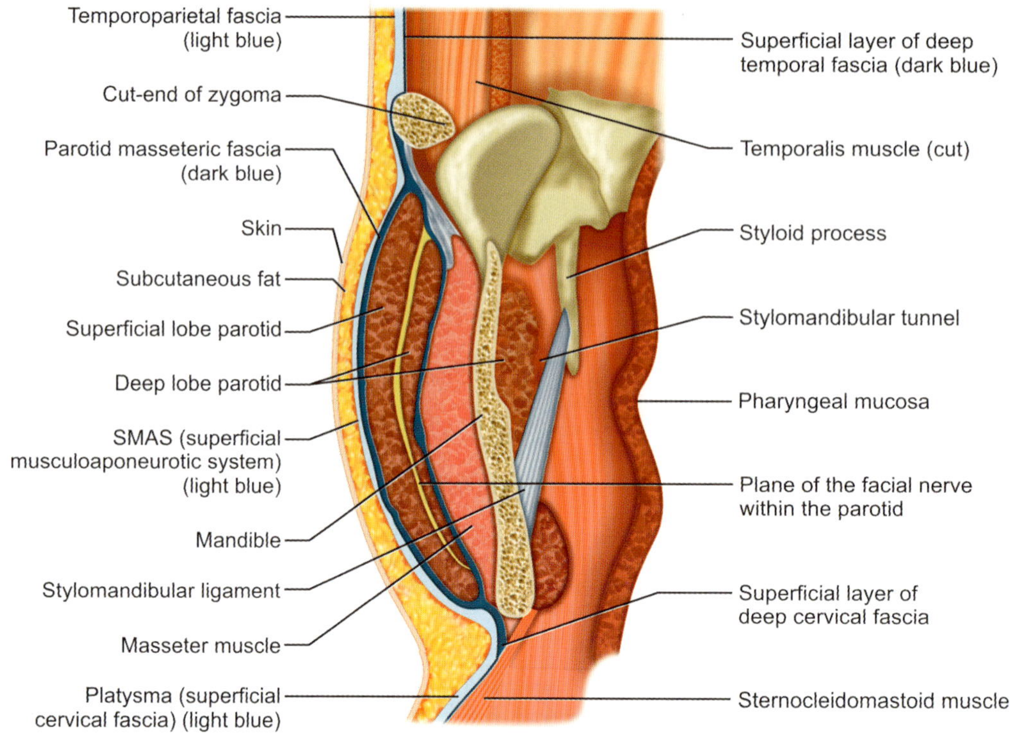

Fig. 21.1: The parotid gland and fascia. The layers of the parotid on coronal section, from superficial to deep: skin, subcutaneous fat, SMAS, parotid fascia, superficial lobe parotid gland, facial nerve branches, deep lobe parotid gland, stylomandibular ligament, parapharyngeal space.

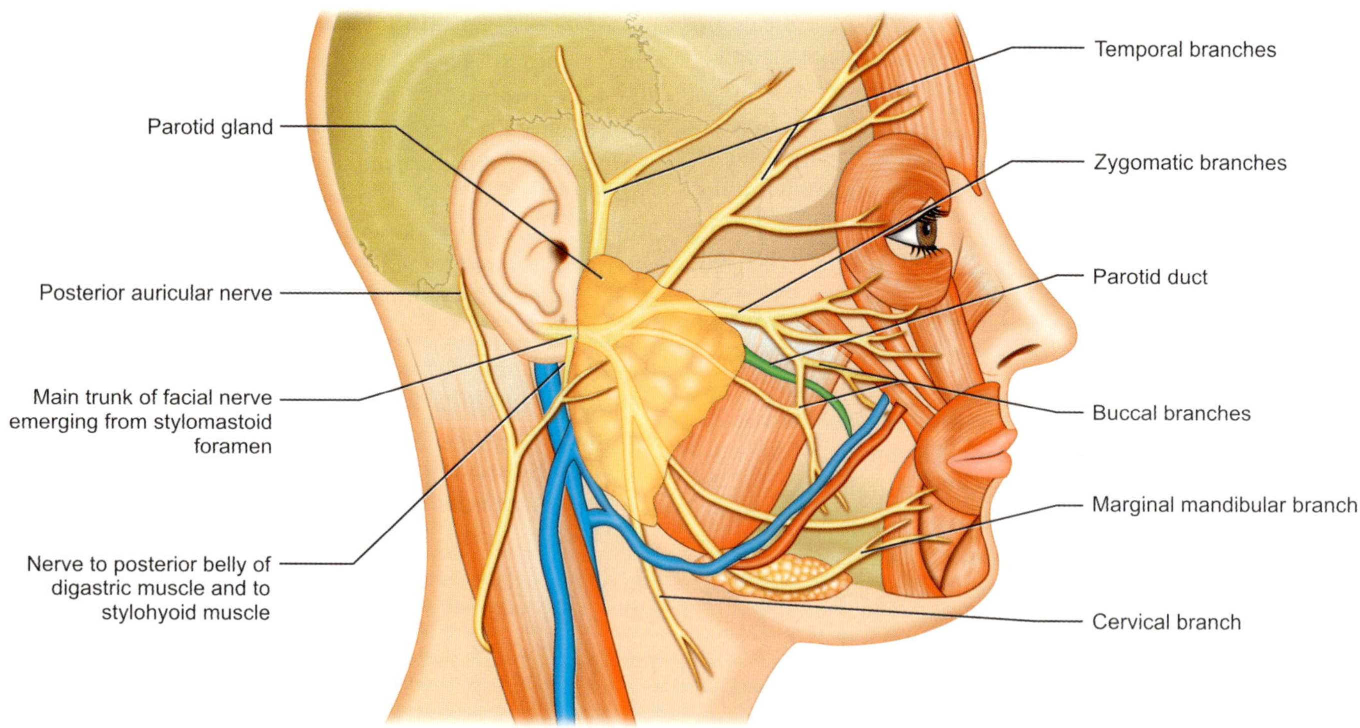

Fig. 21.2: The parotid gland and surrounding anatomy.

surrounding the gland forms a tough condensation at the stylomandibular ligament, which serves to separate the gland from the fascia that separately surrounds the submandibular gland. The fascia also sends septations throughout the substance of the gland, creating lobules and compartments. This can be significant in the setting of an abscess, as there is a tendency for it to be compartmentalized and not easily drained with a single incision. The basic salivary unit is the acinus, composed of acinar cells and surrounded by myoepithelial cells and lymphocytes. The acinar cells are predominantly serous in the parotid gland, and excrete saliva into a central lumen, which is connected to an intercalated duct, and then to a striated duct, and finally an excretory duct. The ducts drain into one another from the separate lobular units in a tree-branch pattern, until finally emptying into the main parotid duct, known as Stenson's duct, after Neils Stenson who described the structure in sheep in 1661.[5] The parotid duct is 4–7 cm long, and leaves the parotid gland at the anterior margin overlying the masseter muscle, and runs anteriorly deep to the SMAS and facial nerves until it pierces the buccopharyngeal fascia and buccinator muscle to empty into the oral cavity. The orifice of Stenson's duct lies in the upper buccal mucosa at approximately the level of the second maxillary molar.

The parotid is described as having a superficial and deep lobe, though there is no true fascial separation of these lobes; instead, the plane of the facial nerve branches running through the parotid establishes the boundary of these lobes. Therefore, a dissection of the superficial parotid occurs lateral to the facial nerve, and the deep lobe medial to the facial nerve. The parotid is sometimes described as having lobular extensions, which arise as the gland extends in various directions to wrap itself around adjacent structures, including the condylar (around the temporomandibular joint [TMJ]), meatal (around the external auditory canal), posterior (over the SCM muscle), glenoid (deep on the vaginal process of the temporal bone), and stylomandibular (extending medially above the stylomandibular ligament) lobules.

The innervation of the parotid gland comes via the auriculotemporal nerve, a branch of the third division of the trigeminal nerve (V3), which provides the sensory innervation. The preganglionic parasympathetic fibers are from the glossopharyngeal nerve, leaving the jugular fossa as Jacobson's nerve forming the tympanic plexus, and then forming the lesser superficial petrosal nerve on the floor of the middle cranial fossa, exiting the skull base through the foramen ovale and synapsing in the otic ganglion, which lies on the medial surface of V3 in the infratemporal fossa. The postganglionic fibers then follow the parotid branches of the auriculotemporal nerve to innervate the gland. The sympathetic innervation is from the superior sympathetic ganglion and follows the course of the external carotid artery branches to the parotid gland.

Vascular Anatomy

The venous drainage from the superficial temporal veins and maxillary veins merges to form the retromandibular vein, which travels within the substance of the parotid gland, deep (medial) to the facial nerve branches. The retromandibular vein exits inferiorly from the parotid gland, and may divide into branches draining anteriorly into the posterior facial vein, which then drains into the internal jugular vein or rarely the anterior jugular vein, or branches draining posteriorly into the external jugular vein.

The external carotid artery travels deep to the posterior belly of the digastric and stylohyoid muscle, along the deep (medial) surface of the parotid gland, and may actually pass through portions of the deep parotid. The terminal branches of the external carotid are the superficial temporal artery and the internal maxillary artery, which branch from the deep surface of the parotid gland, with the superficial temporal artery then taking a more superficial course toward the superior portion of the gland to pass over the zygomatic arch just deep to the temporoparietal fascia (TPF; the continuation of the SMAS/superficial fascia layer), and the internal maxillary artery continues deep to the mandible to pass into the infratemporal fossa between the mandible and the sphenomandibular ligament to enter the pterygopalatine space. Branches from the superficial temporal artery, including the transverse facial artery, pass through the superior portion of gland to the face and the ear, and often parallel branches of the facial nerve.

Nerve Anatomy

The facial nerve exits the skull base at the stylomastoid foramen and then passes through the substance of the parotid gland in an anterior course. The portion of the facial nerve at risk during parotidectomy is responsible for innervation of the muscles of facial expression, the posterior belly of the digastric, and the posterior auricular muscle. The nerve divides shortly after entering the substance of the parotid gland at the pes anserinus into a superior temporofacial trunk, which gives rise to temporal

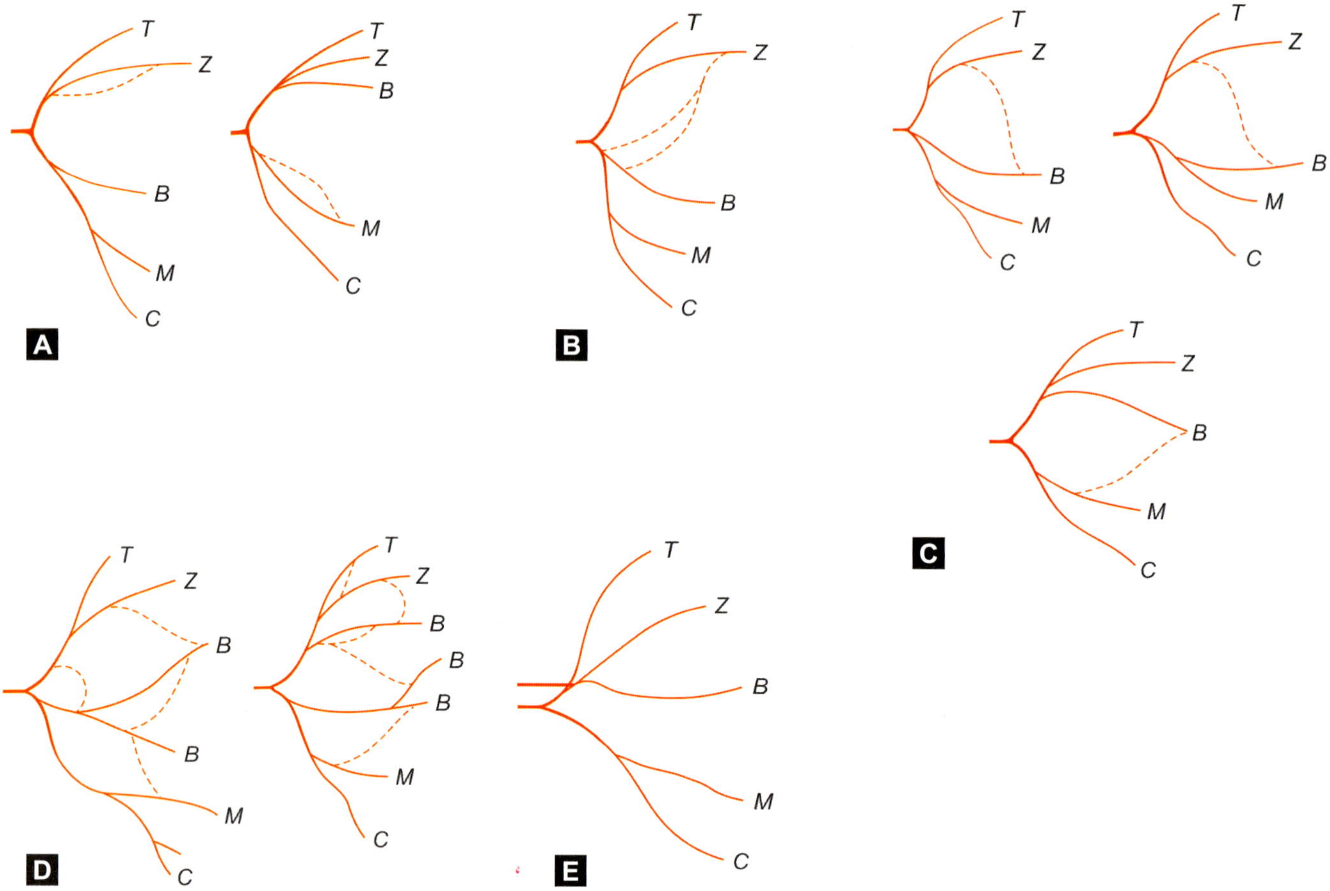

Figs. 21.3A to E: Facial nerve branching patterns. (A) Type I (24%): straight branching, with buccal branch either arising from upper or lower division. (B) Type II (14%): zygomatic loop. (C) Type III (44%): buccal loop. (D) Type IV (14%): multiple variable loops. (E) Type V (3%): two main trunks from temporal bone.
Source: Adapted from Katz and Catalano.[6]

and zygomatic branches, and an inferior cervicofacial trunk, which gives rise to the cervical, marginal, and buccal branches. There are many variations of this branching pattern, and the important principle is that one should not rely on expected patterns, but should trace each nerve and branches out individually until cleared from the specimen (Figs. 21.3A to E).[6] The nerve branches leave the parotid gland through the anterior parotid-masseteric fascia and continue on their course deep to the SMAS to enter the deep surface of the facial muscles they innervate.

PAROTIDECTOMY—INDICATIONS AND CONTRAINDICATIONS

Indications

Superficial parotidectomy: Removal of the lateral parotid lobes with facial nerve dissection:

- Benign parotid neoplasms
- Low-grade malignant neoplasms
- Recurrent sialadenitis or sialolithiasis, not amenable to conservative endoscopic techniques
- Recurrent cysts having failed repeat aspiration and drainage
- Parotid lymph node dissection for cutaneous malignancy

Deep lobe parotidectomy: Removal of the medial parotid lobe with facial nerve dissection:

- Benign parotid neoplasm, limited in size and located medial to the facial nerve

Total parotidectomy: Removal of the lateral and medial parotid lobes, with facial nerve skeletonization:

- Low-grade malignant neoplasm extending medial to the facial nerve
- High-grade malignant neoplasm, with intact facial nerve function

- Extensive benign neoplasm, or recurrent benign tumors

Total parotidectomy with nerve sacrifice: Removal of total parotid gland with involved facial nerve, with identification of proximal and distal nerve segments for grafting

- Malignant neoplasm with facial nerve paralysis

Contraindications

- Incomplete or inappropriate preoperative imaging
- Uncorrected or unevaluated predisposition to bleeding
- Medical comorbidity or contraindication to general anesthesia

SPECIAL CONSIDERATIONS: NERVE MONITORING

It is critically important to be able to assess the function of the facial nerve throughout the procedure, and various methods have been utilized by surgeons. The simplest, most cost-effective, dependable method continues to be direct visual monitoring of the face for stimulation. A simple handheld nerve stimulator can be utilized for the purpose of testing the nerve for stimulation thresholds. In recent decades, continuous electromyographic (EMG) nerve monitoring has been introduced. This monitoring has been demonstrated to have clear benefits for certain types of surgery, e.g. posterior fossa approaches for acoustic neuromas. However, there has been no clear demonstrable benefit for routine superficial parotidectomy.[7] Despite this, facial nerve monitoring during routine parotidectomy has become routine at many centers in the most recent decade. The setup includes two electrode leads placed in each muscle to be monitored (typical monitoring includes the orbicularis oris and orbicularis oculi), which can detect a change in electrical potential as the muscle is depolarized. Ground leads for the muscle electrodes and the stimulator electrode must be placed at a distant site. A monopolar stimulator is utilized to generate an electrical current of set duration, frequency, and magnitude. The setup also includes a video and audio monitor. Two different types of feedback signals can be elicited, in addition to that arising from direct stimulation via the Prass probe.[8] The first are "trains" of prolonged asynchronous low amplitude motor unit activity, which typically signify nerve injury, irritation, or traction. The second are "bursts" of high amplitude synchronous motor unit discharges, which correspond to a single depolarization of the nerve, as from mechanical trauma or electrical stimulation.

Continuous EMG neuromonitoring is not considered the standard of care for parotidectomy, and is currently used as an adjunct tool. If used, the surgeon should not rely on the continuous monitoring to invariably identify the nerve prior to serious inadvertent injury. The surgeon must utilize the information from the monitor as simply another piece of information interpreted in light of the ongoing surgical dissection; instances of transecting the nerve without any indication from a working EMG monitor definitely occur. It is best practice to continue to use standard visual identification of the nerve and visual face-monitoring techniques, with EMG as an additional tool. There may be specific circumstances, such as for recurrent parotid tumors and reoperations in the parotid bed, where electrical nerve stimulators and EMG neuromonitoring have particular utility and benefit.

INSTRUMENTS AND OPERATIVE CONSIDERATIONS

The standard instrument trays utilized in neck dissection surgery are sufficient for parotid surgery, though several specialized instruments should also be considered for inclusion on the set. A set of fine-tipped dissectors is essential for precise dissection around the facial nerve. Some surgeons prefer the McCabe dissector, which has a fine sharp tip, is slightly curved at its tip, has no serrations or teeth, and does not lock, and hence is designed for careful dissection work around nerves and vessels. Though a relatively safe instrument, pitfalls include the sharp tip, which will easily puncture structures if misdirected, and the curved tip, which if opened and closed while dissecting can catch the nerve and pinch it. Other surgeons prefer using fine-tip mosquito or hemostat dissectors, and still others prefer the tip-action and efficiency of using tenotomy scissors for tissue dissection. Though the fineness of the instrument tip aids in the precision of the tissue dissection, it should be borne in mind that increasingly fine tips are sharp and can cause inadvertent injury to the nerve or vessels. Therefore, it is prudent to continuously reassess how fine an instrument tip is necessary to accomplish the dissection maneuvers at hand. Balancing instrument bluntness with dissection precision can certainly enable safer and more efficient surgical practice. In addition, specialized Cummings retractors are especially useful for parotid surgery, as a notch at the end of the retractor can be positioned over the nerve and the curve of the retractor allows the tissue to be distracted up in a lateral trajectory, rather than compressed in on top of the nerve being dissected.

Various types of cautery and coagulation devices are utilized, mainly based on surgeon preference and experience with their use. These include Bovie cautery with either a spatula tip or needle tip; bipolar cautery with various types of hand pieces; ultrasonic-energy shears; or other alternative-energy tissue-sealing devices and hot-knife scalpels (Shaw blades).

The patient should be positioned supine, in reverse Trendelenburg or with the head of the bed elevated 30° (low- or semi-Fowler's position), to assist with hemostasis and edema. The neck should be mildly extended with judicious use of a shoulder roll, and the head should be rotated towards the opposite side. The table tilt and height should be repeatedly adjusted throughout the procedure to optimize the surgeon's and patient's position. The entire hemiface from forehead to chin needs to be visible during the surgery; a convenient surgical drape to maintain sterility and separation of the surgical site from the aerodigestive tract while allowing the face to be visualized is the Ioban Steri-Drap (3M)—or any other sterile transparent adhesive drape can be used, which is laid over the face after the prep, with a hole then cut in the drape over the planned incision.

The patient can be intubated orally with the tube taped to the opposite oral commissure outside of the surgical field. However, the oral endotracheal tube will prevent the jaws from closing fully and being distracted anteriorly during the procedure, which may be important for improving exposure to certain parotid tumors with limited exposure around the mandibular ramus and deep in the parapharyngeal space. Therefore, an alternative consideration is to perform a nasotracheal intubation, and avoid any interference with jaw motion from the endotracheal tube during the procedure.

The anesthesiologist should be reminded that the facial nerve will be monitored, and paralysis of the patient is contraindicated. A member of the surgical team should be positioned appropriately to be able to fully visualize the face throughout the facial nerve dissection.

TECHNIQUE: INCISIONS

The classic skin incision for parotid surgery is the modified Blair incision. This incision was described by Blair in 1912, and modified by Bailey in 1941.[9] The preauricular incision follows the junction of the face and the auricle, following

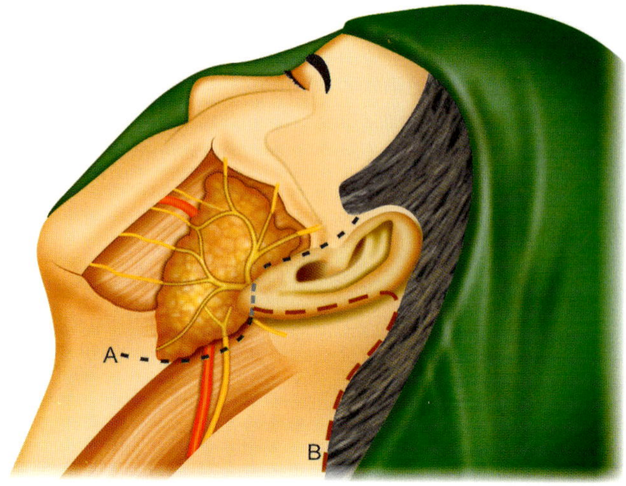

Fig. 21.4: Parotidectomy incisions. (A) The modified Blair incision placed in the preauricular crease down to the lobule, then curves slightly posteriorly on top of the mastoid tip over the SCM muscle and curves gently anteriorly into a neck crease, 2–3 cm below the mandible angle. (B) The facelift incision follows the preauricular crease to the lobule, then curves superiorly behind the ear in the postauricular crease up to the occipital hairline, then inferiorly at the edge of the hairline. (SCM: Sternocleidomastoid muscle).

the incisura and variably hiding the incision behind of or in front of the tragus, then following a preauricular crease to the lobule attachment, at which point the incision gently curves onto the neck over the SCM, aiming to be 2–3 cm below the angle of the mandible and hidden in a neck skin crease (Fig. 21.4). This incision affords excellent visibility of the facial nerve and peripheral boundaries of the parotid gland, and can be easily extended into the neck for a supraomohyoid neck dissection. The incision is well disguised over the face, and is noticeable in the neck only when looking at the oblique or side profile.

Beginning in the 1960s, the rhytidectomy incision began to be utilized for parotid surgery. This incision begins in a preauricular crease identical to the modified Blair incision. When it reaches the lobule, the incision follows the postauricular crease superiorly behind the ear until the occipital hairline is reached, where the incision turns inferiorly and follows the occipital hairline for approximately 6 cm. The benefits of this incision are the avoidance of a more obvious incision on the anterior neck. The incision does afford the visibility to identify and dissect the facial nerve. However, a large skin flap must be elevated, greater retraction is necessary and therefore exposure is not optimal, anterior exposure is limited, and access to the neck is not optimal if a neck dissection is needed. This incision should only be considered in benign, posteriorly located tumors for motivated patients.

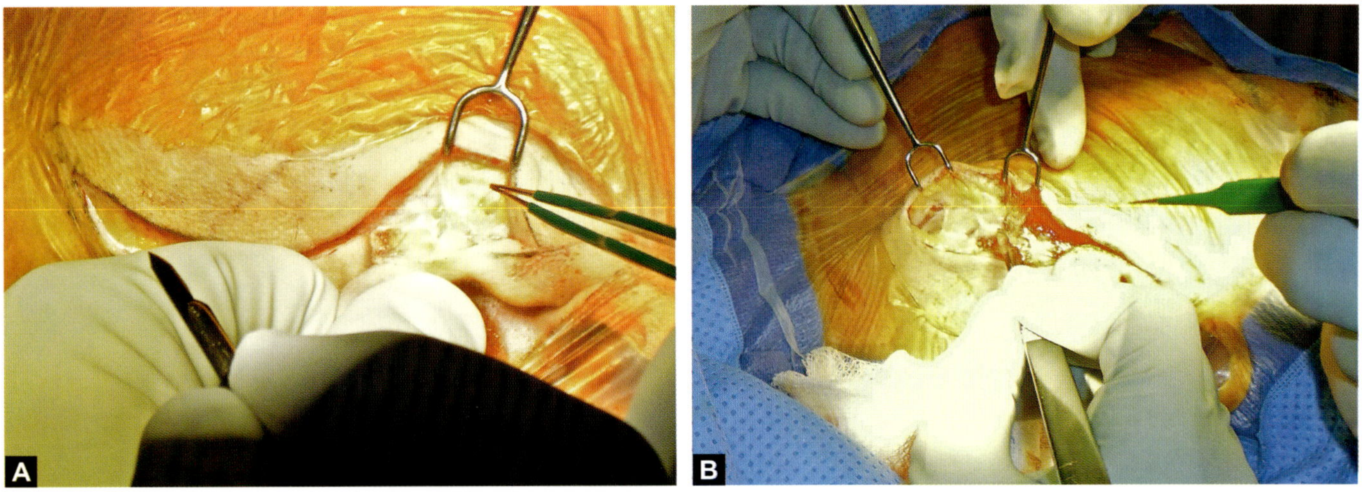

Figs. 21.9A and B: Incision and raising flaps. (A) The incision is made through skin and subcutaneous fat, SMAS, to the parotid fascia. (B) The flap is sharply dissected along the parotid fascia, deep to the SMAS and platysma, being careful to not violate the tumor capsule, until the edge of the tumor or parotid is sufficiently exposed. (SMAS: Superficial musculoaponeurotic system).

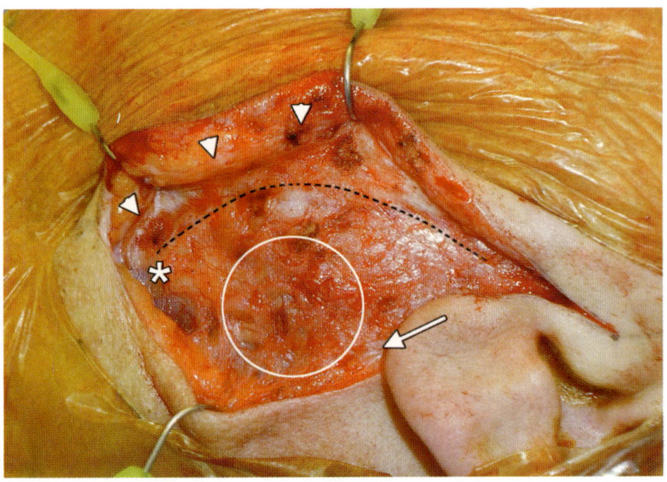

Fig. 21.10: Exposure. The skin flap is reflected to expose the boundaries of the tumor within the parotid gland (marked by solid white line). The skin flap was separated from the parotid fascia in a sub-SMAS/platysma plane (arrowhead marking cut edge of SMAS/platysma, dotted black line marks plane between parotid fascia and SMAS). External jugular vein (asterisk) and great auricular nerve (arrow) are identified. (SMAS: Superficial musculoaponeurotic system).

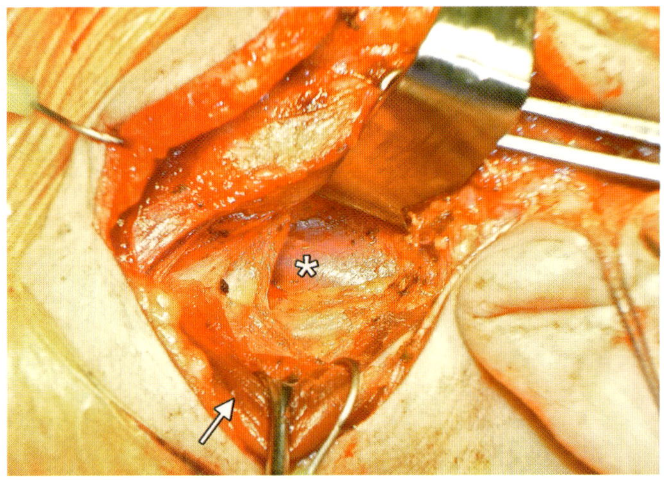

Fig. 21.11: SCM and posterior belly of digastric muscle. The anterior edge of the SCM is dissected and the muscle retracted posteriorly (arrow); the parotid tail is retracted anteriorly with an Allis clamp. Further dissection medially and retraction exposes the posterior belly of the digastric muscle (asterisk). (SCM: Sternocleidomastoid muscle).

dissected first. The tumor specimen is retracted in an anterior direction, and the plane of dissection continues deep to the tumor, identifying the next branch of the facial nerve. The specimen is thus separated from the parotid at the plane of the facial nerve. The buccal branches of the nerve are frequently the most variable in location, and usually both the superior and inferior divisions need to be dissected to identify the small contributions to the buccal branches (Fig. 21.15).

There are many different methods to perform the dissection of the facial nerve branches, and several techniques are described here, though there are many alternatives. A dissector following the course of a nerve branch is spread, and the overlying parotid tissue can be squeezed with a forceps while the assistant observes the face for twitching to ensure the tissue is safe to divide. The tissue can be cut sharply with a #12 blade, a Shaw scalpel, or scissors. Ultrasonic instruments or bipolar cautery may be

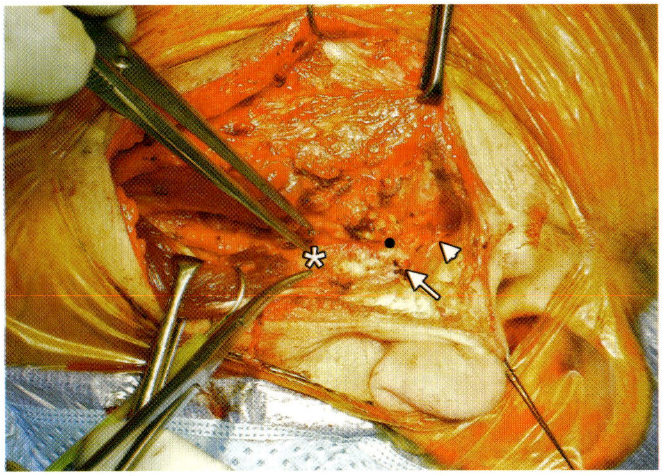

Fig. 21.12: Facial nerve landmarks. The parotid is dissected from the ear perichondrium, identifying the landmarks for localizing the facial nerve, including the tragal pointer (arrowhead), the tympanomastoid groove (arrow), and posterior belly of the digastric (asterisk). The location of the facial nerve can be anticipated (black dot). The dissection is continued along a broad front to maximize the exposure.

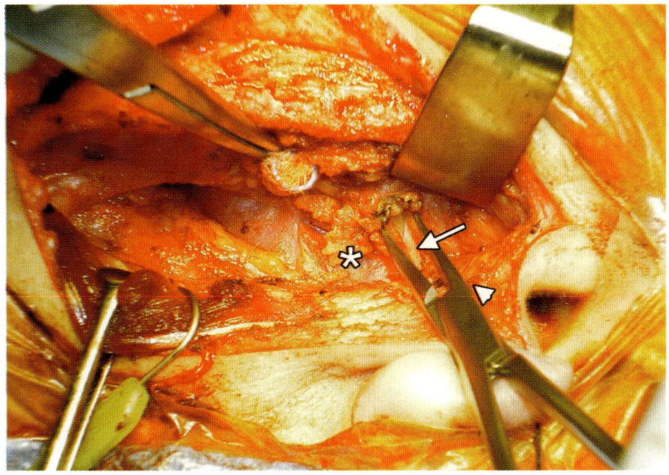

Fig. 21.13: Facial nerve identified. The main trunk of the facial nerve (arrow) is identified superior to the posterior belly of the digastric (asterisk), approximately 1 cm inferior and medial to the tragal pointer (arrowhead).

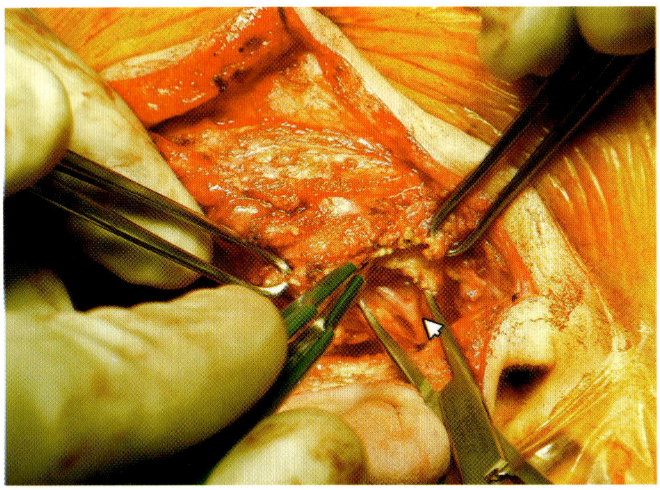

Fig. 21.14: Pes anserinus. The main trunk is followed anteriorly into the parotid gland until the pes anserinus (arrowhead) is identified. At this point the dissection continues based on the location of the tumor—in this case, only the inferior cervicofacial trunk of the facial nerve needs to be dissected to remove the tumor mass.

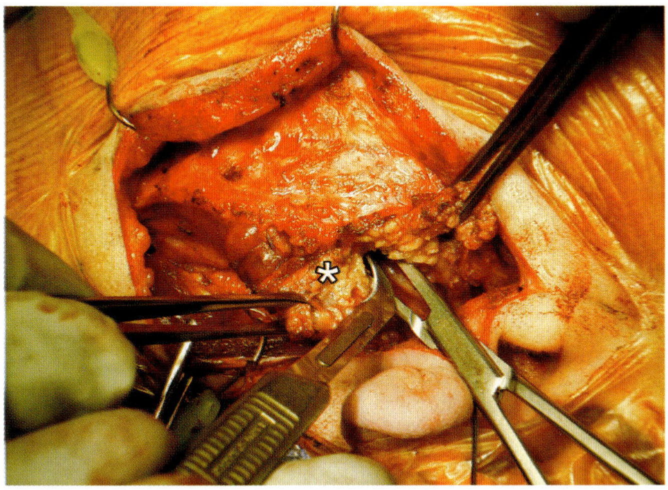

Fig. 21.15: Dissection of nerve branches. The fascia over the nerve is dissected, and the overlying parotid tissue can be divided with bipolar cautery (as depicted in Fig. 21.14), or sharply divided with a #12 blade. The face should be monitored for stimulation of nerve branches. The margin of the tumor (asterisk) is followed with a cuff of normal parotid tissue.

used when appropriate. Much of the tissue to be sharply divided does not require cauterization, as the majority of the parotid tissue does not bleed excessively. When visible vessels are encountered, they are ideally ligated in a controlled manner before being divided. Caution is urged with the use of bipolar cautery or other heated instruments around the nerve, as inadvertent injury is possible; in addition, attempting to control excessive bleeding with the bipolar should be done very carefully and only with the nerve under clear visualization.

Step 8: Branches of the retromandibular vein are often encountered and ligated. The nerve branches are followed to a safe distance around the resection line of the tumor, and as far as the anterior periphery of the gland. The parotid duct should be ligated and divided if necessary (Fig. 21.16).

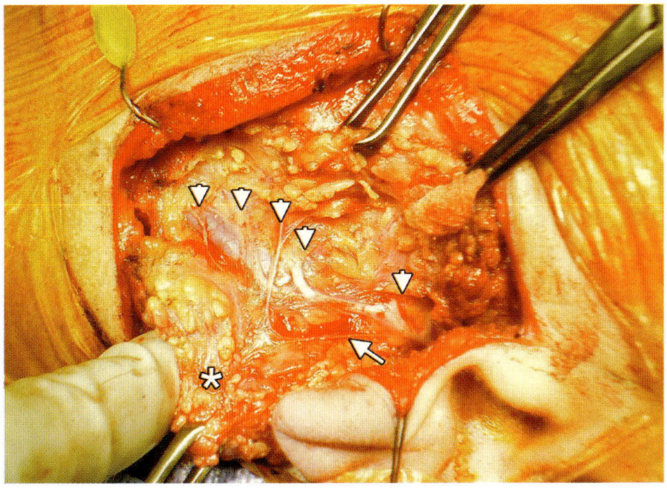

Fig. 21.16: Tumor freed from facial nerve branches. The inferior facial nerve branches (arrowheads) have been successively dissected to the periphery of the parotid, away from the tumor, and the tumor with cuff of normal tissue (asterisk) is retracted inferiorly. The configuration of nerve branches can vary widely; a loop of a buccal branch is seen here (arrow).

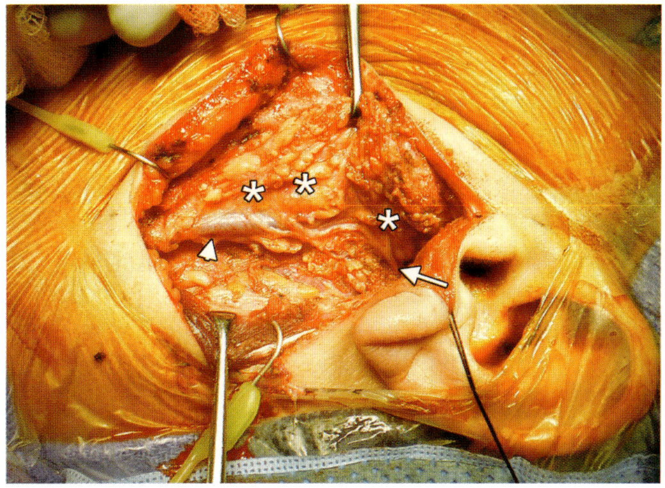

Fig. 21.17: Partial parotidectomy completed. The tumor is removed, the parotid bed is irrigated, hemostasis obtained, and facial nerve function assessed at the main trunk with nerve stimulator. Structures: facial nerve main trunk (arrow), facial nerve branches (asterisks), retromandibular vein (arrowhead).

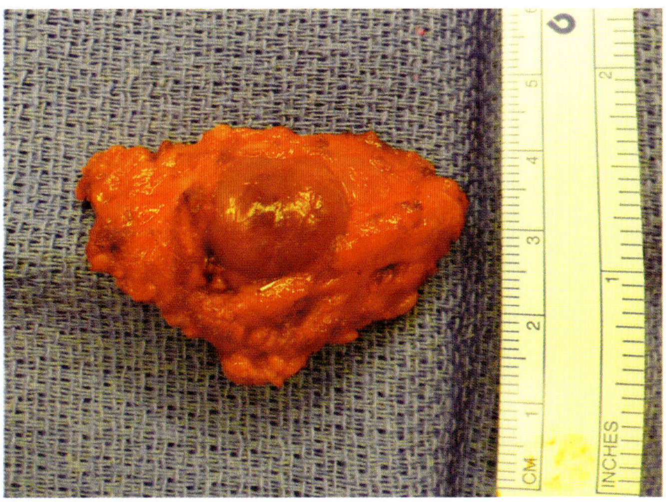

Fig. 21.18: Tumor specimen. Partial parotidectomy specimen, demonstrating a 2-cm cystic tumor surrounded by a margin of normal salivary tissue.

Step 9: The specimen is removed and inspected to determine the adequacy of resection. The main trunk of the nerve can be stimulated to ensure all of the branches to the face remain intact. The wound is irrigated thoroughly, and hemostasis is obtained, with care to avoid cauterization around the nerve (Figs. 21.17 and 21.18).

Step 10: The need for reconstruction can be determined based on the depth of the wound and facial contour, and a SCM flap mobilized as previously described. The preserved SMAS/platysma fascial layer is advanced to cover the remaining parotid tissue and secured with 3-0 Vicryl suture, resuspending the face and potentially preventing the ingrowth of parasympathetic fibers into the dermal sweat glands, which leads to Frey's syndrome. A suction drain is left in the parotid wound bed and brought out through the skin behind the ear. The incision is closed in two layers, with buried 4-0 monocryl in the deep dermal layer, and a 5-0 running cutaneous stitch to perfectly align the epidermal skin edges (Figs. 21.19A to C).

An immediate assessment of facial movement during the extubation process should be done to establish the new baseline of facial nerve function.

A facelift pressure dressing can be placed to help eliminate the dead space in the wound bed and prevent seroma and edema, although it is usually not necessary.

TOTAL PAROTIDECTOMY

Step 1: The steps of the superficial parotidectomy described above are completed with either removal or tethering of the superficial parotid as dictated by the individual tumor. At this point, the lateral surface of the facial nerve and all of its branches within the gland should be visible. The nerve is gently elevated with nerve hooks and the fascial attachments on its deep surface sharply divided with tissue scissors. The nerve should now be completely free from parotid tissue throughout its course.

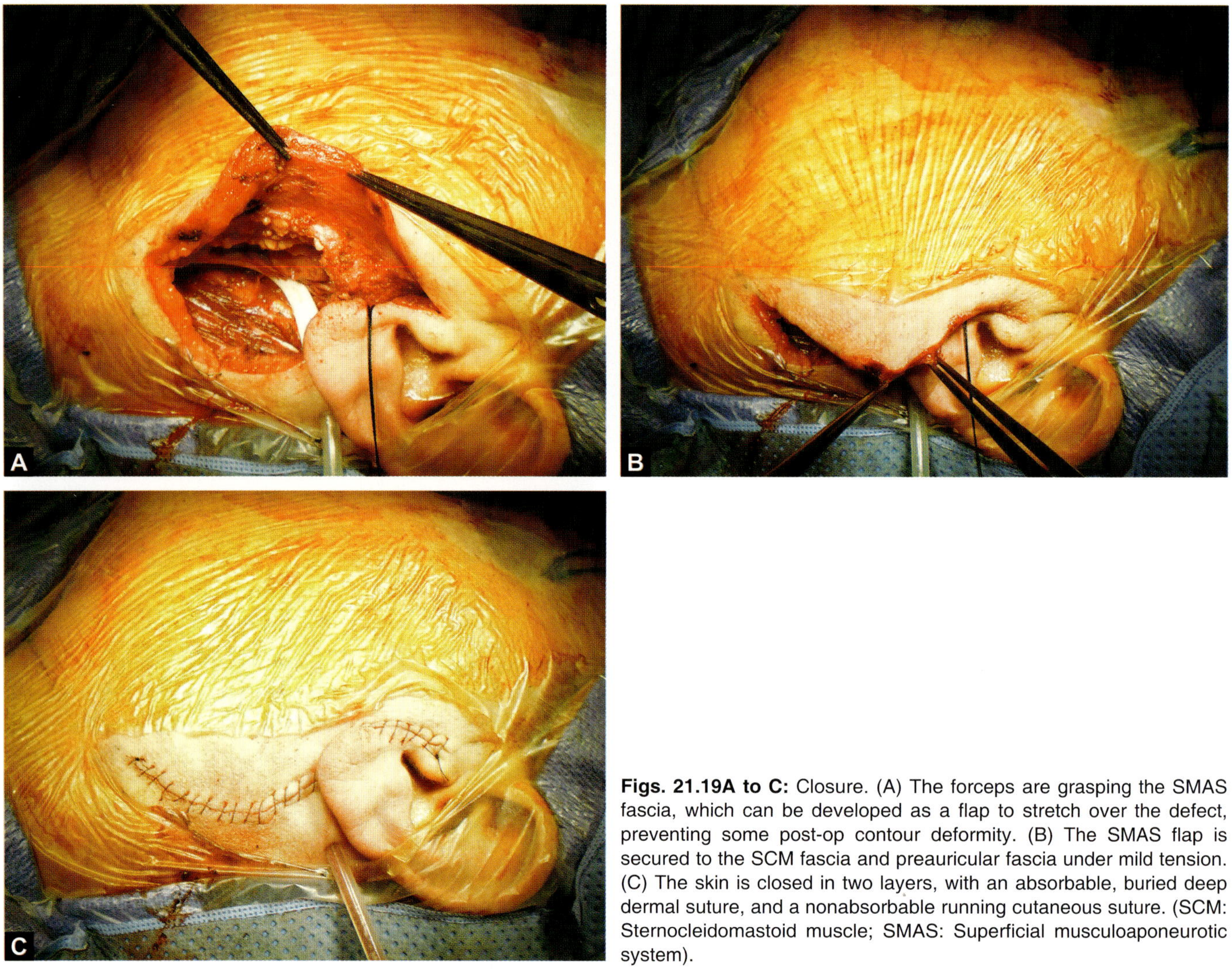

Figs. 21.19A to C: Closure. (A) The forceps are grasping the SMAS fascia, which can be developed as a flap to stretch over the defect, preventing some post-op contour deformity. (B) The SMAS flap is secured to the SCM fascia and preauricular fascia under mild tension. (C) The skin is closed in two layers, with an absorbable, buried deep dermal suture, and a nonabsorbable running cutaneous suture. (SCM: Sternocleidomastoid muscle; SMAS: Superficial musculoaponeurotic system).

Step 2: The dissection of the deep lobe continues by following the parotidomasseteric fascia, freeing the gland from surrounding structures. Inferiorly, the gland is separated from the stylohyoid muscle; anteriorly, it is separated from the masseter muscle; superiorly, it is separated from around the TMJ.

Step 3: Large vessels entering and leaving the deep portion of the gland must be ligated and divided. The external carotid artery is deep and superior to the stylohyoid muscle and typically must be ligated here where it enters the gland. Superiorly, the superficial temporal artery must be ligated where it leaves the gland. Anteriorly, the transverse facial artery should be ligated, while avoiding injuring the zygomatic facial nerve branches it travels with.

Step 4: As the remaining portion of the deep lobe is mobilized from the deep styloid muscles, the internal maxillary artery and veins will be encountered and ligated. Care should be taken to rule out the presence of a loop of the internal carotid artery in this region, to avoid inadvertent injury or ligation. The stylomandibular ligament can be divided, if needed, to improve visibility and bluntly remove any extensions of the gland in the stylomandibular tunnel. At this point, the deep lobe should be freed of all attachments, and the specimen removed from underneath the preserved facial nerve branches.

Step 5: The steps of reconstructing and closing the wound are similar to those discussed previously.

Some temporary weakness of the facial nerve is to be expected whenever this extent of dissection is carried out, and proper attention to eye care is essential in the postoperative setting to avoid eye complications.

COMPLICATIONS

Delayed facial nerve weakness (not present immediately postoperatively, but developing in the next 24 hours) is common, depending on the extent of dissection, is more likely in older patients, and is temporary. Unintentional immediate complete facial nerve paralysis should be very rare. It should be recognized immediately and attempts to perform immediate repair with cable nerve graft interposition should be made. If local anesthetic is used on skin incisions, one must wait for the anesthetic effect to wear off to rule out infiltration as the cause of the nerve dysfunction (for this reason, it is best to avoid or minimize the use of local anesthetic, as there is limited benefit).

Frey's syndrome is the occurrence of sweating from the skin overlying the affected parotid at the time of meals. It is a frequent sequela of parotid injury and was first described by Duphenix in 1757.[10] In 1923 Frey described the pathogenesis of the condition in relation to the auriculotemporal nerve, and in 1932 it was recognized as a sequelae of parotidectomy. The incidence of Frey's syndrome following parotidectomy is reported between 20% and 90%, and some authors suggest this incidence depends on how carefully the symptoms are searched for. Certainly for some patients, the gustatory sweating can be an embarrassing, socially awkward, and frustrating problem. Nonsurgical options for treatment include antiperspirants, anticholinergics, or Botulinum toxin injection. Surgical options include auriculotemporal nerve section, Jacobsen's nerve neurectomy, or interposing tissue between the skin and parotid gland. Consideration may be given at the time of the parotidectomy to preventing the development of this syndrome; a variety of techniques have been described, mostly based on the hypothesis of placing intervening tissue between the parotid bed and the skin to prevent the in-growth of postganglionic parasympathetic nerve fibers into the sweat glands, including a dermal graft, fat graft, SMAS flap, TPF flap, or SCM muscle flap.

Occasionally, sialoceles or salivary fistulas occur; these can be treated with anticholinergics, repeated aspiration/drainage, pressure dressing, or wound packing, and will resolve in time with conservative management. Wound infections are rare, and postoperative antibiotics are not indicated.

Numbness around the earlobe can in general be expected, and patients should be counseled about precautions related to ear piercings and cold weather. The cosmetic appearance of the surgical defect and scar will mature and improve over the first year, and patients should be encouraged to wait before considering any revisions.

REFERENCES

1. Bailey H. The treatment of tumours of the parotid gland with special reference to total parotidectomy. Br J Surg. 1941;28(111):337-46.
2. Kidd HA. Complete excision of the parotid gland with preservation of the facial nerve. Br Med J. 1950;1(4660):989-91.
3. Olsen KD, Moore EJ, Lewis JE. Frozen section pathology for decision making in parotid surgery. JAMA Otolaryngol Head Neck Surg. 2013 ;139(12):1275-8.
4. Janfaza P, Cheney M. Superficial structures of the face, head, and parotid region. In: Janfaza P, et al. (Eds), Surgical Anatomy of the Head and Neck. Cambridge: Harvard University Press; 2011.
5. Lydiatt DD, Bucher GS. The historical evolution of the understanding of the submandibular and sublingual salivary glands. Clin Anat. 2012;25(1):2-11.
6. Katz AD, Catalano P. The clinical significance of the various anastomotic branches of the facial nerve. Report of 100 patients. Arch Otolaryngol Head Neck Surg. 1987;113(9):959-62.
7. Grosheva M, Klussmann JP, Grimminger C, et al. Electromyographic facial nerve monitoring during parotidectomy for benign lesions does not improve the outcome of postoperative facial nerve function: a prospective two-center trial. Laryngoscope. 2009;119(12):2299-305.
8. Yasmine A, Ashram CDY. Intraoperative monitoring of cranial nerves in neuro-otologic surgery. In: Flint P, et al. (Eds), Cummings Otolaryngology Head and Neck Surgery, Fifth Edition. Philadelphia: Mosby; 2010.
9. Terris DJ, Tuffo KM, Fee WE. Modified facelift incision for parotidectomy. J Laryngol Otol. 1994;108(7):574-8.
10. Queiroz Filho W, Dedivitis RA, Abrão Rapoport MD, et al. Sternocleidomastoid muscle flap preventing Frey syndrome following parotidectomy. World J Surg. 2004;28(4):361-4.
11. Cesteleyn L, Helman J, King S, et al. Temporoparietal fascia flaps and superficial musculoaponeurotic system plication in parotid surgery reduces Frey's syndrome. J Oral Maxillofac Surg. 2002;60(11):1284-97.
12. Olsen KD. Superficial parotidectomy. Oper Tech Gen Surg. 2004;6(2):102-14.

CHAPTER 22

Submandibular Gland Excision

Mihir R Patel, Jason G Newman

SURGICAL INDICATIONS—SUBMANDIBULAR GLAND EXCISION

Several disorders result in irreversible histologic changes within the submandibular gland tissue and are indications for submandibular gland excision. Such disorders include sialolithiasis, chronic sialoadenitis, and salivary gland tumors. In the cases of sialolithiasis and chronic sialoadenitis, operative intervention often begins with an exhaustive algorithm of minimally invasive techniques including sialendoscopy.[1] Sialoendoscopy has decreased the need for submandibular gland excision secondary to sialoadenitis, and a recent study identified sialolithiasis as the indication for submandibular gland excision in 38% of cases.[2] Submandibular gland tumors accounted for 47% of the cases in another series with benign tumors diagnosed in 67% (n = 28) and malignant tumors in 33% (n = 14).[3] In the submandibular gland, pleomorphic adenoma accounts for 30% to 60% of all neoplasia and 75% of all benign tumors.[3,4] Adenoid cystic carcinoma is the most common malignant neoplasm of the submandibular gland, followed by mucoepidermoid carcinoma.[5]

Tumors clinically manifest as painless, discrete, firm, mobile masses below the inferior border of the mandible. Benign masses of the submandibular gland are difficult to clinically distinguish from those that are malignant, although malignancies tend to be larger and may have faster clinical doubling times.[6] Pain is a poor clinical prognosticator and has been reported in up to 30% of patients with malignant tumors.[7] Fixation to the overlying skin and limited mobility are indicative of malignancy, identified in only 3% of submandibular tumors.[8] Ipsilateral weakness of the marginal mandibular branch of the facial or hypoglossal nerve or lingual nerve hypesthesia suggests perineural invasion and is a late clinical sign almost exclusive to malignancy.

Differential diagnosis of a submandibular mass that has no features of malignancy should include lymphadenopathy, vascular malformation, and plunging ranula. Infectious and noninfectious granulomatous disease, such as sarcoidosis and tuberculosis, may also present with swelling and mass in the submandibular region.[9] Hematologic malignancies, including Hodgkin and non-Hodgkin's lymphoma, may manifest as submandibular swellings.

Radiologic evaluation of a submandibular mass is indicated after a thorough history and examination. Ultrasound is advocated as an initial noninvasive modality that can assist in determining benign from malignant pathology. Ultrasound fine-needle aspiration biopsy may help analyze superficial salivary gland lesions with the same precision as computed tomography (CT) and magnetic resonance imaging (MRI).[10] In determining the exact anatomic location of submandibular masses (intraglandular versus extraglandular). MRI provides slightly higher accuracy rates than contrast-enhanced CT.[11,12] CT may have some benefit in detecting early cortical erosion of the mandible and identifying regional metastatic disease.[11] In the preoperative evaluation of high-grade salivary gland tumors, positron emission tomography/CT has shown superiority to CT alone in both diagnosis and staging.[13]

SURGICAL TECHNIQUE—SUBMANDIBULAR GLAND EXCISION

The patient is placed in the supine position, and general anesthesia is achieved via orotracheal intubation. Cervical

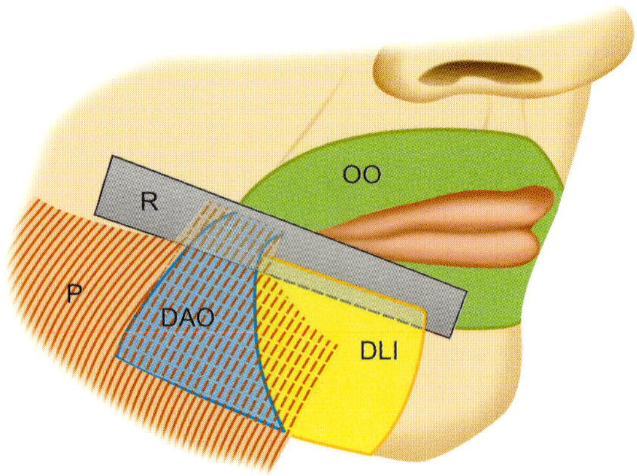

Fig. 22.1: Lower lip facial mimetic muscles. (OO: Orbicularis oris; R: Rhisorius; P: Platysma; DAO: Depressor anguli oris; DLI: Depressor labii inferioris).

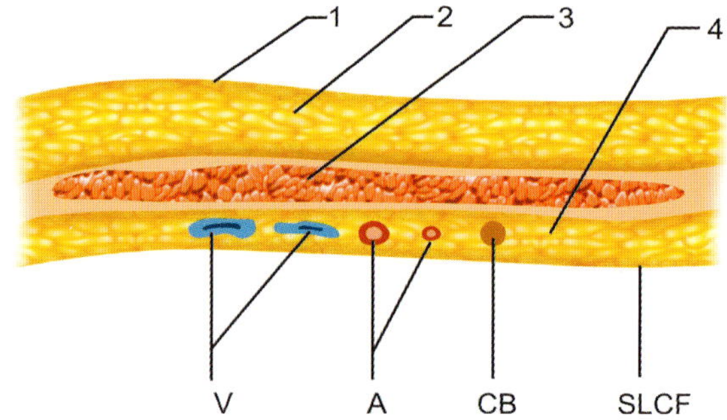

Fig. 22.2: Layers of the neck with neurovascular structures over the inferior submandibular gland. (1: Skin; 2: External fatty layer; 3: SMAS and platysma; 4: Internal fatty layer; V: Anterior jugular vein tributaries; A: Submental artery branches; CB: Cervical branch of facial nerve; SLCF: Superficial layer of cervical fascia).

extension is aided with a shoulder roll. Placing the head of the bed at a 20°–35° incline provides further extension and reduces venous pressure and thus venous bleeding. After adjusting the table, it is important to palpate the occiput to ensure that the head is resting on a circular foam pillow and not suspended in the air. The head is then rotated slightly (10°–20°) opposite to the side of the lesion to facilitate exposure of the submandibular gland. The anterior neck is prepared with povidone-iodine and draped in the standard sterile fashion. Preincision antibiotics are administered at this time with 10 mg of IV dexamethasone, which anesthesia literature has shown to reduce postoperative emesis. The patient remains unparalyzed throughout the procedure to monitor for nerve activity.

The incision line is placed in a neck crease that begins approximately 3 cm below the gonion (angle of the mandible) and ends at the point 4 cm below the mandible at the first premolar (tooth number 21 on the left, 28 on the right). This incision runs a course toward the inferior edge of the hyoid bone, a palpable landmark that provides important anatomical information during the procedure. The incision placement also minimizes injury to the marginal mandibular and cervical branches of the facial nerve. The entire skin incision is made and taken through the superficial cervical fascia that is confluent with the platysma. The platysma originates from the superficial fascia over the pectoral and deltoid muscles and is contiguous with the superficial muscular aponeurotic system layer in the face and the temporoparietal fascia layer of the scalp. The muscle inserts onto the mandible while interdigitating with the depressor muscles of the lip (Fig. 22.1). For this reason, the corner of the lip will depress while using the bovie to cut the platysma, leading the inexperienced surgeon to believe the marginal mandibular branch of the facial nerve is being harmed. The platysma is innervated by the cervical branch of the facial nerve and back stimulation from the cervical nerve to the marginal mandibular branch can emulate this phenomenon as well.

A subplatysma skin flap is elevated superiorly, taking care to keep the superficial layer of the deep cervical fascia down. The subplatysma flap is secured with a 2-0 silk suture to the drapes with a Kelley clamp to keep the field of dissection exposed. Elevation of the superficial layer of the deep cervical fascia begins at the greater cornu of the hyoid bone, which is palpable. This simplifies identification of the digastric tendon and provides a safe level at which to elevate the superficial layer of the deep cervical fascia. A mosquito clamp is used to create an opening in the fascia at the hyoid and dissection proceeds posteriorly toward the angle of the mandible to identify the submandibular gland, the anterior facial vein, and the marginal mandibular branch of the facial nerve.

The marginal mandibular branch of the facial nerve is located in the subplatysma plane within the fatty layer that is immediately superficial to the superficial layer of the deep cervical fascia, which invests the submandibular gland (Fig. 22.2). A common source of confusion is that the cervical branches tend to be superficial, innervate the platysma, and stimulation of the cervical branch mimics movement from marginal mandibular nerve stimulation. Anatomical cadaveric studies by Dingman in 1962 identified the course of the marginal mandibular nerve in relation to the lower border of the mandible and the facial artery at the antegonial notch.[14] Dingman observed that posterior to the facial artery, the marginal mandibular branch runs above the inferior border of the mandible in 81% of the specimens.[14] In the remaining 19%, the marginal branch formed a downward arc up to 1.0 cm below the inferior border of the mandible.[14] In 98% of the specimens, the main branch of the nerve is superficial to the facial artery at the antegonial notch.[14] Anterior to the notch, the nerve was not observed traveling below the inferior border of the mandible. In 1979, Conley remarked that his experience identified the course of the marginal mandibular nerve to be 1–2 cm below the inferior border of the mandible in almost every instance.[15] Conley noted that live dissection with the neck extended displaces the marginal mandibular caudad while in cadavers the tissues have contracted and the rigidity prevents this natural displacement.[15] In our experience, following the course of the anterior facial vein toward the antegonial notch with a McCabe nerve dissector best identifies the nerve (Fig. 22.3). The nerve courses just superficial to the vein and the facial artery will be encountered as dissection proceeds toward the antegonial notch. Once the nerve is identified, it may be traced anteriorly along its course toward the depressor anguli oris, depressor labii inferioris, mentalis, and part of the orbicularis and risorius. The marginal mandibular nerve is displaced or tethered to the superior subplatysma flap with a Vicryl stitch.

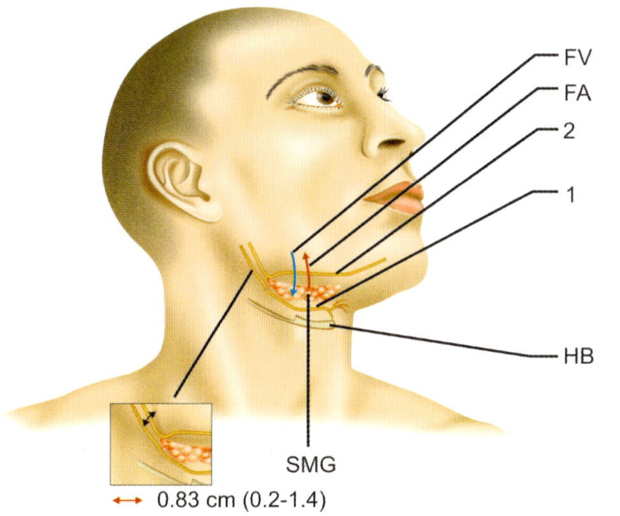

Fig. 22.3: Identifying the marginal mandibular branch of the facial nerve. (FV: Facial vein; FA: Facial artery; 2: Marginal mandibular branch; 1: Cervical branch; HB: Hyoid bone; SMG: Submandibular gland).

An alternative to this approach is to raise a subplatysma flap that includes the superficial layer of the deep cervical fascia, thus exposing the submandibular gland and facial vessels and protecting the facial nerve. The facial vein is more superficial and encountered first. The vein is ligated below the level of the marginal mandibular branch and then displaced cephalad. An identical maneuver is performed for the facial artery (Figs. 22.4A and B).

The identified digastric tendon is then traced posteriorly to expose the posterior belly of the digastric muscle (Fig. 22.5). This maneuver mobilizes the inferior aspect of the submandibular gland, which is then traced anteriorly to expose the mylohyoid. The anterior border of the mylohyoid is retracted medially to expose the connective tissue where the lingual and hypoglossal nerves

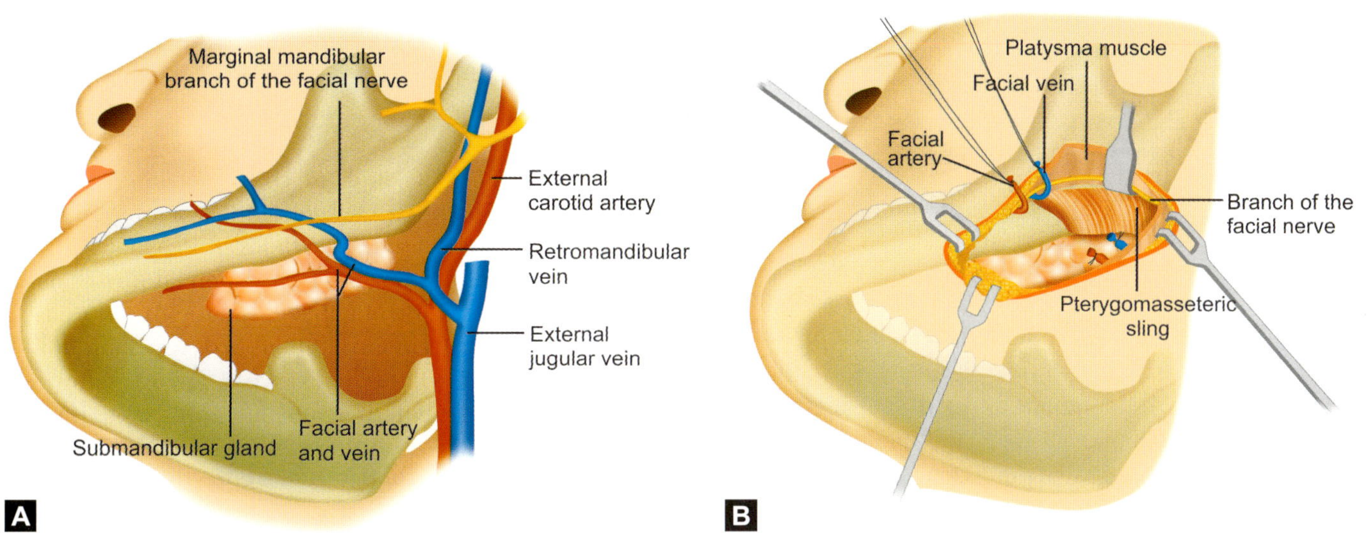

Figs. 22.4A and B: The vein is ligated below the level of the marginal mandibular branch and then displaced cephalad. An identical maneuver is performed for the facial artery.

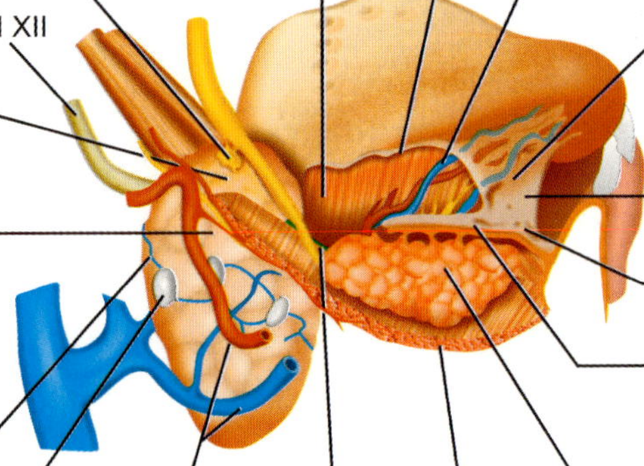

Fig. 22.5: The identified digastric tendon is then traced posteriorly to expose the posterior belly of the digastric muscle.

are found overlying the hyoglossus muscle (Fig. 22.6). The lingual and hypoglossal nerve run parallel to each other in the submandibular triangle, but in different planes. The lingual nerve is superficial and cephalad to the hypoglossal nerve and is exposed with gentle use of a kitner (i.e. pusher or peanut). The nerve and artery to the mylohyoid is encountered along the lateral border of the mylohyoid prior to its sacrifice. The lingual nerve is verified with identification of the submandibular ganglion. The lingual nerve, a branch of V3, joins the chorda tympani nerve before passing between the medial pterygoid muscle and the ramus of the mandible. The course continues obliquely to the side of the tongue over the superior constrictor and styloglossus (Fig. 22.6). From here the lingual nerve passes between the hyoglossus and deep part of the submandibular gland where the submandibular ganglion is suspended by the nerve. (The lingual nerve then courses inferiorly, crossing the duct of the submandibular gland to supply sensation to the anterior two-thirds of the tongue and transmits taste via the chorda tympani.) The submandibular ganglion is ligated along with the submandibular gland duct with suture ligature. The submandibular gland duct courses above the mylohyoid muscle along the lateral aspect of the hyoglossus and genioglossus muscles toward the floor of the mouth. Once the submandibular ganglion and duct are ligated, the proximal facial artery is the final major structure keeping the gland in place. Care is taken to dissect out the facial artery as it loops over the submandibular gland as it courses toward the external carotid. At this point, the proximal facial artery is divided and ligated, releasing the submandibular gland from the floor of mouth. Care is taken to achieve adequate hemostatsis and Valsava maneuver request from anesthesia to identify small vessels that require bipolar cautery. The wound is then irrigated with saline and a small drain is placed, such as #7 Jackson Pratt drain, left to bulb suction until removal. The incision is closed, beginning with 3-0 Vicryl sutures to approximate the platysma for the deep layer. The intermediate layer is closed with 4-0 Vicryl running suture through the subcutaneous layer followed by meticulous closure of the skin.

SURGICAL COMPLICATIONS—SUBMANDIBULAR GLAND EXCISION

The postoperative scar is visible and may sometimes become worse with hypertrophy or keloid. The marginal mandibular branch of the facial nerve, which lies in the subplatysmal plane overlying the gland, is the most commonly injured nerve in submandibular gland excision by the transcervical approach. Damage to the nerve, which has been reported to occur in 1–7.7% of cases,[16] may result in drooling from the corner of the mouth and asymmetry of the mouth angle. Other nerve injuries include injury

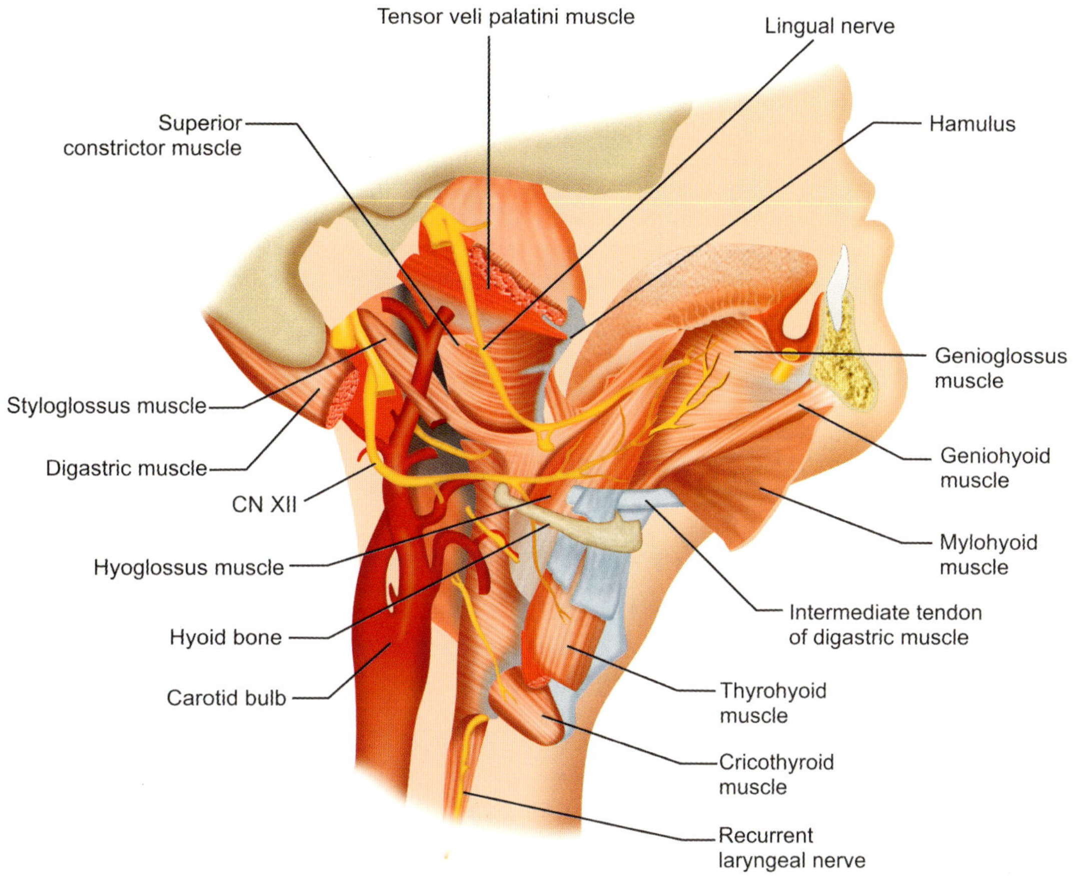

Fig. 22.6: The anterior border of the mylohyoid is cut medially to expose the connective tissue where the lingual and hypoglossal nerves are found overlying the hyoglossus muscle.

to the lingual and hypoglossal nerves; these nerves are rarely injured at the hands of an experienced surgeon and injury affects 1.4% and 2.9% of patients, respectively.[16] In recent series with over 100 submandibular glands excised, postoperative hematomas are seen in 2–10%, risk of infection is between 2% and 9.3%, and salivary fistula occurs in 2%.[2,17]

REFERENCES

1. Nahlieli O, Nakar LH, Nazarian Y, et al. Sialoendoscopy: a new approach to salivary gland obstructive pathology. J Am Dent Assoc. 2006;137:1394-400.
2. Springborg LK, Møller MN. Submandibular gland excision: long-term clinical outcome in 139 patients operated in a single institution. Eur Arch Otorhinolaryngol. 2013: 270(4):1441-6.
3. Yilmaz M, Akil F, Yener HM, et al. Submandibular gland excision: 10-year outcome. Otolaryngology; 2013;3(138):2.
4. Alves FA, Perez DE, Almeida OP, et al. Pleomorphic adenoma of the submandibular gland: clinicopathological and immunohistochemical features of 60 cases in Brazil. Arch Otolaryngol Head Neck Surg. 2002;128(12):1400-3.
5. Salama AR. Robert AO. Clinical implications of the neck in salivary gland disease. Oral Maxillofac Surg Clin North Am. 2008;20(3):445-58.
6 Spiro RH. Salivary neoplasms: overview of a 35-year experience with 2,807 patients. Head Neck Surg. 1986;8(3):177-84.
7. Spiro J, Spiro RH. The neck: diagnosis and surgery. St. Louis: Mosby; 1994. pp. 295-306.
8. Terhaard CH, Lubsen H, Van der Tweel I, et al. Salivary gland carcinoma: independent prognostic factors for locoregional control, distant metastases, and overall survival: results of the Dutch head and neck oncology cooperative group. Head Neck. 2004;26(8):681-92 [discussion 692-93].
9. Rapidis AD, Stavrianos S, Lagogiannis G, et al. Tumors of the submandibular gland: clinicopathologic analysis of 23 patients. J Oral Maxillofac Surg. 2004;62(10):1203-8.
10. Yousem DM, Kraut MA, Chalian AA. Major salivary gland imaging. Radiology. 2000;216(1):19-29.
11. Chikui T, Shimizu M, Goto TK, et al. Interpretation of the origin of a submandibular mass by CT and MRI imaging. Oral Surg Oral Med Oral Pathol Oral Radiol Endod. 2004; 98(6):721-9.

12. Koyuncu M, Sesen T, Akan H, et al. Comparison of computed tomography and magnetic resonance imaging in the diagnosis of parotid tumors. Otolaryngol Head Neck Surg. 2003;129(6):726-32.
13. Jeong HS, Chung MK, Son YI, et al. Role of 18FFDGPET/CT in management of high-grade salivary gland malignancies. J Nucl Med. 2007;48(8):1237-44.
14. Dingman RO, Grabb WC. Surgical anatomy of the mandibular ramus of the facial nerve based on the dissection of 100 facial halves. Plast Reconstr Surg. 1962;29:266.
15. Baker DC, Conley J. Avoiding facial nerve injuries in rhytidectomy anatomical variations and pitfalls. Plast Reconstr Surg. 1979;64(6):781-95.
16. Chang YN, Chuan-Hsiang K, Yaoh-Shiang L, et al. Comparison of the intraoral and transcervical approach in submandibular gland excision. Eur Arch Otorhinolaryngol. 2013;270(2):669-74.
17. Preuss SF, Klussmann JP, Wittekindt C, et al. Submandibular gland excision: 15 years of experience. J Oral Maxillofac Surg. 2007;65(5):953-7.

CHAPTER

23 Tumors of the Parapharyngeal Space

Courtney B Shires, Jonathan Giurintano, Jason G Newman

INTRODUCTION

The parapharyngeal space is one of the most anatomically complex areas of the head and neck.[1] A potential space in the deep neck, the parapharyngeal space is most commonly imagined as an inverted pyramid, with a base consisting of the skull base and its apex at the greater cornu of the hyoid bone. Laterally, the space is bounded by the mandibular ramus, parotid gland, and medial pterygoid muscle; medially, the space is bounded by the superior pharyngeal constrictor muscle. The prevertebral fascia and cervical vertebrae form the posterior boundary. As the superior pharyngeal constrictor muscle is distensible, tumors of the parapharyngeal space tend to grow medially and inferiorly within the potential space to present as a pharyngeal or neck mass. While only 0.5% of all reported head and neck tumors are located within the parapharyngeal space, its complex anatomical relationships allow a wide variety of tumors. A variety of surgical approaches are reported in the literature for access to this highly complicated space, including transoral, transcervical, transmandibular, and transparotid approaches.

ANATOMY

A potential space in the deep neck, the parapharyngeal space is most commonly imagined as an inverted pyramid, with a base consisting of the skull base and its apex at the greater cornu of the hyoid bone. Medially, the pyramid is bound by the buccopharyngeal fascia of the superior pharyngeal constrictor muscle, and the lateral boundary is formed by the mandibular, parotid gland, and medial pterygoid muscle (Figs. 23.1 to 23.3). The pyramid may be divided into two subdivisions, the prestyloid and poststyloid (Fig. 23.4), by the tensor veli palatini muscle. This muscle originates at the styloid process,

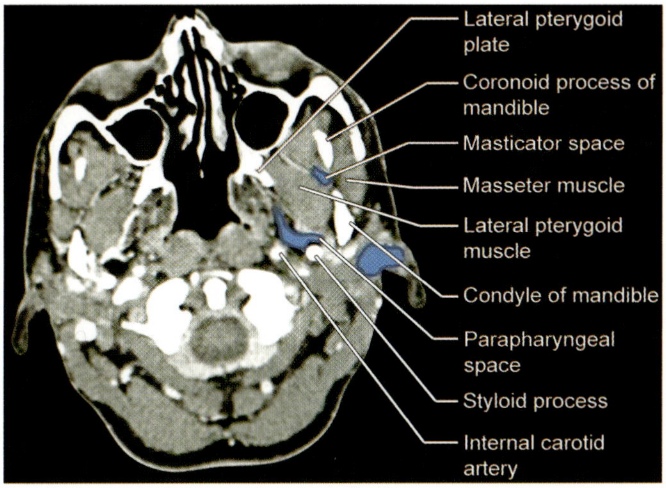

Fig. 23.1: Inferior parapharyngeal space in the axial plane.

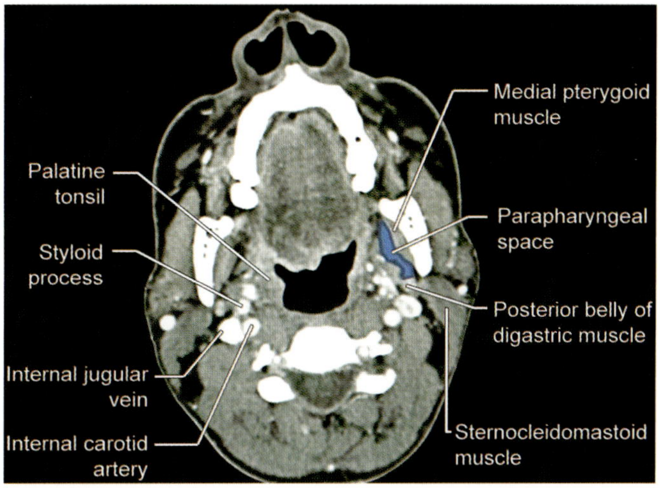

Fig. 23.2: Superior parapharyngeal space in the axial plane.

running through the parapharyngeal space to insert in the lateral pterygoid plate. The prestyloid compartment is located anterolaterally and contains the deep lobe of the parotid gland as well as many minor structures, including adipose tissue, small vascular structures, lymph nodes, and minor nerves. The more important structures traversing the parapharyngeal space are found in the more posteromedially located poststyloid compartment, including the carotid sheath, glossopharyngeal nerve (CN IX), vagus nerve (CN X), and accessory nerve (CN XI) as they exit the jugular foramen, as well as the hypoglossal nerve (CN XII) and cervical sympathetic chain as it lies posterior to the carotid sheath.

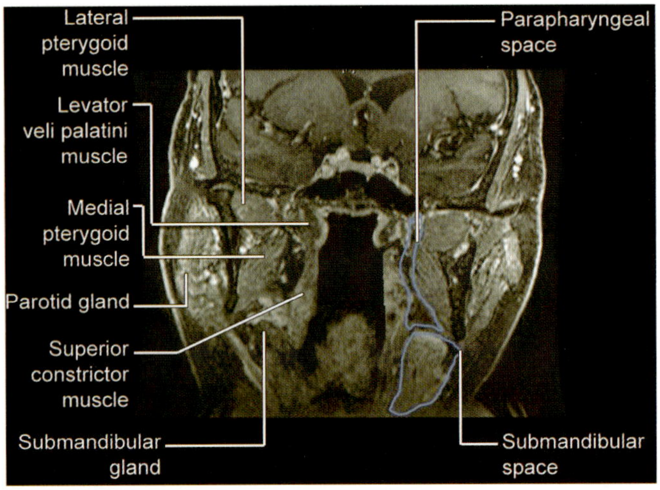

Fig. 23.3: Parapharyngeal and submandibular spaces in the coronal plane.

PRESENTATION

Parapharyngeal space tumors may present in various manners depending on the location of the tumor and adjacent structures involved. For tumors involving the prestyloid compartment, patients will often present with an asymptomatic bulging of the lateral wall of the oropharynx. These masses may first be noticed by a clinician on routine physical examination, or if the tumor reaches at least 2.5 to 3 cm in diameter, the patient's swallowing and breathing may be affected, with trismus, dysphonia, Eustachian tube dysfunction, and obstructive sleep apnea reported as presenting symptoms.[2] A related mass may or may not be present in the parotid gland or within the lateral neck itself. Tumors involving the poststyloid compartment are more often symptomatic given the cranial nerves and sympathetic plexus traversing this space. For example, tumors arising from the vagus nerve may present with vocal cord paralysis, tumors affecting the hypoglossal nerve may present with unilateral tongue weakness, and tumors originating in the cervical sympathetic chain may produce Horner's syndrome (ptosis, myosis, and anhydrosis). As the presenting symptoms of parapharyngeal space tumors are often nonspecific, we must rely on imaging for diagnosis.

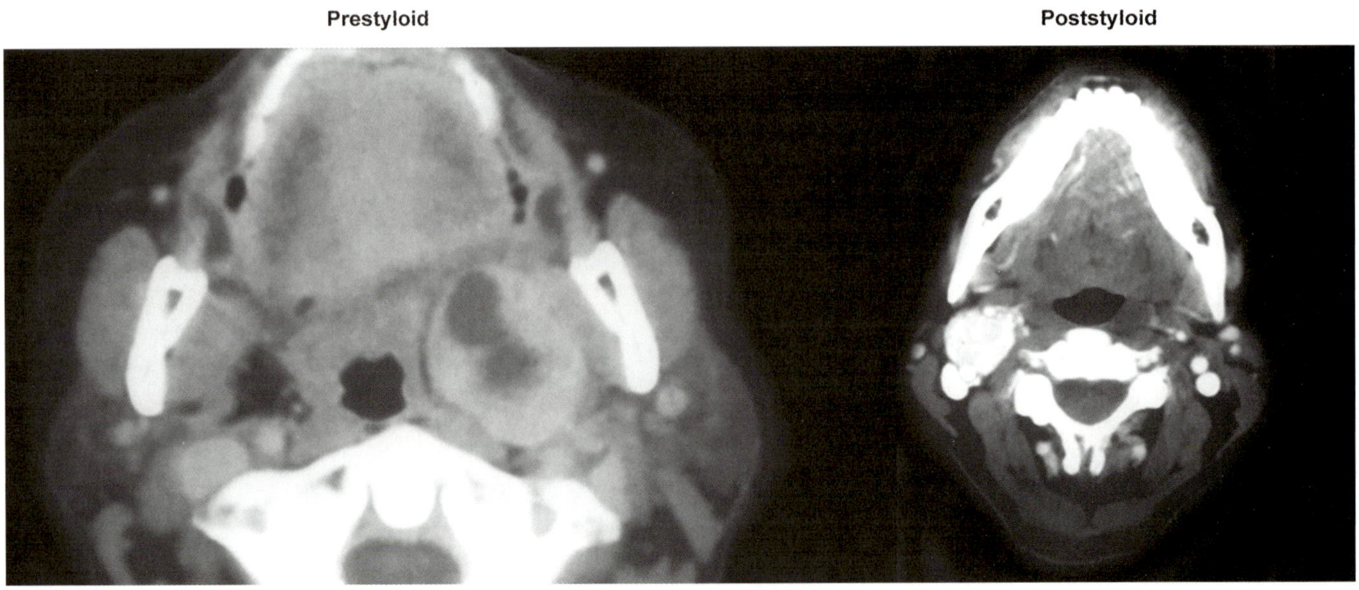

Fig. 23.4: The prestyloid and poststyloid divisions of the parapharyngeal space.

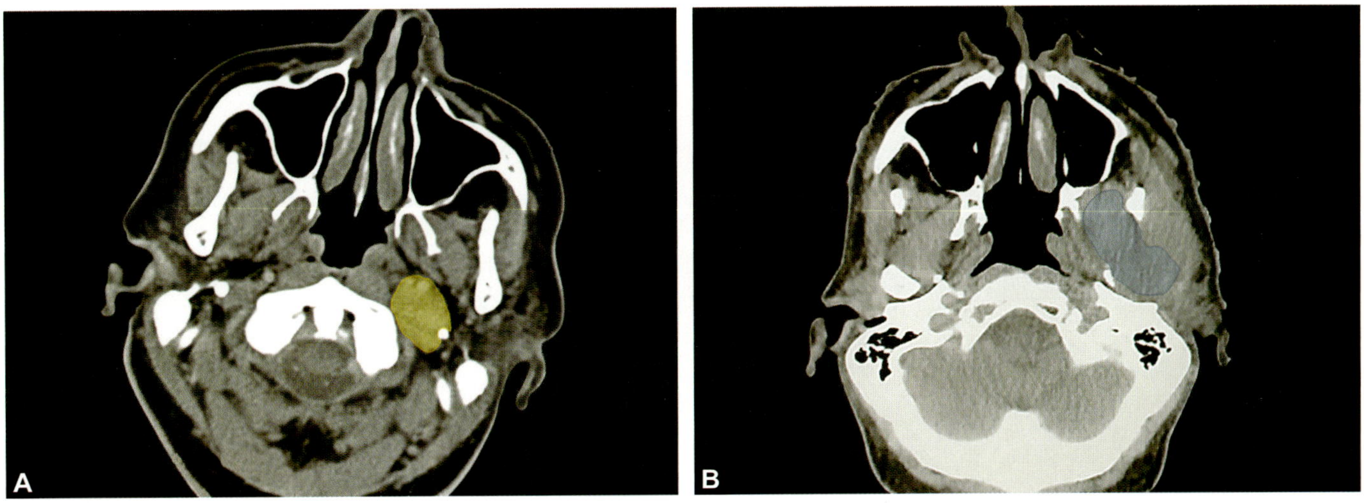

Figs. 23.5A and B: CT scans in the axial plane demonstrating (A) left prestyloid mass (shaded yellow), a schwannoma of the vagus nerve, and (B) left poststyloid mass (shaded blue), hepatocellular carcinoma metastatic to the parapharyngeal space. Note its relationship to the styloid process.

EVALUATION

Because the parapharyngeal space is a potential space, workup of a suspected parapharyngeal space mass must include imaging studies to determine if the tumor is pre- or poststyloid, and to determine the nature of the neoplasm (tumor size, invasion of adjacent structures, or presence of lymphadenopathy). Computed tomography (CT) scan and magnetic resonance imaging (MRI) with gadolinium are the preferred study for imaging tumors of the parapharyngeal space. As MRI is superior to CT in the imaging of soft tissue structures, MRI better demonstrates the tumor's relationship to the deep lobe of the parotid gland; in addition, T1 imaging sequences define the tumor–fat interface, and T2 imaging sequences demonstrate the tumor margin and tumor–muscle interface. CT scanning is quicker, less expensive and often adequate. To report that a lesion originated in the parapharyngeal space, the lesion must be completely surrounded by parapharyngeal space fat.[3] Distinguishing whether the tumor is located in the pre-styloid or poststyloid compartment is of utmost importance, as it helps narrow the differential diagnosis of the tumor type, and it serves as the guide for planning the surgical approach to the tumor (Figs. 23.5A and B). Biopsy by fine-needle aspiration (FNA) (often necessitates CT guidance) may be used to aid in the preoperative diagnosis of the tumor; sometimes the tumor's characteristics on imaging provide sufficient information, lessening the need for obtaining a tissue diagnosis.

For tumors that appear vascular on CT or MRI, angiography may be considered. For patients with suspected paragangliomas, one should ask if the patient has had palpitations, flushing, hypertension, or a family history of paragangliomas. If a secreting paraganglioma is suspected, catecholamines should be examined in a 24-hour urine specimen. Pheochromocytomas should always be sought and excised before paragangliomas to avoid intraoperative hypertensive crisis.[4]

TUMORS

Comprising only 0.5% of all head and neck neoplasms, tumors of the parapharyngeal space may be primary neoplasms, metastases from distant sites, or extensions of neoplasms from adjacent structures. In diagnosing neoplasms of the parapharyngeal space, the location of the neoplasm in either the prestyloid or poststyloid component should be established.

1. *Prestyloid compartment*: As the deep lobe of the parotid gland is situated within the prestyloid compartment, tumors located in the prestyloid parapharyngeal space are most often salivary in origin. The most common neoplasm of the parotid gland is the pleomorphic adenoma, and as such the most common neoplasms in the prestyloid compartment are pleomorphic adenomas arising in the deep lobe of the parotid gland, growing through the stylomandibular tunnel into the parapharyngeal space. Although pleomorphic adenomas are the most prevalent neoplasm in the

Table 23.1: Benign and malignant lesions reported in the parapharyngeal space.

BENIGN			MALIGNANT		
	Prestyloid	Poststyloid		Prestyloid	Poststyloid
Angiomyxolipoma		*	Adenocarcinoma	*	
Arteriovenous malformation		*	Adenoid cystic carcinoma	*	
Branchial cleft cyst	*	*	Carcinoma ex-pleomorphic adenoma	*	
Hemangioma		*	Carotid body tumor		*
Internal carotid aneurysm		*	Fibrosarcoma	*	*
Lipoma	*	*	Hemangiopericytoma		*
Lymphangioma	*	*	Leiomyosarcoma	*	*
Lymphoid hyperplasia	*	*	Liposarcoma	*	*
Myoepithelioma	*		Lymphoepithelial carcinoma	*	
Neurilemmoma		*	Lymphoma	*	*
Neurofibroma		*	Malignant meningioma		*
Osteolipoma	*	*	Malignant mixed tumor	*	
Paraganglioma		*	Metastatic (breast, hepatocellular, renal, thyroid)	*	*
Pleomorphic adenoma	*		Mucoepidermoid carcinoma	*	
Rhabdomyoma	*	*	Neurofibrosarcoma		*
Schwannoma		*	Neurogenic sarcoma		*
Teratoma	*	*	Osteosarcoma	*	*
Warthin's tumor	*		Salivary duct carcinoma	*	
			Squamous cell carcinoma	*	*

prestyloid parapharyngeal space, multiple other tumor types are documented in the literature (Table 23.1).[4,5]

2. *Poststyloid compartment*: With cranial nerves IX, X, XI, and XII, and the sympathetic plexus traversing the poststyloid parapharyngeal space, tumors originating in this space are largely neurogenic. The most common neurogenic neoplasm of the poststyloid space is the schwannoma (neurilemmoma), which is often found to affect the vagus nerve and sympathetic chain. These tumors are typically benign and slow growing, and they generally do not affect the nerve from which they originate. Neurofibromas, associated with Type I neurofibromatosis (von Recklinghausen disease), may be found in the poststyloid compartment in these select patients. Unlike schwannomas, neurofibromas are not encapsulated and often affect their nerve of origin. The most symptomatic of the poststyloid space tumors are paragangliomas, which most commonly arise from the nodose ganglion of the vagus nerve, the carotid body, or the jugular bulb. Paragangliomas arise from paraganglia cells, special chemoreceptor cells located along the major vessels whose function is part of the sympathetic nervous system. Paragangliomas, which are most often found in the parapharyngeal space, are carotid body tumors and glomus vagale tumors.

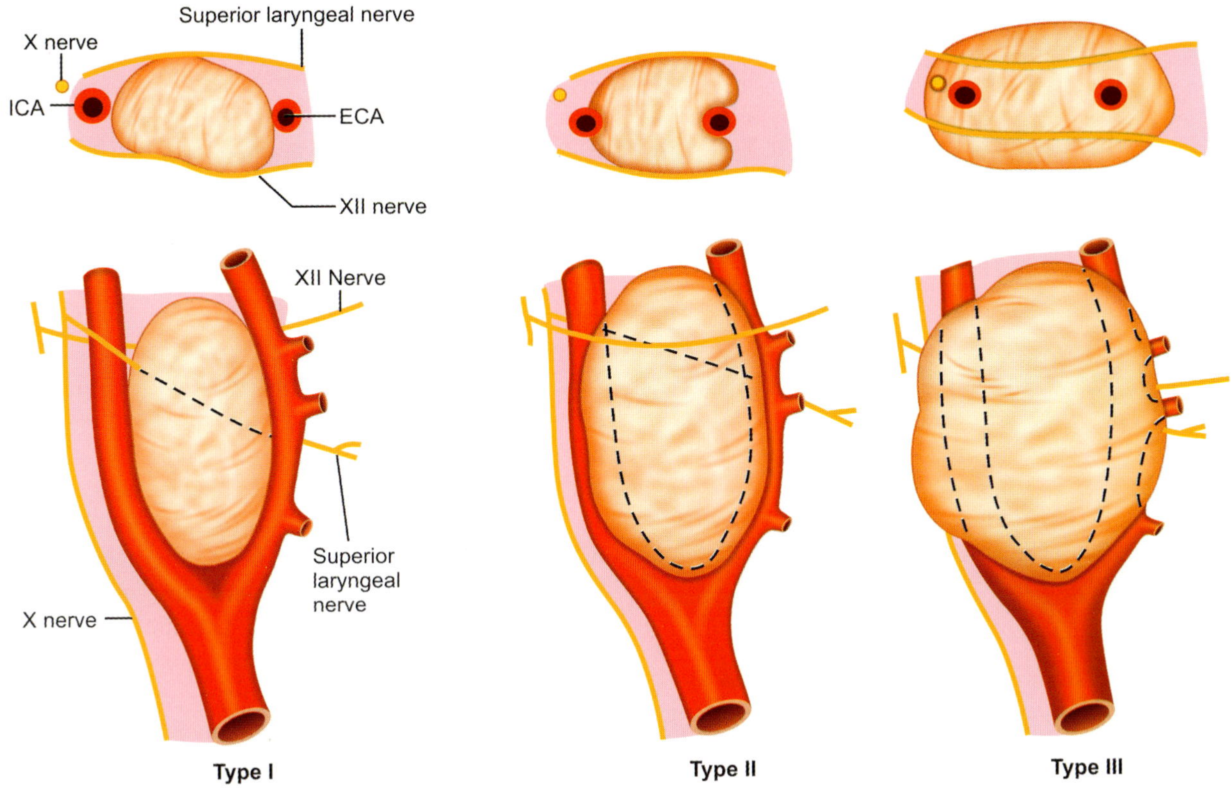

Figs. 23.6: Shamblin classification of carotid body tumor.

Carotid Body Tumors

Accounting for more than half of paragangliomas, carotid body tumors originate from the carotid body, which is located at the bifurcation of the carotid artery. Carotid bodies serve as chemoreceptors whose function is to aid in the regulation of breathing and blood pressure. In characterizing carotid body tumors, Shamblin et al. created a classification system for relating the carotid body and its relationship to the carotid artery (Fig. 23.6).[6] Shamblin classification divides carotid body tumors into three groups: Shamblin I tumors are minimally attached to the carotid artery and easily resectable. Shamblin II tumors partially surround the carotid artery and are more adherent to the vessel adventitia layer than Shamblin I tumors. In Shamblin III tumors, the carotid bifurcation is encased by tumor, and the tumor actually invades into the muscularis layer of the artery. While Shamblin I and II tumors are candidates for surgical resection, attempt at dissection of Shamblin III tumors results in violation of the carotid wall. As such, Shamblin III tumors require sacrifice of the affected internal carotid artery with reconstruction by a vascular surgeon. The Shamblin classification is often used as a predictor of vascular morbidity, with Shamblin I tumors carrying the least risk and Shamblin III tumors carrying the greatest risk of postoperative morbidity. For Shamblin III tumors, radiation therapy and stereotactic radiosurgery (gamma knife) are often used as lower morbidity alternatives to major vascular reconstructive surgery. On imaging, carotid body tumors are identified by the presence of the "lyre sign," the classic splaying of the internal and external carotid arteries at the bifurcation by the tumor (Fig. 23.7).

Glomus Vagale Tumors

Arising in the paraganglia tissue associated with the superior, inferior, and middle vassal ganglia along the descent of the vagus nerve, glomus vagale tumors are often discovered as asymptomatic masses located posterior to the carotid artery, although some patients may present with neural deficits (vocal cord paralysis or dysphagia). Glomus vagale tumors can be separated into three stages depending on involvement of the skull base: Stage I tumors lie in the parapharyngeal space and do not involve the jugular foramen, Stage II tumors invade the jugular foramen but do not cause bony destruction, and Stage III

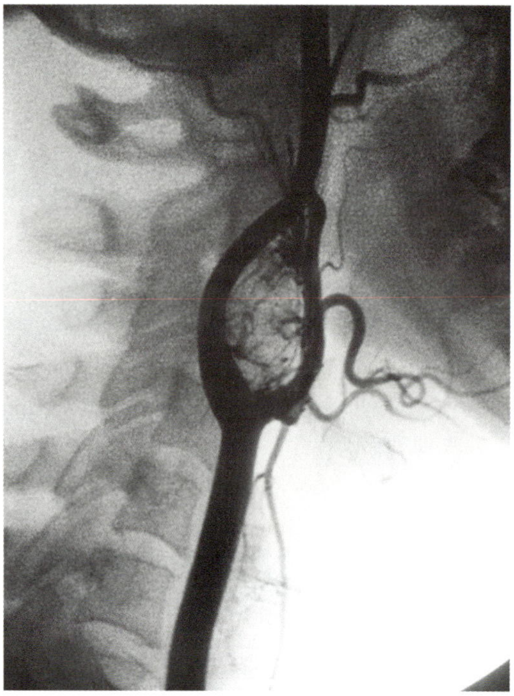

Fig. 23.7: Angiogram of carotid body tumor. These are found between the carotid bifurcation and cause splaying of the internal carotid artery and external carotid artery, resulting in the lyre sign.

tumors invade the jugular foramen with destruction of the bony skull base and possible involvement of the carotid canal. Because the tumor originates from the vagus nerve itself, excision creates a high vagal injury, resulting in vocal cord paralysis. For this reason, a type I thyroplasty is often performed in conjunction with glomus vagale tumor resection.[7]

SURGICAL APPROACHES

Depending on the tumor type, location, and characteristics, there are multiple different surgical approaches to the parapharyngeal space. Approaches include transoral, transcervical, transcervical submandibular, transcervical transparotid, transmandibular, or any combination of these approaches. Occasionally, a patient has multiple comorbidities inhibiting surgery, extensive carotid body tumors with failure of balloon occlusion test, or refusal of surgery.[5] These patients may be followed routinely with imaging or considered for radiation There is also debate whether benign, asymptomatic, incidentally found parapharyngeal space masses require excision, and observation certainly should be considered. Although surgical techniques have been established and morbidity has been minimized, there are still risks to surgical excision. For patients who are surgical candidates, they are described here.

Transoral Approach

The parapharyngeal space is an anatomically difficult and challenging space to access intraorally. In the 1920s, the transoral approach was one of the most common approaches, but by the 1960s open neck surgery was the standard of care.[8,9] With the advent of transoral robotic surgery (TORS), the transoral approach is gaining popularity in resecting smaller parapharyngeal space tumors, particularly tumors located in the prestyloid parapharyngeal space. O'Malley et al. described the first series of 10 patients treated with TORS for parapharyngeal space tumors in 2010.[10]

Tumors that may be considered for removal via TORS are prestyloid benign tumors. Lesions not appropriate for TORS are those displacing the internal carotid artery medially, tumors with significant extension into the stylomandibular tunnel, lesions involving the bony skull base, paragangliomas, or FNA-proven malignancies.[11] TORS resection of salivary gland tumors with parotid involvement is controversial. Although FNA or open biopsy of prestyloid masses has traditionally been discouraged, some perform CT-guided transfacial FNA prior to TORS.[11]

For this approach, the oral endotracheal tube is either secured along the dorsal tongue with the mouth gag or sutured to the buccal mucosa or nasolabial groove. The Crowe–Davis mouth retractor is placed, slightly displacing the tongue to the contralateral side. The 0° endoscope is advanced to place the operative site in view. The spatula tip cautery is placed in the trocar ipsilateral to the tumor and the 5-mm Maryland dissector is placed in the trocar contralateral to the lesion. A relaxed U-shaped incision is made in the mucosa from the soft palate to the posterior floor of the mouth (Figs. 23.8A to C). Care is taken to not enter the tumor with the incision. The medial pterygoid tendon is visualized laterally and the constrictor muscle is located medially. If needed to expose the extent of the tumor, the medial fibers of the medial pterygoid muscle are divided. Gentle, slow blunt dissection around the tumor with the Maryland dissector, cautery tip, suction tip, and finger is then used to deliver the tumor. The tumor capsule is then inspected for any breach. The wound is irrigated. The mucosa is closed with 3-0 Vicryl in horizontal mattress sutures. A Penrose drain may be placed in the incision and removed on postoperative day 1.[11]

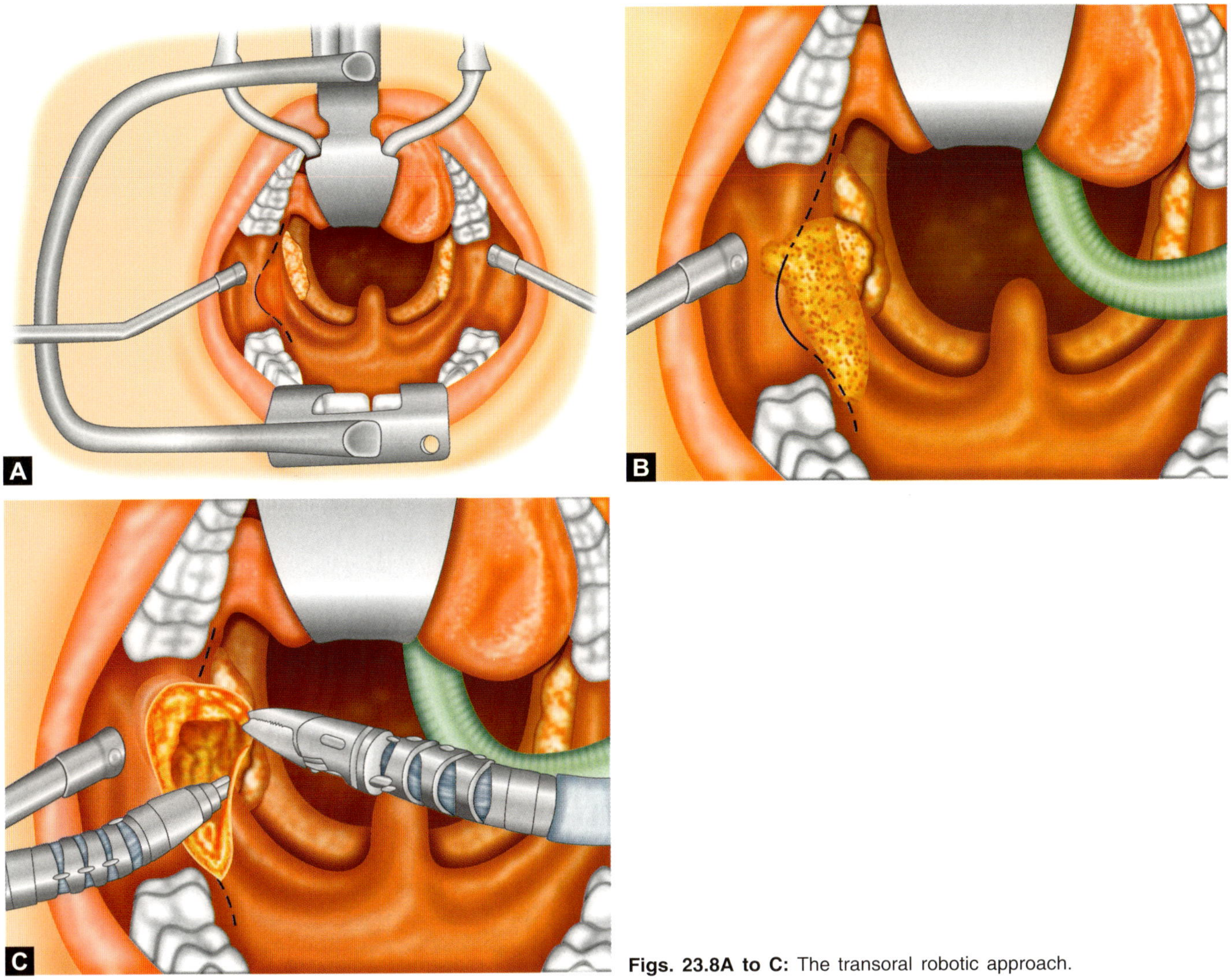

Figs. 23.8A to C: The transoral robotic approach.

Transcervical Approach

The transcervical approach should be used for paragangliomas, poststyloid masses, and large prestyloid masses that are not adherent to the parotid gland (fat is seen between the mass and parotid gland on imaging). Most tumors of the prestyloid parapharyngeal space can be approached via a cervical incision. Unlike the poststyloid tumors, there is usually no need to dissect the submandibular space for small prestyloid tumors.

An incision is made in a natural skin crease of the neck from just below the mastoid tip to the greater cornu of the hyoid bone. This should be at least two finger widths inferior to the mandible. Subplatysmal flaps are raised. The sternocleidomastoid muscle is delineated and retracted laterally. The carotid sheath is identified. Vessel loops are placed around the common carotid artery and internal jugular vein to ensure control of the vessels in the event of inadvertent injury. The hypoglossal nerve is identified as it crosses the carotid arteries and passes deep to the mylohyoid muscle. The vagus nerve is found in the carotid sheath between the internal carotid artery and the internal jugular vein. Intense inflammation of surrounding tissues may be noted if preoperative embolization has been performed (Fig. 23.9).

For carotid body tumors, the carotid bifurcation is identified. The external carotid artery may need to be transected and ligated to assist with dissection of the internal carotid artery.

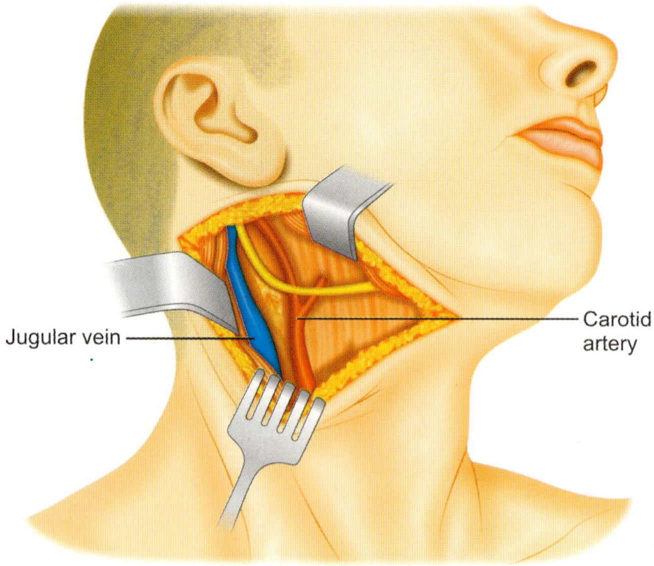

Fig. 23.9: Transcervical approach—transverse incision at level of hyoid, submandibular gland removed or retracted, incision through the fascia deep to the submandibular space. Increase exposure by releasing digastric, stylohyoid, styloglossus from hyoid, cut stylomandibular ligament, mandibulotomy.

For glomus vagale tumors or schwannomas of the vagus nerve, the vagus nerve is dissected from inferior to superior. Gentle dissection is continued superiorly, separating the tumor from the carotid artery. Rarely, with a schwannoma, it may be possible to remove the tumor from out of the underlying nerve and leave the nerve intact. However, usually the nerve is transected once dissection has been accomplished superior and inferior to the tumor. A Type I thyroplasty is performed to prevent aspiration, dysphagia, and dysphonia.

Schwannomas of the superior cervical ganglion will arise deep to the carotid artery bifurcation. The carotid artery is retracted, exposing the tumor. If the tumor cannot be removed from within the native nerve, the sympathetic chain is transected above and below the tumor. Horner's syndrome is expected postoperatively.

Transcervical Submandibular Approach

The transcervical approach is the most commonly used surgical approach to the prestyloid parapharyngeal space, as it allows for sufficient access to the tumor while allowing for access to the vascular and neural structures. The submandibular space also has open communication with the parapharyngeal space, as there is no fascia separating these two spaces.[3] This facilitates removal of parapharyngeal space tumors through the submandibular space.

The parapharyngeal space is approached through a Risdon incision located in a natural skin crease of the upper neck. Dissection is taken down through the platysma, and subplatysmal flaps are elevated. The anterior border of the sternocleidomastoid and posterior belly of the digastric muscle are identified, and dissection is taken superiorly toward the submandibular gland. The marginal mandibular branch of the facial nerve is identified in the fascia overlying the submandibular gland. The fascia is divided inferiorly and retracted superiorly to protect the marginal mandibular nerve. The facial vein may be divided and elevated, which should protect the marginal mandibular nerve. The lingual nerve is found superior to the hypoglossal nerve, deep to the mylohyoid muscle, and superficial to the styloglossus muscle. The gland is mobilized and retracted anteriorly, allowing exposure of the apex of the prestyloid parapharyngeal space. With the tumor identified, blunt dissection may be used to excise the tumor from surrounding tissues. A finger can palpate the mandible laterally and the constrictors medially. If further exposure is needed to access the tumor, the stylomandibular ligament may be divided to facilitate anterior displacement of the mandible, or the styloid muscles and posterior belly of the digastric muscle may be divided. The hypoglossal nerve passes deep to the digastric muscle and should be identified before dividing this muscle. The submandibular gland may be removed for further exposure after ligation of the submandibular duct, submandibular ganglion, and feeders from the facial artery posterosuperiorly and inferiorly. With the tumor removed, a drain is placed, the wound is closed in layers, and a pressure dressing applied.

Transcervical Submandibular Approach with Mandibulotomy

If the transcervical submandibular approach fails to provide enough access for tumor resection, the mandible may be dislocated anteriorly, or a mandibulotomy may be performed. Tumors, which may require a mandibulotomy, include malignant tumors, tumors of significant size, tumors adjacent to the skull base, or tumors related to vascular structures.

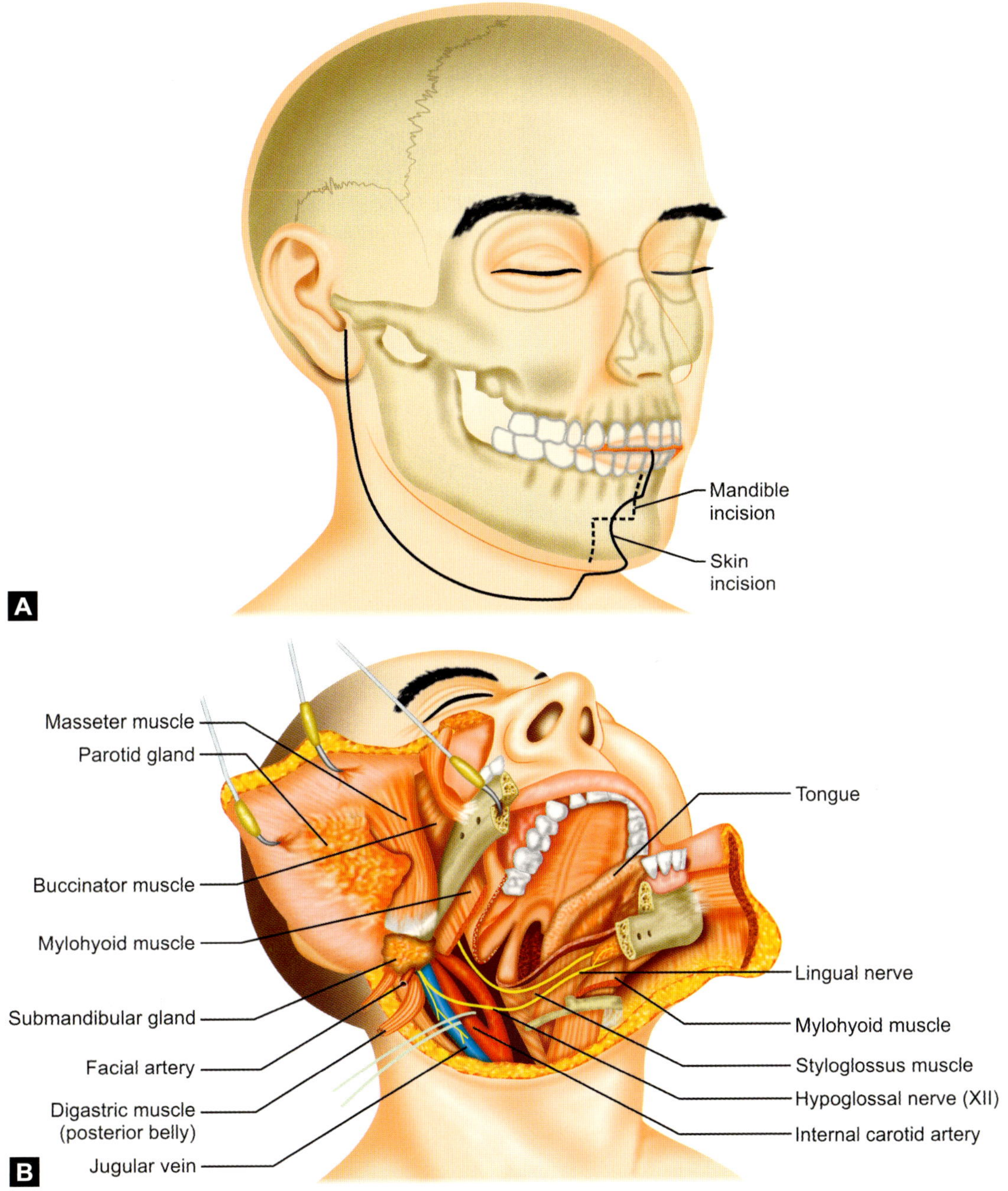

Figs. 23.10A and B: Planned skin incision for transcervical submandibular approach with mandibulotomy. This is marked from the mastoid tip through a skin crease of the neck toward the hyoid bone to the midline, carried superior to the submental crease, curved around the mentum to the mental crease, and carried superiorly through the midline lower lip.

An incision is planned from the mastoid tip through a skin crease of the neck toward the hyoid bone to the midline, carried superior to the submental crease, curved around the mentum to the mental crease, and carried superiorly through the midline lower lip (Fig. 23.10A). It is often not necessary to include the superior extent of this incision. The transcervical approach is performed as described above (Fig. 23.10B).

There are a variety of locations in which to create a mandibulotomy (Fig. 23.11). A vertical parasymphyseal mandibulotomy between the first premolar and canine is often used to preserve the integrity of the inferior alveolar

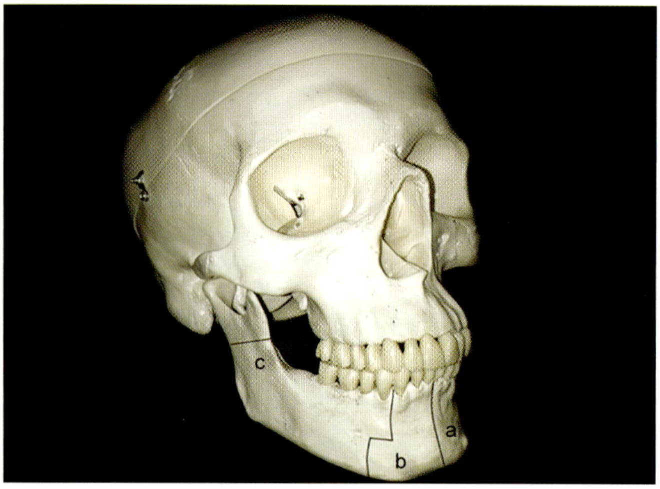

Fig. 23.11: Locations in which to create a mandibulotomy: (a) median mandibulotomy between the two central incisors, (b) stair-step or vertical parasymphyseal mandibulotomy between the first premolar and canine, and (c) horizontal mandibulotomy of the ascending ramus above the lingula.

nerve. If even further exposure is necessary, a second horizontal mandibulotomy of the ascending ramus above the lingula may be performed and the mandible reflected superiorly. Some surgeons prefer to create a median mandibulotomy between the two central incisors. Whichever technique is used, plates should be aligned and bent prior to making bone cuts to ensure proper placement of plates after resection is complete. Screws are placed; the screws and plates are then removed and set aside for use at the end of the case.

After the transcervical approach is complete, the periosteum on either side of the planned mandibulotomy is elevated and an oscillating saw is used to create the mandibulotomy. The cautery is used to incise the floor of the mouth from the mandibulotomy along the alveolar lingual sulcus to the anterior tonsillar pillar. The muscles attached to the mandible (anterior belly of the digastric muscle and mylohyoid) are divided to permit lateral retraction of the mandible. Care is taken to preserve the lingual and hypoglossal nerves. If the tumor in the parapharyngeal space is not visible, extension of the oral incision along the anterior tonsillar pillar is performed. The tonsil and upper constrictor muscles are retracted medially for access toward the skull base.

After tumor excision, the mandible is reconstructed with previously bent plating, hemostasis is assured, and the soft tissue wound is closed in layers. Watertight closure of the mouth is important to prevent orocutaneous fistula. The vermilion border should be realigned in its native position. A Jackson Pratt drain may be placed and brought out through the cervical incision.

Approach requiring a mandibulotomy inherently carries increased risk of morbidity, and a temporary tracheostomy may be required for postoperative airway protection. Risks include postoperative airway edema and the presence of postoperative malocclusion.

Transcervical Transparotid Approach

If the lesion is in continuity with the deep lobe of the parotid gland and no intervening fat is noted on imaging, the transparotid approach should be used to protect the facial nerve. The transcervical transparotid approach is often utilized for deep lobe parotid neoplasms that are growing into the parapharyngeal space. Unlike the transcervical with submandibular approach, the transcervical with transparotid approach provides exposure and protection of the facial nerve.

A modified Blair incision is made starting superior and anterior to the tragus, carried inferiorly in a preauricular skin crease, curved around the earlobe, and continued in a curvilinear fashion to the submandibular area. The preauricular skin is elevated, keeping fat on the undersurface of the skin and fat on the superficial surface of the parotid gland. The posterior border of the parotid gland is then dissected from the cartilaginous external auditory canal. At the inferior portion of the incision, subplatysmal flaps are elevated. The sternocleidomastoid and digastric muscles are identified. Branches of the greater auricular nerve entering the parotid gland are transected. Just inferior to the tragal pointer, the common trunk of the facial nerve is identified. The nerve exits the stylomastoid foramen just medial to the insertion of the digastric muscle onto the mastoid tip. The branches of the facial nerve are gently dissected, traveling anterior from the main trunk. The branches are preserved while the parotid parenchyma is divided. Once the superficial lobe of the parotid gland has been removed and the branches of the facial nerve identified, gentle dissection is used to separate tumor from the deep parotid lobe (Figs. 23.12A and B).

This approach can also be combined with the mandibulotomy approach. The transcervical transparotid approach is not sufficient for tumors that extend to the infratemporal fossa or through the skull base; thus, in cases requiring exposure of these regions, the addition of an infratemporal fossa approach is needed.[12]

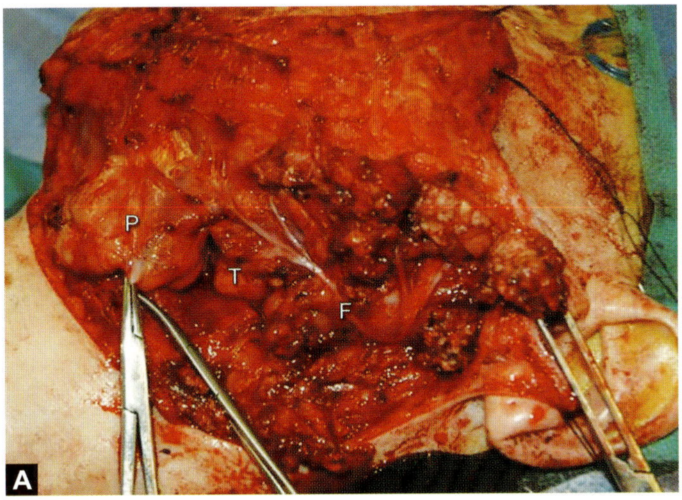

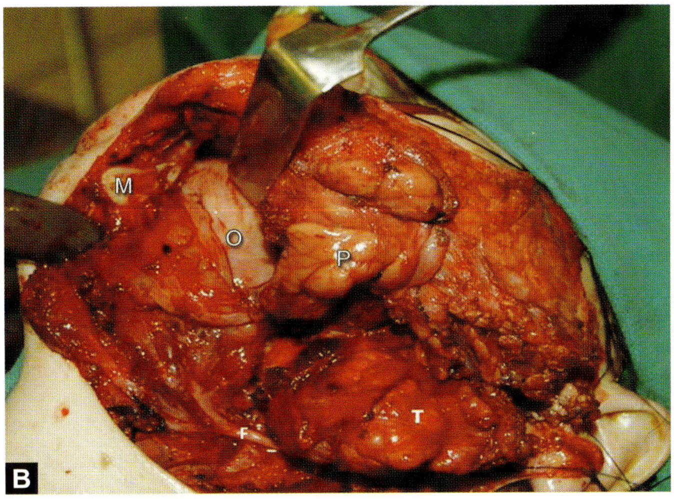

Figs. 23.12A and B: Transparotid approach to a prestyloid mass. (A) The facial nerve (F) is dissected, the parotid (P) retracted forward, and prestyloid tumor (T) is visible. (B) Tumor (T) is mobilized from deep to the facial nerve (F). The superficial parotid lobe (P), oral tongue (O), and midline mandibulotomy (M) are visible.

SUMMARY

The parapharyngeal space is an anatomically complex space described as an inverted pyramid, with a base consisting of the skull base and its apex at the greater cornu of the hyoid bone. It may be divided into two separate compartments, a prestyloid and poststyloid compartment. Tumors located in the prestyloid compartment are most often salivary gland in origin, and tumors located in the poststyloid compartment are typically neural in origin. Appropriate physical examination and imaging studies are imperative for preoperative diagnosis and surgical planning. Various surgical approaches to the parapharyngeal space exist, with care taken to avoid damage to vital structures such as cranial nerves VII, IX, X, XI, and XII, the sympathetic plexus, and the carotid artery.

REFERENCES

1. Som PM, Biller HF, Lawson W, et al. Parapharyngeal space masses: an updated protocol based upon 104 cases. Radiology. 1984;153:149-56.
2. Lawson VG, LeLiever WC, Makerewich LA, et al. Unusual parapharyngeal lesions. J Otolaryngol. 1979;8(3):241-9.
3. Harnsberger HR, Osborn AG, Ross J, et al. Diagnostic and Surgical Imaging Anatomy: Brain, Head and Neck, Spine. Macdonald AJ (Ed). Salt Lake City: Amirsys; 2007. pp. 140.
4. Myers EN, Johnson JT. Management of tumors of the parapharyngeal space. In: Myers EN (Ed). Operative Otolaryngology—Head and Neck Surgery. Philadelphia, PA: Saunders Elsevier; 2008:657-66.
5. Rant V, Sinnathuray AR, McClean G, et al. Metastatic breast carcinoma in the parapharyngeal space. J Laryngol Otol. 2001;115:750-2.
6. Shamblin WR, ReMine WH, Sheps SG, et al. Carotid body tumor (chemodectoma): clinopathologic analysis of ninety cases. Am J Surg. 1971;122:732-9.
7. Urguhart A, Johnson J, Myers E, et al. Glomus vagale: paraganglioma of the vagus nerve. Laryngoscope. 1994;104(4): 440-5.
8. New GB. Mixed tumors of the throat, mouth, and face. JAMA. 1920;5:732-6.
9. Work WP. Tumors of the parapharyngeal space. Trans Pac Coast Otoophthalmol Soc Annu Meet. 1964;45:72-82.
10. O'Malley BW Jr, Quon H, Leonhardt FD, et al. Transoral robotic surgery for parapharyngeal space tumors. ORL J Otorhinolaryngol Relat Spec. 2010;72:332-6.
11. Rassekh Ch, Weinstein GS, Loevner LA, et al. Transoral robotic surgery for prestyloid parapharyngeal space masses. Oper Techn Otolaryngol. 2013;24:99-105.
12. Shahinian H, Dornier C, Fisch U. Parapharyngeal space tumors: the infratemporal fossa approach. Skull Base Surg. 1995;5(2):73-81.

CHAPTER

24 Surgery for Carotid Body Paraganglioma

Gina D Jefferson, Jacqueline Wulu, Barry L Wenig

INTRODUCTION

Carotid body tumors (CBTs), also known as carotid body paraganglioma or chemodectoma, are uncommon vascular masses found at the bifurcation of the common carotid artery into the external and internal carotid arteries. Carotid body tumors are the most common type of paragangliomas of the head and neck occurring at a rate of about 1:30,000.[1] Other types of paragangliomas include glomus tympanicum, vagal paraganglioma, and glomus jugulare.[2] Paragangliomas are neuroendocrine tumors developed from the stem cells of the neural crest. The carotid body contains chemoreceptors that regulate respiration and blood pH by adjusting the sympathetic response to hypoxia.[3,4] Hypoxic conditions are theorized to contribute to the development of CBTs due to glandular enlargement as a compensatory mechanism to improve hypoxemia. The carotid body is made up of three cell types that produce neurochemicals[5] that can be secreted in functional tumors signaling the release of catecholamines, although the majority are nonfunctional tumors. Functional CBTs occur in about 1–3% of cases.[2]

EPIDEMIOLOGY

Carotid body tumors may arise sporadically or occur secondary to genetic predisposition. These tumors are discovered during mid-adult life and can manifest unilaterally or bilaterally. Familial forms of CBTs occur in about 10–25% of cases and can develop due to de novo genetic mutations, chromosomal abnormalities, or familial syndromes such as multiple endocrine neoplasia type II or neurofibromatosis type I.[4,5] Heritable paraganglioma are mapped to at least four different chromosomal loci, and the four types associated with CBT have a dominant mode of inheritance.[5] These patients have a higher incidence of multiple paraganglioma tumors including the locations of the adrenal gland when the tumor is called pheochromocytoma, the temporal bone, or the mediastinum. Those presenting with CBTs who are found to have germ line mutations should undergo screening for other tumors.[4] In addition to the multicentricity of familial paraganglioma, there is a higher incidence for familial CBTs to occur bilaterally. Familial tumors also tend to present earlier in life.[4]

The morbidity of CBTs is related to their ability to grow very large and infiltrate the surrounding area prior to causing symptoms that prompt medical consultation. Carotid body tumors are usually benign but have the potential to compress major vasculature and cranial nerves and constrict nearby structures. The rate of malignant of CBTs is estimated at 10% with an increased risk in young patients harboring hereditary tumors.[5,6] Malignant tumors are not defined by histopathology, as there is no described feature such as hypercellularity, nuclear pleomorphism, extracapsular spread, or lymphovascular invasion that predicts malignant behavior of CBT.[4,6] Nodal or distant disease are currently diagnostic criteria for malignancy, although metastasis may ultimately occur several years after removal of the primary CBT. Metastasis may arise within the cervical lymph nodes or more distantly within bone, liver, and lung.[4,5]

PRESENTATION

Carotid body tumors are indolent and painless. They are often discovered incidentally. The most common sign is a pulsatile neck mass that moves within the medial and lateral plane.[5] Carotid body tumors typically grow in a longitudinal direction towards the skull base and may also result in a submucosal pharyngeal mass.[4] Tumors larger than 5 cm are those that typically have the ability to cause peripheral cervical neuropathy, cranial nerve injury, or disruption to the sympathetic chain.[2]

Secretory or functional CBTs are associated with symptoms related to the release of catecholamines including episodic hypertension, tachycardia, palpitations, syncope, seizures, hypokalemia, facial flushing, and stroke.[7] Patients with functional tumors may also experience hypotension after tumor removal because of an immediate reduction in the amount of catecholamines circulating in the blood.[7] Preoperative determination of this type of CBT is determined by measuring plasma and urine levels of catecholamines. Secretory tumors are associated with preoperative malignant hypertension, postoperative hypotension, and stroke in addition to cranial nerve damage.[7]

SURGICAL ANATOMY

The carotid body is composed of glandular tissue measuring 2–6 mm in diameter that is derived from mesodermal and ectodermal neural crest cells.[5] It is located within the periadventitia on the posteromedial side of the carotid artery bifurcation.[8] The gland is supplied by the external carotid, vertebral artery, and vasa vasorum with its greatest supply often coming from the ascending pharyngeal artery.[3,5] Its innervation is derived from the glossopharyngeal nerve.

The carotid artery branches from the aorta in the mediastinum to ascend into the neck running medial to the internal jugular vein that both run within the carotid sheath accompanied by the vagus nerve. The vagus nerve is posterolateral to the carotid artery. The carotid sheath shares the visceral layer of the pretracheal fascia that surrounds the thyroid gland.

The superficial root of the ansa cervicalis crosses the lateral surface of the common carotid to join with the inferior root of the ansa cervicalis. The superior belly of the omohyoid muscle traverses the common carotid, while the anterior border of the sternocleidomastoid (SCM) muscle lies superficial to the carotid bifurcation. The bifurcation of the common carotid occurs at the fourth cervical vertebrae and at the inferior border of the hyoid bone. The internal carotid artery (ICA) lies posterior to the external carotid artery and branches within the skull, while the external carotid artery (ECA) provides eight named branches supplying the face and the neck. The hypoglossal nerve runs superficial to the ECA.

RADIOGRAPHIC EVALUATION

The history and physical examination may point to the diagnosis of a CBT and imaging studies serve as confirmation. Initially, neck mass evaluation is often radiographically conducted using computed topography (CT) scans with contrast. Characteristically, CBTs accumulate contrast on CT scan and when 5 cm or greater will demonstrate the Lyre sign, or widening at the carotid bifurcation, thereby increasing the distance between the external and internal carotid arteries.[5] CT scan is also useful in determining if bone erosion is present.

An MRI scan with gadolinium provides further detail differentiation between tumor and other soft tissues of fat and muscle as well as demonstrate intracranial extent. Moreover, there are characteristic findings of CBT on MRI scan. Carotid body tumors present with a unique pattern on T2-weighted imaging with areas of hyperintensity in contrast to muscle. There is also a characteristic "salt and pepper" appearance of paraganglioma that represents the flow voids within the vascular tumor on T2-weighted imaging.[4,6]

Nuclear imaging studies such as the octreotide scan, meta-iodobenzylguanidine (MIBG) scan and even PET scan may aid in the examination for the presence of additional paragangliomas. The octreotide scan utilizes octreotide radiolabeled with indium 111 or technetium 99. Octreotide is an analog of somatostatin that can bind to somatostatin receptors that are present in greater density in neuroendocrine tumors like paragangliomas, neuroblastomas, and carcinoid tumors for example. Studies have demonstrated >94% sensitivity for neuroendocrine tumors and 75% specificity in the head and neck for tumors >1 cm in size.[9] Meta-iodobenzylguanidine scan utilizes a radioisotope similar in molecular structure to norepinephrine and therefore concentrates in adrenal and extra-adrenal paraganglia.[10] Finally, with the discovery of various paraganglioma genotype, defining imaging phenotype may occur through choice of PET radiotracer; however, several radiotracers remain either difficult to obtain or investigational.[10,11]

Angiography further evaluates the carotid vasculature and cerebral circulation.[4] Angiography will also identify large arteries supplying the enhancing vascular lesion. Locating feeder arteries is essential in preoperative procedures such as stenting and embolization. Arteriography is also beneficial for embolization procedures prior to surgical resection as well as performing a balloon occlusion test to determine if the patient can tolerate carotid artery ligation

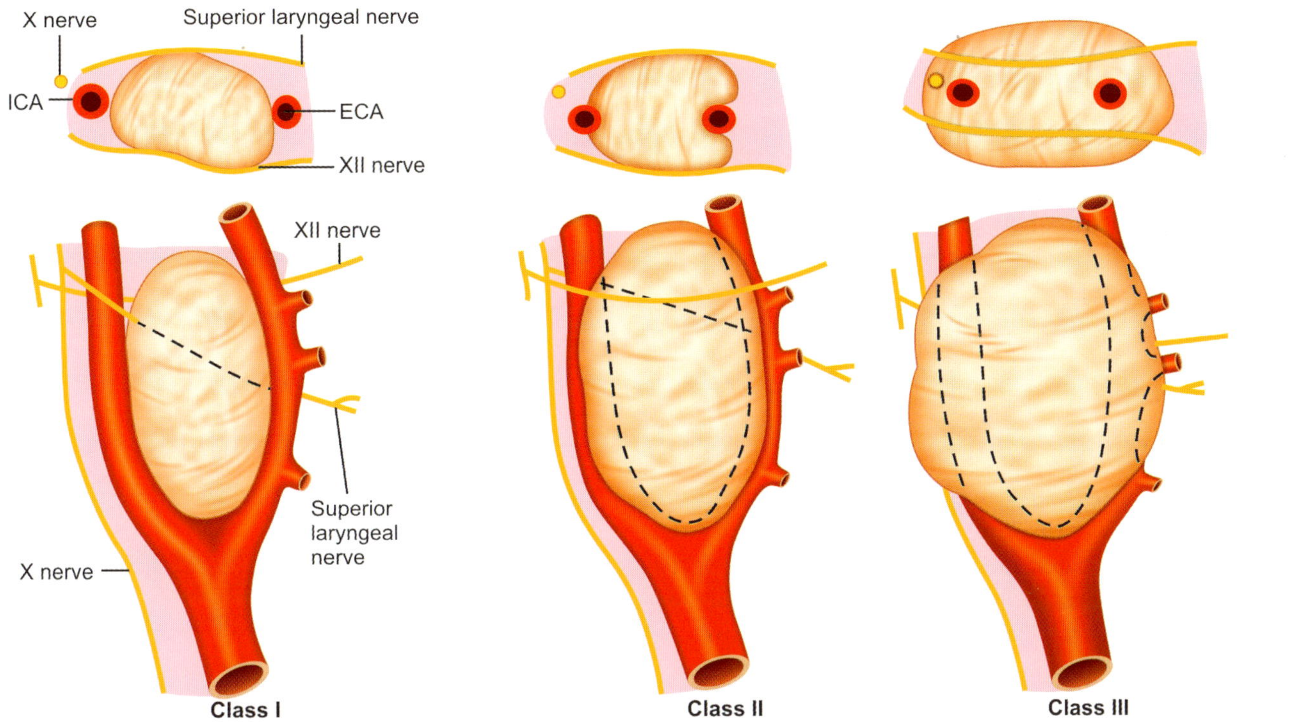

Fig. 24.1: Shamblin classification of carotid body tumors for difficulty of surgical resection. Class I tumors are localized and easily resected. Class II tumors adhere to or partially surround the carotid arteries. Class III completely surrounds or encases at least one of the arteries.

or requires revascularization or reconstruction when the CBT resection results in interruption of the carotid artery integrity.[12]

FURTHER EVALUATION

Due to possible function of CBTs and secretion of catecholamines leading to adverse sequelae, patients should undergo at a minimum urine catecholamine levels that may prompt administration of α- and β-adrenergic blocking medications prior to resection. Great care is required while resecting functional CBTs given that manipulation may lead to increased catecholamine release and thereby result in intraoperative hypertension and potentially a cerebrovascular adverse event.[6]

MANAGEMENT

Surgical Management

Surgical excision is the recommended treatment modality for CBTs. Surgical removal presents a great challenge because the tumor is highly vascular and also places cranial nerves at risk of injury.[5,13,14] The Shamblin classification system (Fig. 24.1) was established to determine anticipated surgical morbidity related to the involvement of the tumor with respect to the carotid arteries.[3] Carotid body tumors are classified into three groups according to preoperative imaging or gross examination. Shamblin class I tumors minimally adhere to either vessel, while Shamblin class II tumors are attached more to the adventitia and incompletely encase the external and internal carotid vessels. Tumors that are attached completely to the carotid bifurcation are classified as Shamblin class III. Class II and III tumors are usually >5 cm in diameter and class III tumor excision results in the greatest complications.[5,14] Class I tumors are associated with the fewest complications and are more easily resected.[5,14] Thus, the anticipated severity of postexcision sequelae can be discussed at length with the patient and adjuvant management planned accordingly. Due to the asymptomatic nature of CBTs and their indolent process, tumors are often identified when their growth results in Shamblin class II or III classification.[4,5,14]

Some surgeons elect to embolize the CBT prior to surgical resection to decrease tumor vascularity and intraoperative blood loss. This aspect of management remains controversial as many argue that embolization obscures the subadventitial plane of dissection, making excision more difficult. Preoperative embolization does not change the risk of injury to nerves.[3] Embolization is often recommended when resecting tumors 5 cm in size or greater of Shamblin class II or III. Preoperative embolization also places patients at an increased risk of stroke with an incidence of about 10% due to embolization material obstructing vessels other than the intended target.[4]

Another technique for reducing intraoperative blood loss and potentially reducing tumor size is stent blockade of blood flow into the tumor from feeding vessels, thereby decreasing tumor vascularity and indirectly tumor size. The use of preoperative covered stents in the carotid artery system is a simple procedure that may also decrease the risk of stroke. Covered stents permit coverage of the many smaller vascular branches that may not undergo satisfactory embolization.[1] Patients undergoing preoperative stent placement often achieve better outcomes and avoid neovascularization and inflammatory responses when the surgical resection is performed within 48 hours of stenting.[1] Carotid stenting may significantly benefit patients with class III tumors where there is an increased risk of stroke due to ICA manipulation for excision.[7] Stenting combined with embolization procedures may prove most advantageous for patients undergoing planned resection of large CBTs involving the skull base or Shamblin class II or III tumors, given periosteal or adventitial invasion. Of note, stent placement does mandate antiplatelet therapy with both aspirin and clopidogrel initially tapered to a single drug 1–6 months following stent insertion for at least 6 months up to an indefinite time period.[15]

Patients with Shamblin class III tumors may also undergo surgical shunting between the common carotid and ICA to decrease the risk of bleeding, stroke, and mortality prior to resection of the tumor.[16] This technique allows for continuous cerebral perfusion. A shunt tube connecting the common carotid to the internal carotid allows for easier resection of the CBT and the involved vessel.[16] Proper shunt placement can be confirmed with ultrasound of the ICA. The shunt is removed after resection and a saphenous vein graft is used for the bypass graft between the common carotid and internal carotid. Potential risks of shunting include stroke due to embolization of atherosclerotic plaques and thrombosis. Intravenous heparin is given to prevent thrombosis and preoperative imaging studies are performed to identify potential areas with atherosclerotic plaques that may dictate performance of endarterectomy.[16]

Patients with bilateral CBTs should have the smaller tumor resected first because its removal places the patient at a less risk for complications. Should complications such as cranial nerve injury arise that cause the patient dysfunction and poorer quality of life, radiation therapy is an option for managing the contralateral tumor.[3]

Surgical Approaches

Several methods are described in the literature to afford access to the parapharyngeal space for resection of tumors. The most common method employed in these reports is excision via a transcervical approach.[13] Further extension of the transcervical approach includes anterior dislocation of the mandible facilitated by division or resection of the styloid process, stylohyoid, and posterior digastric musculature. Likewise, the transcervical approach combined with other approaches may also prove advantageous depending upon involved or intimately related structures to the parapharyngeal space. These combined approaches include transcervical-transparotid, transcervical-transmastoid, and transoral-transcervical. Most relevant for CBTs is the transcervical-transmastoid approach. Finally, mandibulotomy may augment the transcervical approach for some larger, >8 cm CBTs.[13]

The transcervical approach utilizes a transverse skin incision in a natural skin crease at the level of the carotid bifurcation approximated by palpation of the inferior border of the hyoid bone (Figs. 24.2A to C). Subplatysmal skin flaps are subsequently elevated. The investing neck fascia overlying the anterior aspect of the SCM muscle is incised while continuously rolling the SCM posteriorly in order to fully expose the carotid sheath. Exposure of the superior aspect of the sheath is facilitated by level II lymphadenectomy. This also permits pathologic evaluation of lymph nodes to determine if the CBT is malignant.[4,6] Additional superior access is gained by division of the investing fascia of the submandibular gland in order to retract the gland superiorly.

The most important step in tumor removal is superior and inferior control of the blood vessels. This includes identification of the internal jugular vein, common, and internal carotid arteries and placing vessel loops on each. The inferior carotid sheath is now circumferentially freed in order to achieve immediate control of the vessel should bleeding with further dissection ensue. At this point, identification and dissection is performed of the spinal accessory, hypoglossal and vagus nerves. Dissection of

Section 7

Surgery for Skin Cancer

Section Editor: ***Genevieve A Andrews***

Chapters

CHAPTER 25

Surgical Management of Nonmelanoma Cutaneous Malignancies of the Head and Neck

Vijay A Patel, Genevieve A Andrews

INTRODUCTION

Nonmelanoma skin cancer (NMSC) is the most common type of malignancy worldwide, with over 3.5 million new cases recorded each year.[1] The incidence of nonmelanoma skin cancer is increasing annually.[2] NMSC encompasses a heterogeneous group malignancies including the more common basal cell carcinoma (BCC) and cutaneous squamous cell carcinoma (cSCC) as well as the less frequent Merkel cell carcinoma (MCC) and dermatofibrosarcoma protuberans (DFSP). Ultraviolet radiation is the most common risk factor for the majority of NMSCs (BCC, cSCC, MCC), although external beam irradiation and arsenic ingestion have also been implicated in the development of BCC and cSCC. In addition, chronic inflammation and industrial carcinogens have been linked with increased incidence of cSCC. Immunosuppression is a significant risk factor for the development of cSCC and MCC. Human papillomavirus and polyomavirus infection have also been implicated in the development of cSCC and MCC, respectively.[3,4] The biologic behavior of these cutaneous lesions can be characterized by size extent, location, and histologic differentiation. If NMSC is not properly diagnosed and treated in the early stages, high morbidity and substantial disfigurement can occur due to extensive local invasion. In general, regional and distant spread of NMSC is uncommon except for in MCC, which has a remarkably high rate of lymphatic spread.[5]

Basal Cell Carcinoma

Basal cell carcinoma is the most common type of cancer, with incidence estimates ranging from 124 cases per 100,000 persons per year United States.[6] BCC is a malignant neoplasm derived from basal keratinocytes of the epidermis and surrounding adnexal structures. The vast majority of NMSCs are BCCs, and there appears to be no known precursor lesions. The preferred treatment modality is either Mohs micrographic surgical or wide local excision, with 4- to 10-mm margins depending on the risk level of the tumor. One prospective study compared cure rates of wide local excision (defined as taking the recommended clinical margins with histological examination using a "bread-loafing" technique to assess deep and lateral margins +/- circumferential peripheral margin assessment) versus Mohs surgery and showed no significant difference in recurrence rates after resection of primary BCC (4.1% versus 2.5%, respectively). However, Mohs surgery did show significantly better recurrence rate after resection of recurrent BCC compared with wide local excision (2.4% versus 12.1%, respectively).[7] Generally, BCCs of the central face, especially the nose and eyelids, are treated with Mohs surgery rather than wide local excision because of its tissue sparing advantage. Intraoperative frozen section margin assessment is recommended in conjunction with wide local excision for high-risk BCC, although permanent section margin assessment postoperatively is also acceptable if wider margins than recommended are taken and reconstruction is delayed, or if circumferential peripheral and deep margins after recommended margins are obtained and reconstruction is delayed.[8] Radiation therapy is recommended in the postoperative setting for tumors with adverse features such as extensive perineural invasion or positive margins unable to be cleared with further surgery. Radiation therapy as the primary treatment modality is typically reserved for patients with unresectable lesions and those who are poor surgical candidates. If surgery and radiation are unacceptable treatment options for locally advanced

BCC, treatment with the Food and Drug Administration-approved hedgehog inhibitor vismodegib is a possibility. BCC rarely metastasizes via blood or lymphatics (0.003–0.05%).[9] However, in the rare situation in which BCC has metastasized to lymphatics or distantly, lymphadenectomy and vismodegib, respectively, can be used.

Cutaneous Squamous Cell Carcinoma

Cutaneous squamous cell carcinoma accounts for 20% of NMSCs and is the second most common cutaneous malignancy, with an age-adjusted incidence of 49.6–139.8 per 100,000 persons per year in the United States.[10] The majority of cSCCs arise in the head and neck, and certain cervicofacial regions are more prone to recurrence after treatment of cSCC, such as the ear and lip skin.[11] cSCC is a malignant neoplasm derived from epidermal keratinocytes. Unlike BCC, cSCC can develop from precursor and in situ lesions. The principal precursor entity, actinic keratosis, is the most common premalignant cutaneous lesion. The preferred treatment for cSCC is Mohs surgery or wide local excision with 4–6-mm surgical margins or ≥1-cm margins for very high risk cSCC. One systematic review of the literature found similar recurrence rates at 3% for Mohs surgery and 5.4% for wide local excision.[12] Radiation therapy as a primary treatment modality is generally reserved for unresectable lesions and nonsurgical candidates. It is also used as postoperative therapy for patients with cSCC at high risk for recurrence. Follow-up is strongly recommended with complete lymph node and skin examinations every 3–6 months for the first 2 years and 6–12 months thereafter.

Merkel Cell Carcinoma

Merkel cell carcinoma is a rare, aggressive cutaneous tumor derived from cells at the dermal-epidermal junction. Merkel cells are of neuroendocrine origin and are usually found on mucous membranes and skin and function as mechanoreceptor complexes. A polyomavirus has been implicated in the pathogenesis of approximately 80% of MCCs, although the exact mechanism of carcinogenesis remains unknown.[13] Imaging can be useful in identifying and quantifying the extent of disease. Radiographic evidence of nodal disease should be confirmed with a fine-needle aspiration biopsy or core biopsy. Immune panel using CK-20 and TTF1 should be tested on lymph nodes to help establish the diagnosis of node positive MCC. Wide local excision with sentinel lymph node biopsy (SLNB) is the treatment modality of choice for primary localized tumors within the head and neck, with 1–2 cm margins peripherally, and a deep margin to and likely including the next uninvolved fascia layer. It has been reported that 55% of patients have lymph node metastases at presentation or develop them shortly thereafter.[14] Hence the importance of evaluation of the draining lymph node basin cannot be overstated. Radiation to the primary site and draining lymph node basin should be considered for head and neck MCC patients as postoperative therapy even when the SLNB is negative due to the higher rate of false-negative sentinel lymph nodes in head and neck MCC compared to other body sites.[15] Local recurrence rate after surgery followed by postoperative radiation for MCC of all sites has been reported as 10.5% versus 52.6% without postoperative radiation.[14] Chemotherapy is used primarily for metastatic disease as its role in local and regional disease remains undefined. Distant metastases at presentation or on follow-up occur in about 31% of patients, most commonly in distant lymph nodes, with distant skin, lung, central nervous system, and bone occurring in order of decreasing frequency.[14] About 30% of MCC patients treated with intent to cure had local recurrence.[14] Due to frequent recurrence, vigilant follow-up is strongly recommended every 3–6 months for the first 2 years and 6–12 months thereafter.

Dermatofibrosarcoma Protuberans

Dermatofibrosarcoma protuberans is one of the less common types of nonmelanoma skin cancer, with an estimated incidence of 4.2–4.5 cases per million persons per year in the United States.[16] DFSP is a low-grade fibroblastic sarcoma of the dermis and is characterized by a translocation event between chromosomes 17 and 22, resulting in overexpression of platelet-derived growth factor receptor β. About 14% of DFSP lesions are found in the head and neck region and growth is typically indolent, with local recurrence sometimes occurring decades later.[17] Diagnosis of any questionable lesion requires a high level of clinical suspicion, thorough history, complete skin and lymph node examination, and deep subcutaneous punch or incisional biopsy with the appropriate immune panel confirmation (CD34 positive and factor XIIIa negative). Poor prognostic factors include high mitotic rate and fibrosarcomatous change. The preferred treatment for DFSP is surgical excision, traditionally with wide local excision, with more recent studies advocating Mohs surgery.

Due to the propensity for DFSP to invade with irregular and frequently deep, subclinical finger-like extensions, peripheral margins of 2–4 cm and deep margins including the fascia layer deep to the deepest involved tissue layer should be removed when feasible. Some form of complete peripheral and deep margin assessment is necessary prior to a complex definitive reconstruction. Definitive radiation can be used for unresectable DFSP or in patients who are not fit for surgery. Postoperative radiation therapy is typically reserved for patients with unresectable positive margins or after surgery for recurrent disease. Imatinib mesylate remains an option for patients who have unresectable, recurrent, and/or metastatic DFSP with the (17;22) translocation. Studies have reported local recurrence rates ranging from 0% to 60% after standard surgical excision. However, a recent review of the literature using more recent surgical techniques showed a pooled local recurrence rate of 7.3% for wide local excision and 1% for Mohs surgical excision.[18] The incidence of regional and distant metastases is low at approximately 1% and 4%, respectively. The lung is the primary site of distant spread. Vigilant follow-up of the primary site is recommended every 6–12 months with biopsies of any suspect lesions as clinically indicated.

TREATMENT

The purpose of treatment is total tumor eradication with the smallest recurrence risk, using the most morbidity-minimizing and cost-effective method acceptable to the patient. Surgery remains the mainstay of treatment, with excellent overall cure rates. The choice of treatment approach primarily depends on the location of the tumor, age and health status of the patient, and associated risk factors for tumor recurrence. Mohs surgery is useful for select high-risk BCC, cSCC, and DFSP, particularly in areas where tissue sparing is extremely advantageous, such as on the nose or eyelid.

Preoperative Evaluation

A careful and thorough evaluation involving a complete medical history, physical examination, adequate tissue biopsy, and radiological imaging if appropriate is instrumental in the process of surgical planning for primary resection of a head and neck malignancy. The physical examination should include careful visual observation of the patient, a full neurologic assessment of the cranial nerves, and evaluation of any suspect lesions or lymph nodes. Clinical presentation and skin lesion appearance often are very helpful in diagnosing the type of nonmelanoma skin cancer. However, biopsy is recommended for definitive diagnosis. NMSCs can be excisionally biopsied with narrow margins using a simple elliptical incision. For thin lesions (e.g. Bowen disease or superficial BCC), a partial shave biopsy would be ideal as it provides a larger surface area of malignant cells. For thicker lesions, a punch biopsy is more appropriate given that deeper cells are included in the histological examination. In addition, a punch biopsy is a reasonable alternative when excision is impractical due to size or location of a lesion. Signs and symptoms that imply advanced tumor stage include tumor fixation, which suggests tumor invasion into periosteum and possibly into bone deep to the tumor, and cranial nerve dysfunction, which suggests significant perineural invasion at the skull base. Bone invasion is best visualized with computed tomography (CT) with contrast. Widened and enlarged cranial nerve foramina, which suggest advanced cranial nerve involvement at the skull base, can also be visualized via CT scan. Generally, both soft tissue and perineural involvement are best visualized on magnetic resonance imaging, although in many situations, CT delineation of soft tissues is adequate for determining extent of disease. Physical examination and imaging studies are the modes of detecting metastatic lymph nodes. However, in the case of MCC, sentinel lymph node biopsies are also recommended to detect subclinical disease. Appropriate consultations (ophthalmology, neurosurgery, and plastic surgery) as well as multidisciplinary evaluations should be pursued as appropriate for advanced tumors. Recommendations regarding the avoidance of aspirin and nonsteroidal anti-inflammatory medications as well as temporary discontinuation of anticoagulants like warfarin are individually addressed with each patient to avoid bleeding problems during surgery.

Indications

There are several indications for wide local excision over Mohs surgery for primary resection of cutaneous malignancies of the head and neck. First, patients with advanced NMSCs involving underlying bone are not candidates for Mohs surgery, as bone cannot be frozen to immediately check the margins. Second, wide local excision should be used in patients whose NMSCs are very extensive; those with invasion of the parotid gland or facial nerve, for example, require composite resection

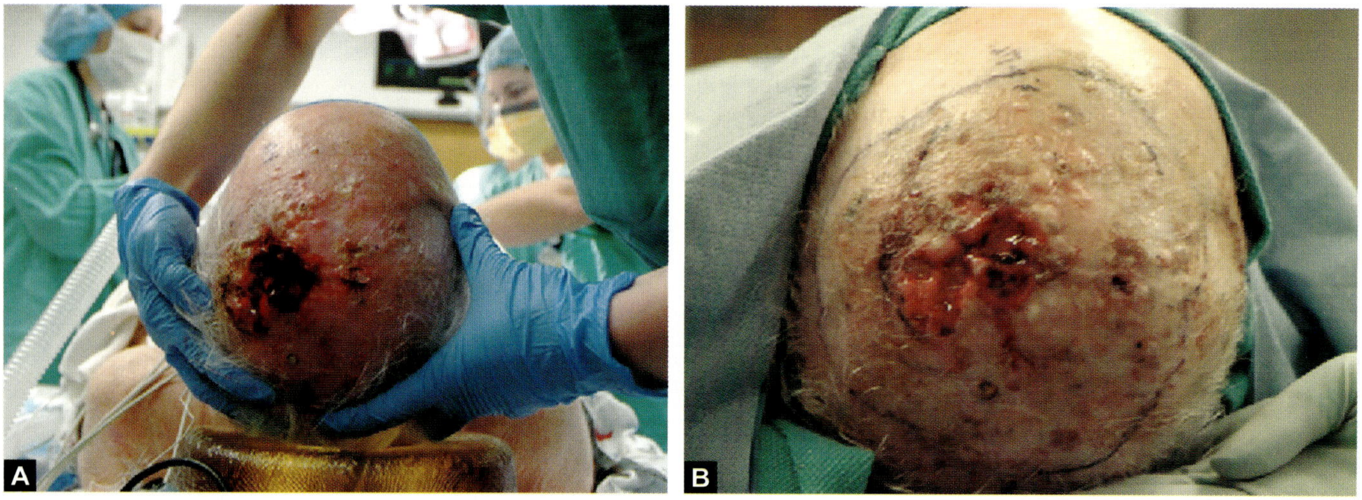

Figs. 25.1A and B: Multifocal cutaneous squamous cell carcinoma (cSCC) of the scalp. (A) This patient is an elderly man with indolent B-cell lymphoma and a significant history of unprotected sun exposure who was referred by a Mohs surgeon for management of multifocal well moderately differentiated cSCC of the scalp. Note the cluster of ulcerated lesions on the left side of the scalp with additional nodular lesions on the vertex, anterior, and posterior aspects of the scalp, which were biopsy-proven to be cSCC. (B) Due to the diffusely abnormal appearance of the scalp skin and the close proximity of the cSCC lesions, the margins of resection are marked approximately 1 cm around the conglomerate cSCC scalp lesions and abnormal-appearing scalp skin.

of more than just the skin and subcutaneous tissue. Also, if a complicated and/or immediate reconstruction after primary surgical resection is needed, these patients are often better served by wide local excision by a head and neck surgeon with intraoperative frozen section margin assessment. Finally, access to a Mohs trained surgeon may be unrealistic for many patients with nonmelanoma cutaneous malignancies of the head and neck.

Surgical Technique

Local anesthesia with or without IV sedation is used during primary resection of cutaneous malignancies whenever possible. However, there are several factors that would prompt one to use general anesthesia, such as length of procedure, patient anxiety and ability to cooperate, and the necessity for complicated resections or reconstructions. The resection is done under clean conditions. Perioperative antibiotics are not recommended if the patient is healthy.[19] The appropriate tumor-specific surgical margins around the circumference of the tumor are measured and marked. Surrounding induration and erythema are considered part of the tumor, and as such, the surgical margin is measured from these features, if present (Figs. 25.1A and B). If appropriate, a primary closure ellipse or flap closure is designed around the marked margins parallel to relaxed skin tension lines. For high-risk NMSCs, temporary coverage with a skin graft, biological dressing, or sterile dressing is recommended until final margins are proven to be negative. Subcutaneous injection is then performed along marked skin, using a local anesthetic containing epinephrine. The skin is then incised circumferentially around the lesion. The dissection is carried through the subcutaneous fat tissues to an adequate depth (Fig. 25.2). The peripheral skin margins (including the subcutaneous tissue and deep fascia edge) of high-risk NMSCs can be taken prior to amputation of the specimen so that when frozen section evaluation is requested, it can be performed during the completion of the resection to minimize operative time and patient exposure to general anesthesia (Fig. 25.3). When excising the deep aspect of the NMSC, the fascial boundary deep to the deepest tissue layer involved by tumor is exposed or taken with the specimen for margins, with variations depending on the specific tumor type and depth of penetration into the deepest tissue layer (Fig. 25.4). The specimen is then marked with sutures while it is still attached to the patient to ensure correct orientation (Fig. 25.5). Finally, the specimen is amputated and further deep margins are taken for high-risk tumors (Fig. 25.6). The frozen-section specimens are labeled in relation to their orientation within the defect and surrounding anatomy. The specimen is examined ex vivo in the operating room to identify any areas of concern for a close margin. An appropriate width and depth of additional margin in this region of concern can then be taken from the patient. For complicated composite resections in which multiple

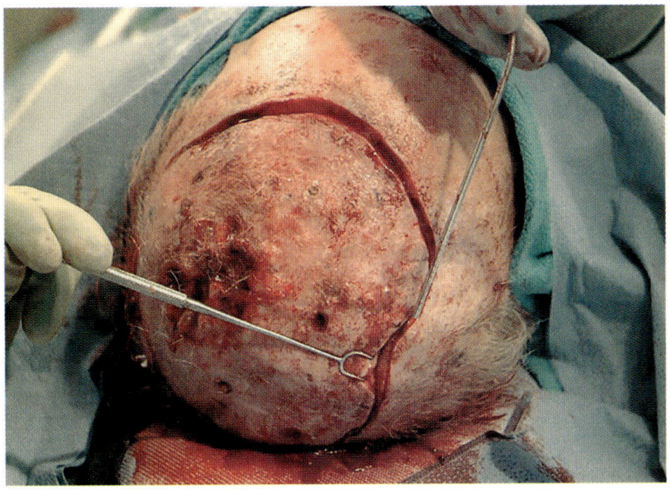

Fig. 25.2: Peripheral incisions are made through the skin, subcutaneous tissue, and galea aponeurosis with a 15-blade scalpel under general anesthesia.

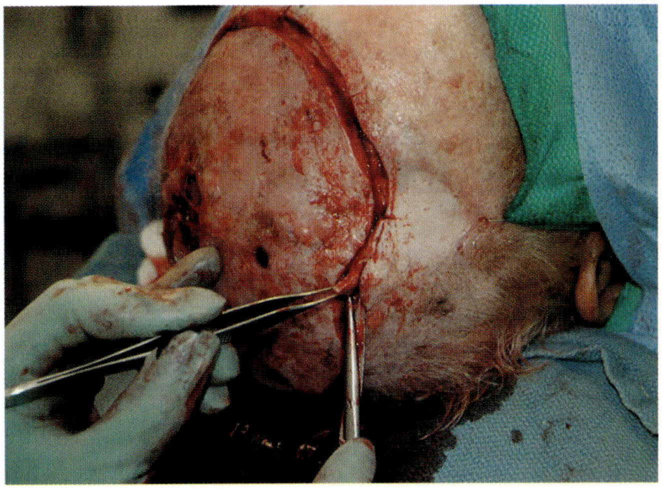

Fig. 25.3: Prior to resection of the deep aspect of the specimen, 1–2 mm, complete peripheral margins are taken from the patient sent to pathology for intraoperative frozen section margin assessment.

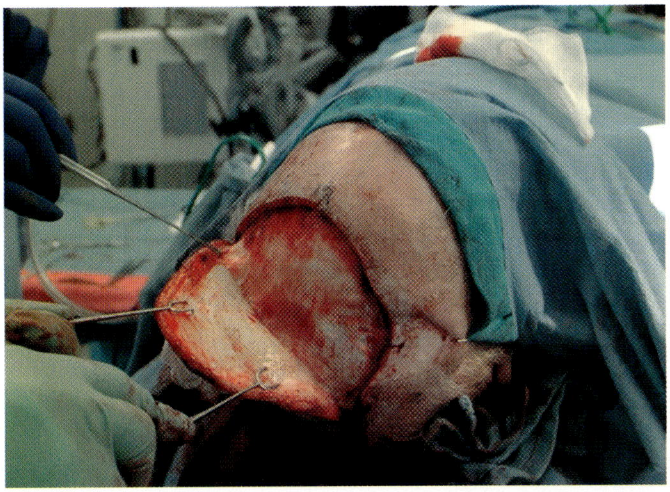

Fig. 25.4: The deep scalp resection is performed starting anteriorly where the cutaneous squamous cell carcinoma (cSCC) nodule was palpably the most superficial in the subgaleal plane. As the resection proceeds toward the thickest cSCC lesions, the galea is closely inspected and frequently palpated for irregularities that would suggest invasion into the galea.

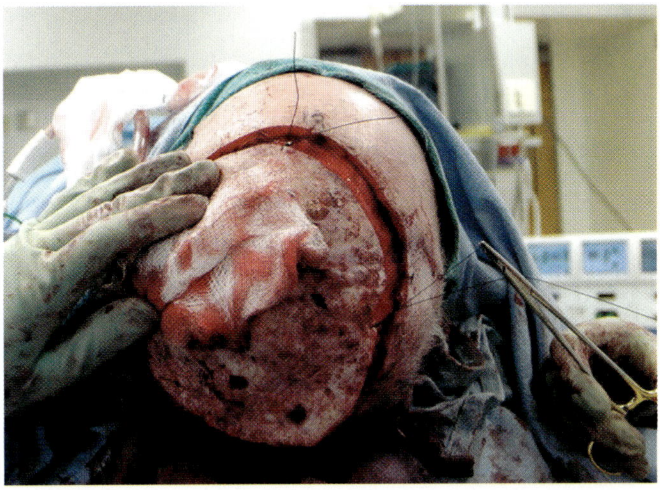

Fig. 25.5: Prior to complete amputation of the circular scalp specimen, marking stitches are placed anteriorly and right laterally to ensure correct orientation once the specimen is disconnected from the patient. This is particularly important for the pathologist's description of the specimen given the possibility that a permanent (formalin-fixed) pathologic margin can return as positive or close requiring targeted reexcision in that area.

structures are removed, the specimen is properly oriented for the pathologist personally. The wound is thereafter appropriately reconstructed or covered in a sterile fashion, as appropriate (Figs. 25.7A to C). Should a margin return as positive after a complex reconstruction, the flap touching the positive margin would need to be further resected to prevent tumor seeding of the flap. Thus for high-risk NMSCs in need of significant undermining of local or regional tissue for reconstruction, the patient is often best served by returning to the operating room 1-2 weeks later for delayed reconstruction or reexcision, depending on the final pathologic margin status.

Complications

Complications are uncommon and not unique to excisions of NMSCs. They include wound infection, dehiscence, seroma, and site-specific complications, such as facial

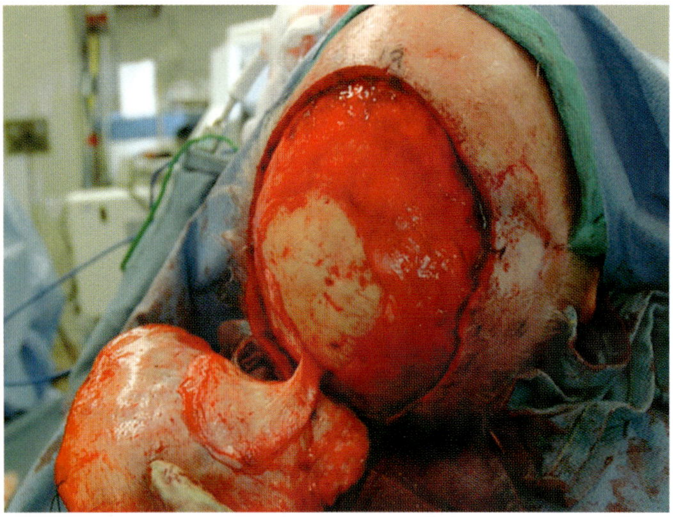

Fig. 25.6: The main scalp specimen is amputated deeply. Note that the periosteum was excised deep to the left scalp where the cutaneous squamous cell carcinoma lesions were the thickest due to irregularity and color change of the galea in this region. The underlying periosteum and calvarium is smooth without evidence of erosion.

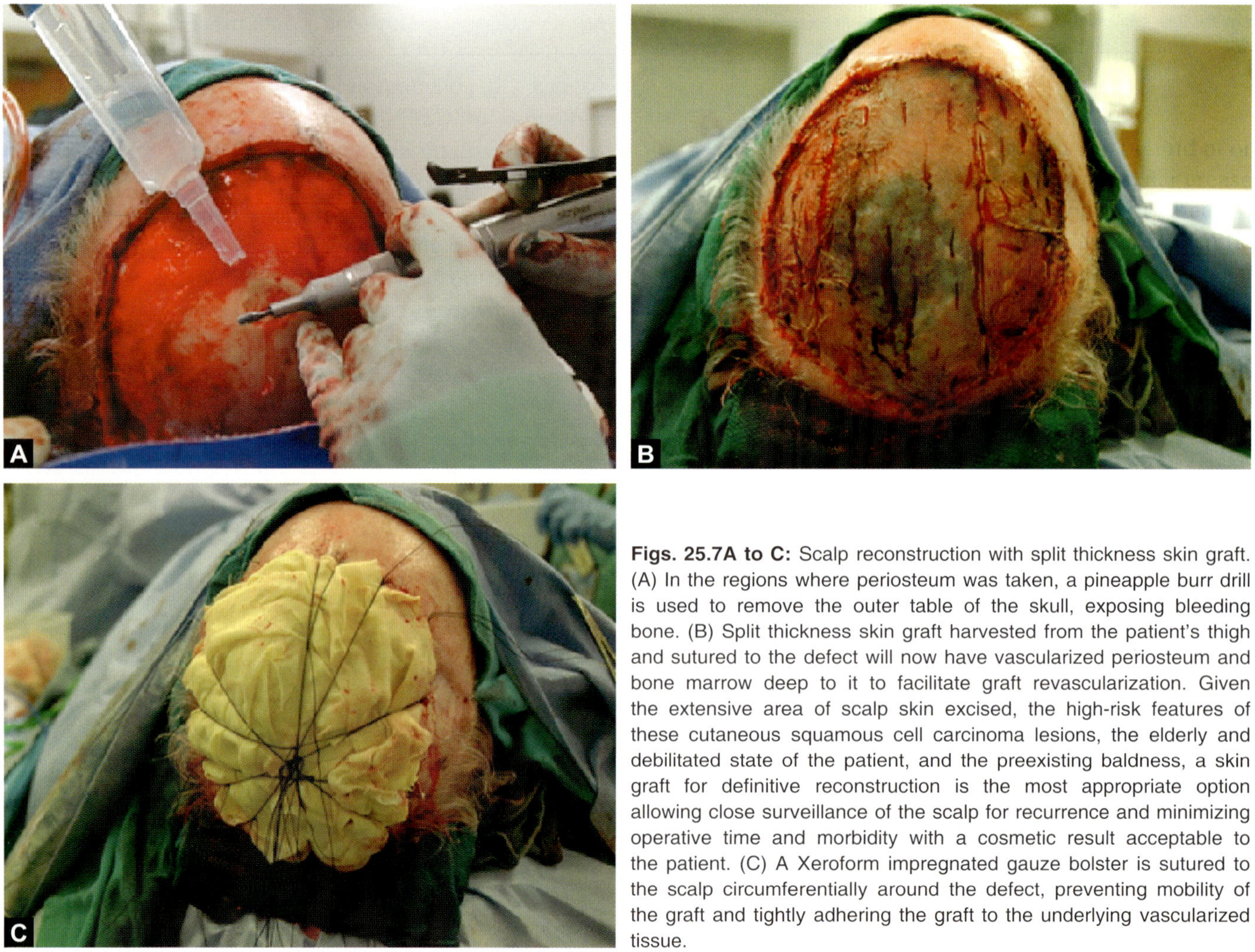

Figs. 25.7A to C: Scalp reconstruction with split thickness skin graft. (A) In the regions where periosteum was taken, a pineapple burr drill is used to remove the outer table of the skull, exposing bleeding bone. (B) Split thickness skin graft harvested from the patient's thigh and sutured to the defect will now have vascularized periosteum and bone marrow deep to it to facilitate graft revascularization. Given the extensive area of scalp skin excised, the high-risk features of these cutaneous squamous cell carcinoma lesions, the elderly and debilitated state of the patient, and the preexisting baldness, a skin graft for definitive reconstruction is the most appropriate option allowing close surveillance of the scalp for recurrence and minimizing operative time and morbidity with a cosmetic result acceptable to the patient. (C) A Xeroform impregnated gauze bolster is sutured to the scalp circumferentially around the defect, preventing mobility of the graft and tightly adhering the graft to the underlying vascularized tissue.

nerve injury. Unsightly scars and cosmetic deformity may occur but should be minimal with careful and proper preoperative planning. Incomplete resection occurs rarely when the recommended surgical margins are resected. To minimize the probability of recurrence, preoperative evaluation should focus on elucidating tumor extension into deep structures such as the parotid gland and bony external auditory canal via CT scan, as complete resection in these situations could be significantly complex, possibly involving parotidectomy and lateral temporal bone resection.

Postoperative Care

The patient as well as immediate family members and/or caretakers are provided with instructions containing explanations on proper wound care. Wounds that have skin grafts are usually dressed with a bolster dressing that is left in place for 1–2 weeks after the procedure and must be kept dry. Antibiotics are often prescribed for the duration of any packing or bolster to minimize bacterial colonization and resultant toxicity or infection. Postoperative lifestyle instructions, for example, regarding alcohol consumption, driving and exercise restrictions, and bowel regimen should be explained to the patient to optimize wound healing and for maximum patient comfort and safety during the recovery period. A follow-up appointment usually is made about 1–2 weeks postoperatively to remove sutures and skin graft dressings. Patients should be followed routinely to check for recurrent disease by the surgeon and/or a dermatologist. Because patients who develop NMSC are more prone to develop additional NMSC in the future compared to the general population, these patients should be seen by a dermatologist for whole body skin screenings routinely. In addition, patients should perform skin self-examinations routinely. Instructions on sun protection strategies, including protective clothing, hats, and sunscreen to reduce exposure to ultraviolet radiation, should be given to the patient.

CONCLUSION

Although overall the burden of NMSC measured in terms of morbidity and mortality is relatively modest, the direct costs are quite substantial, owing to its high incidence worldwide. In the United States Medicare population alone, NMSC is among the five most costly cancers to treat. Surgical management remains the preferred modality for treatment of cutaneous malignancies of the head and neck. The head and neck surgeon is frequently presented with cutaneous lesions in his or her clinical practice, the majority of which are NMSCs. These cases will often be quite advanced or aggressive upon presentation. With thoughtful preoperative planning, thorough surgical technique, and adequate follow-up, optimal results with function, cosmesis, and oncological control can be successfully achieved.

REFERENCES

1. Rodgers HW, Weinstock MA, Harris AR, et al. Incidence estimated of nonmelanoma skin cancer in the United States. Arch Dermatol. 2006;146:283-7.
2. DeVesa SS, Blot WJ, Stone BJ, et al. Recent cancer trends in the United States. J Natl Cancer Inst. 1995;87(3):175-82.
3. Nindl I, Gottschling M, Stockfleth E. Human papillomavirus and non-melanoma skin cancer: Basic virology and clinical manifestations. Disease Markers. 2007;23:247-59.
4. Feng H, Shuda M, Chang Y, et al. Clonal integration of a polyomavirus in human Merkel cell carcinoma. Science. 2008;319:1096-100.
5. Santamaria-Barria JA, Boland GM, Yeap BY, et al. Merkel cell carcinoma: a 30-year experience from a single institution. Ann Surg Oncol. 2013;20(4):1365-73.
6. Chuang TY, Popescu A, Su WP, et al. Basal cell cacrcinoma: a population-based incidence study in Rochester, Minnesota. J Am Acad Dermatol. 1990;22413-7.
7. Mosterd K, Krekels GA, Nieman FH, et al. Surgical excision versus Mohs micrographic surgery for primary and recurrent basal-cell carcinoma of the face: a prospective randomized controlled trial with 5-years' follow-up. Lancet Oncol. 2008;9:1149-56.
8. National Comprehensive Cancer Network Clinical Practice Guidelines in Oncology. 2010. Retrieved February 9, 2014 from www.nccn.org.
9. von Domarus H, Stevens PJ. Metastatic basal cell carcinoma. Report of five cases and review of 170 cases in the literature. J Am Acad Dermatol. 1984;10(6):1043-60.
10. Karia PS, Han J, Schmults CD. Cutaneous squamous cell carcinoma: estimated incidence of disease, nodal metastasis, and deaths from disease in the United States, 2012. J Am Acad Dermatol. 2013;68(6):957-66.
11. Rowe DE, Carroll RH, Day CL. Prognostic factors for local recurrence, metastasis, and survival rates in squamous cell carcinoma of the skin, ear, and lip. Implications for treatment modality selection. J Am Acad Dermatol. 1992;26(6):976-90.
12. Lansbury L, Bath-Hextall F, Perkins W, et al. Interventions for non-metastatic squamous cell carcinoma of the skin: systematic review and pooled analysis of observational studies. BMJ. 2013;347:f6153.

13. Kuwamoto, S. Recent advances in the biology of Merkel cell carcinoma. Hum Pathol. 2011;42(8):1063-77.
14. Medina-Franco H, Urist MM, Fiveash J, et al. Multimodality treatment of Merkel cell carcinoma: case series and literature review of 1024 cases. Ann Surg Oncol. 2001;8(3):204-8.
15. Willis AI, Ridge JA. Discordant lymphatic drainage patterns revealed by serial lymphoscintigraphy in cutaneous head and neck malignancies. Head Neck. 2007;29(11):979-85.
16. Criscione VD, Weinstock MA. Descriptive epidemiology of dermatofibrosarcoma protuberans in the United States, 1973 to 2002. J Am Acad Dermatol. 2007;56(6):968-73.
17. Mendenhall WM, Zlotecki, RA, Scarborough MT. Dermatofibrosarcoma protuberans. Cancer. 2004;101(11):2503-8.
18. Bogucki B, Neuhaus I, Hurst EA. Dermatofibrosarcoma protuberans: systematic review. Dermatol Surg. 2012;38(4):537-51.
19. Johnson JT, Yu VY, McGrew L. Infectious Diseases and Antimicrobial Therapy of Ears, Nose, and Throat, 1st edn. Philadelphia, PA: WB Saunders;1997. pp. 587-619.

CHAPTER 26

Surgical Management of Cutaneous Melanoma of the Head and Neck

Marcus J Magister, Irina M Chaikhoutdinov, Genevieve A Andrews

INTRODUCTION

The incidence of melanoma has steadily risen over time and was estimated to be the fifth most common cancer diagnosed in the United States in 2013, excluding basal and squamous cell skin cancer.[1] It was estimated that there were 76,250 newly diagnosed cases of melanoma with an additional 61,300 cases of melanoma in situ.[1] Among dermatologic cancers, melanoma represents < 5% of cases but accounts for more than half of all skin cancer-related mortality. In 2013, over 9,400 deaths were expected as a result of cutaneous melanoma.[1]

Cutaneous melanoma is caused by an aberrant proliferation of epidermal melanocytes. Melanocytes, which are embryologically derived from neural crest cells, are found in numerous tissues including skin, mucosa, and uvea. Melanoma can develop from precursor or acquired nevi in a step-wise progression of hyperplasia, dysplasia, and invasion.[2] The precursor lesions to melanoma include dysplastic (atypical) nevi, congenital nevi, and lentigo maligna (melanoma in situ).[3] Ultraviolet (UV) radiation has long been associated with the development of melanoma. Those who are fair skinned and redheaded are at increased risk for developing melanoma.[4] The strongest predictive factors for the development of melanoma include multiple atypical nevi, previously diagnosed melanoma, and a family history of melanoma.[4] Alterations in CDKN2A, a gene that encodes the tumor suppressors p16 and p19, have been associated with both sporadic and hereditary tumors, including melanoma and nonmelanoma malignancies, and are among the most common mutations found in melanoma.[4]

TREATMENT

Surgery is the primary treatment modality of cutaneous melanoma that has not spread distantly. Surgical treatment includes wide local excision (WLE) and, when pathologic lymph nodes are present, removal of the lymph nodes that drain the relevant cutaneous region. In the absence of clinically positive lymph nodes, WLE is often accompanied by sentinel lymph node biopsy (SLNB). SLNB for cutaneous melanoma, first described for melanoma by Morton et al. in 1992,[5] is the precise identification of a cutaneous melanoma's first draining lymph node(s), the sentinel lymph node(s) (SLN) (Figs. 26.1A and B). SLN identification is achieved using lymphoscintigraphy ± single-photon emission computerized tomography–computerized tomography (SPECT-CT) (Figs. 26.2A to D) and perilesional blue dye injection, with subsequent excisional biopsy to accurately diagnose subclinical, microscopic lymph node metastases. When found, patients with positive SLNs are selected to go on to have completion lymphadenectomy. In the final report of the multicenter selective lymphadenectomy (MSLT-1) trial, SLNB with subsequent completion lymphadenectomy for sentinel node positivity was found to significantly increase the 10-year disease-free survival in patients with melanomas of Breslow depth > 1.20 mm (71.3% for the SLNB with lymphadenectomy group versus 64.7% for the nodal observation group).[6] Despite the efficacy of primary surgical management for cutaneous melanoma without distant spread, surgery may not always be a viable option due to medical comorbidities or patient preference. One study of 42 patients with lentigo maligna (melanoma in situ) of the head and neck who were treated

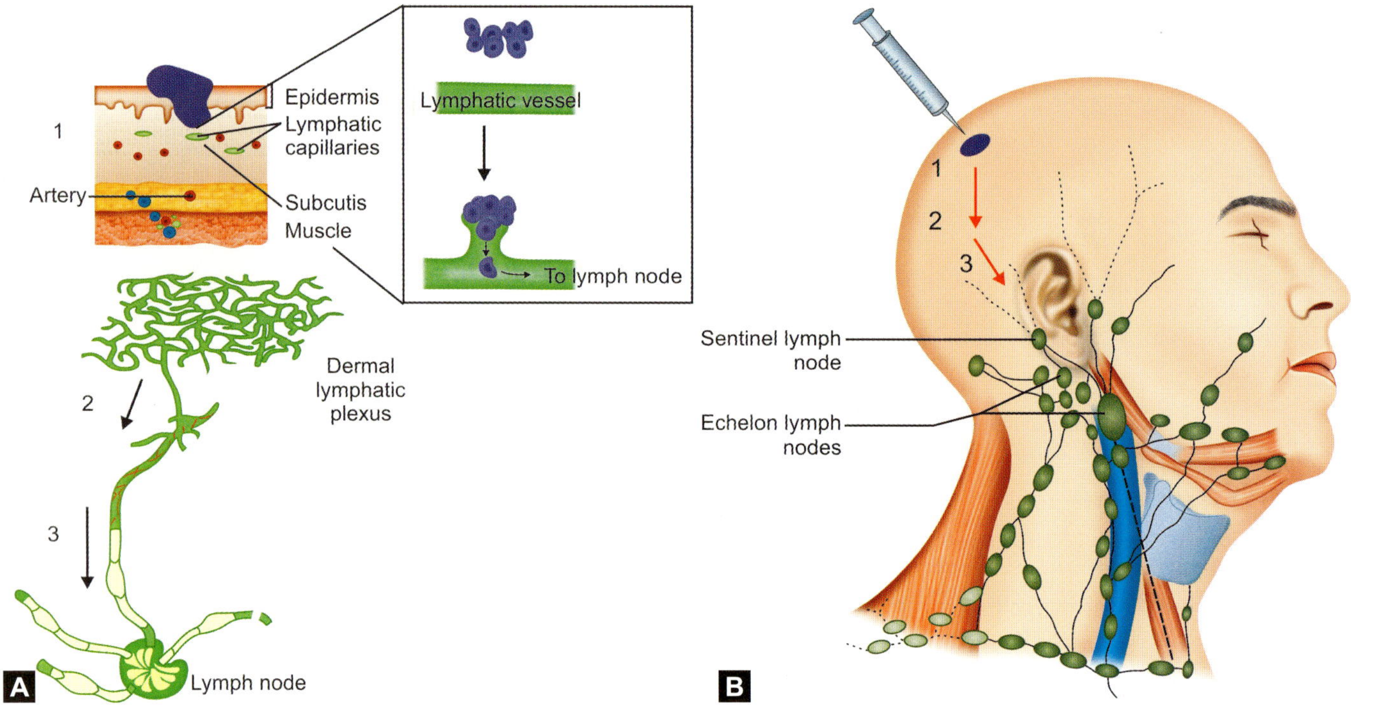

Figs. 26.1A and B: (A) The process of cutaneous melanoma lymph node metastases. (1) New lymphatic vessels sprout toward the tumor in response to both cytokines secreted from the tumor and interstitial fluid hypertension. The new lymphatics facilitate intraluminal access of tumor cells to the dermal lymphatic capillary plexus.[5a] (2) Tumor cell-containing lymph fluid flows from within the thin-walled lymphatic capillaries to the collecting lymphatic vessels, which are deeper in the tissues. (3) The lymph fluid is then filtered in the first draining lymph node, called the sentinel lymph node (SLN). It is here that a metastatic tumor cell can be deposited and grow. This is the lymph node targeted in the SLN biopsy. (B) This procedure utilizes intradermal injection of blue dye and radiotracer around the perimeter of the cutaneous melanoma to map the lymph node basin draining the skin lesion, and essentially retrace the path of lymph node potential metastases. After the lymphatic fluid reaches the SLN, it passes through it and on into the efferent lymph vessels to the next echelon of nodes. The flow then continues on to several more echelons of nodes, with ultimate coalescence of the lymphatic vessels into the thoracic duct in the left upper neck, where the lymph fluid is recirculated in the cardiovascular system.

with fractionated radiation reported a 0% recurrence at an average follow-up of 23 months.[7] Thus, in the uncommon situation of lentigo maligna in a patient who is not a surgical candidate, radiotherapy may be considered as lone treatment with curative intent.

In addition to surgical management of nondistantly metastatic melanoma, various adjunctive therapies have been investigated. These include systemic chemotherapies, vaccines, radiation therapy, and immunotherapies. Of the systemic therapies mentioned, only immunotherapy with interferon-α2b (IFN-α2b) and its pegylated form have been Food and Drug Administration-approved in the postoperative setting for use in melanoma patients with stage IIB and III disease, which corresponds to very thick melanomas and regionally metastatic melanoma, respectively.[8] In the Society for Immunotherapy of Cancer 2013 consensus statement, it was recommended that all patients with stage IIB and III cutaneous melanoma receive some form of IFN-α2b in addition to standard surgical therapy due to a significant improvement in relapse-free survival by about 30%, with the evidence being strongest for stage III patients.[8-12] Postoperative radiotherapy is recommended for local control after WLE for desmoplastic neurotropic melanoma.[13] Postoperative radiation to the nodal basin after cervical lymphadenectomy for regionally metastatic melanoma is also recommended. Radiation is specifically recommended in the postlymphadenectomy setting for patients found to have ≥2 positive nodes and/or a ≥2 cm melanoma deposit in a node based on the eligibility criteria for a trial, which showed significantly decreased lymph node recurrence in melanoma patients treated with postoperative radiation compared to the group who did not receive postoperative radiation, although there was no difference in overall survival.[14]

The goal of treatment of distantly metastatic (stage IV) melanoma is primarily focused on prolonging and

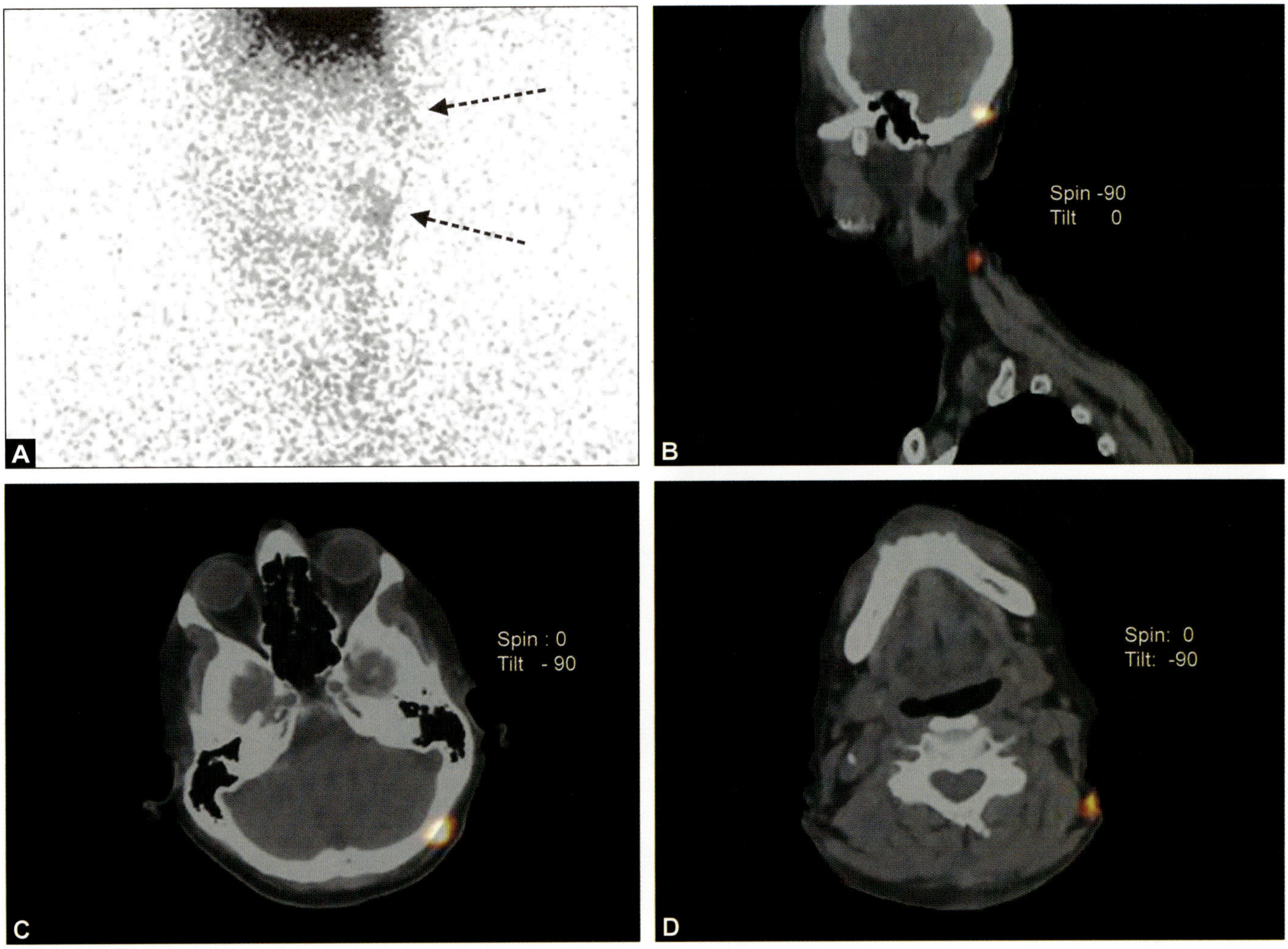

Figs. 26.2A to D: Lymphoscintigraphic and single-photon emission computerized tomography–computerized tomography (SPECT-CT) images from a patient with a scalp melanoma, clinical stage T2b N0 M0. (A) Anteroposterior lymphoscintigraphic view taken 40 minutes postintradermal injection of 0.25 mCi technetium 99m sulfur colloid in four quadrants (12, 3, 6, and 9 o'clock positions) of a 7.9-cm cutaneous melanoma of the scalp showing two areas of radiotracer localization in the left suboccipital and level Va lymph node basins (see arrows); the dense area of radioactivity above these is the location of the primary tumor and injection sites. (B) Sagittal view of fused SPECT-CT images showing a 1.2 × 0.4 cm left suboccipital sentinel lymph node. Axial views of fused SPECT-CT images demonstrate (C) a left suboccipital sentinel lymph node, as well as (D) a 0.5 × 0.5 cm left level Va sentinel lymph node.

maintaining quality of life, rather than curing disease. Metastatectomy can be performed for certain patients with low-volume disease. However, in cases where patients are not surgical candidates, systemic chemotherapy and radiation are often used to palliate symptoms. Vemurafenib is often used when the BRAFV600 mutation is identified in the melanoma of patients with distantly metastatic disease since it was shown to have a complete response rate of 48% in this patient population.[15] Other drugs recommended for various clinical scenarios for metastatic melanoma include IL-2, ipilimumab (anti-CTLA4 monoclonal antibody), and traditional cytotoxic chemotherapeutics (usually dacarbazine).[8] Even with the best current therapies available, 2-year survival rates for stage IV melanoma have been reported to be around 20%.[16] Ipilimumab is currently being investigated in the neoadjuvant setting in stage III melanoma patients, and preliminary data show an improvement in progression-free survival.[17]

PREOPERATIVE EVALUATIONS

The first step in the evaluation of head and neck melanoma is obtaining a complete history and physical examination pertinent to the lesion in question. Specific inquiry

Table 26.1: Preoperative evaluation of cutaneous melanoma of the head and neck.

History & physical examination	Risk factors: • Personal or family history of melanoma • History of intermittent, intense exposure to UV radiation • Multiple benign or atypical nevi • Red or blonde hair, fair complexion ABCDE criteria[18] • Asymmetry, border irregularity, color variation, Diameter >6 mm, and evolution of the lesion • Over 80% of cutaneous melanomas meet ≥ 2 ABCDE criteria Ulceration
Biopsy	Excisional (preferred) • Full skin thickness • Excision of entire lesion with 1–3-mm margin Incisional/punch (if lesion is not amenable to excisional biopsy) • Full skin thickness • Partial excision through the thickest portion of the lesion
Clinical lymph node examination	If suspicious on physical examination +/- imaging • If abnormal proceed with FNA with or without ultrasound guidance – A positive FNA obviates the need for SLNB and complete lymphadenectomy should be performed – If FNA negative proceed with SLNB, if indicated (Table 26.3)

(FNA: Fine needle aspiration; SLNB: Sentinel lymph node biopsy)

should be made for the presence of any personal or family risk factors and demonstration of the "ABCDE" criteria (Table 26.1).[18] Following an adequate history and physical examination, any lesion suspicious for melanoma should undergo biopsy. An excisional biopsy is the preferred method of obtaining a pathologic specimen and is ideal for small to moderately sized lesions. An incisional or punch biopsy is a full-thickness biopsy where only a portion of the lesion is removed; this can be useful for large lesions or for lesions in cosmetically sensitive areas where a histopathologic diagnosis should be made before taking wider margins. A shave biopsy is a partial thickness biopsy, which should only be used when the clinical suspicion of melanoma is low. WLE should not be performed in the absence of a histopathologic diagnosis.

A basic evaluation for regional and distant metastases should be performed when there is a suspicion for cutaneous melanoma of the head and neck by inspecting for satellite lesions in the skin surrounding the melanoma and palpating all draining lymph node basins. Should any suspicious satellite lesions or clinically positive lymph nodes be identified, additional studies are warranted. When examining the regional lymphatic system of the head and neck, it is important to remember the various patterns of lymphatic drainage found within this region of the body. Depending on the specific location of the primary cutaneous melanoma within the head and neck, lymphatic metastases can develop in the anterolateral cervical lymph nodes, the parotid gland and lateral cervical lymph nodes, the posterolateral cervical lymph nodes with or without mastoid and suboccipital lymph nodes, or a combination of these drainage basins.[19] Thus, all these lymph node basins should be palpated in the basic evaluation for regional metastases. If any lymph nodes are found to be palpably enlarged, fine-needle aspiration (FNA) biopsy with or without ultrasound guidance should be performed to confirm regional metastasis (Table 26.1). For those patients with signs or symptoms suspicious for distant metastatic disease at the time of presentation, imaging of these areas utilizing plain films, CT, positron emission tomography (PET)-CT, or magnetic resonance imaging (MRI) should be used to complete clinical staging. If SLNB is to be performed, lymphoscintigraphy, with SPECT-CT as a helpful adjunct, is typically done in the morning of the SLNB but can be performed as early as 24 hours prior to SLNB (Figs. 26.2A to D).[20,21] The information obtained from the lymphoscintigraphy ± SPECT-CT is combined with intraoperative studies such as intradermal injection of isosulfan blue dye and hand-held gamma probes to accurately identify all SLNs.

The tumor-node-metastasis (TNM) staging system of cutaneous melanoma is based upon the thickness of the biopsied melanoma, the presence or absence of ulceration and mitotic bodies, and the number and location of metastasis to regional or distant sites (Table 26.2).[16] Localized disease is categorized as prognostic stage I or II depending on the above histopathologic features. The presence of nodal metastasis or satellitosis (in-transit metastasis) yields stage III disease, and distant metastasis yields stage IV disease.[16] Determining the clinical stage of disease prior to treatment is essential to accurately discuss patients' prognoses as survival rates decrease with increased tumor thickness and presence of metastases.[16]

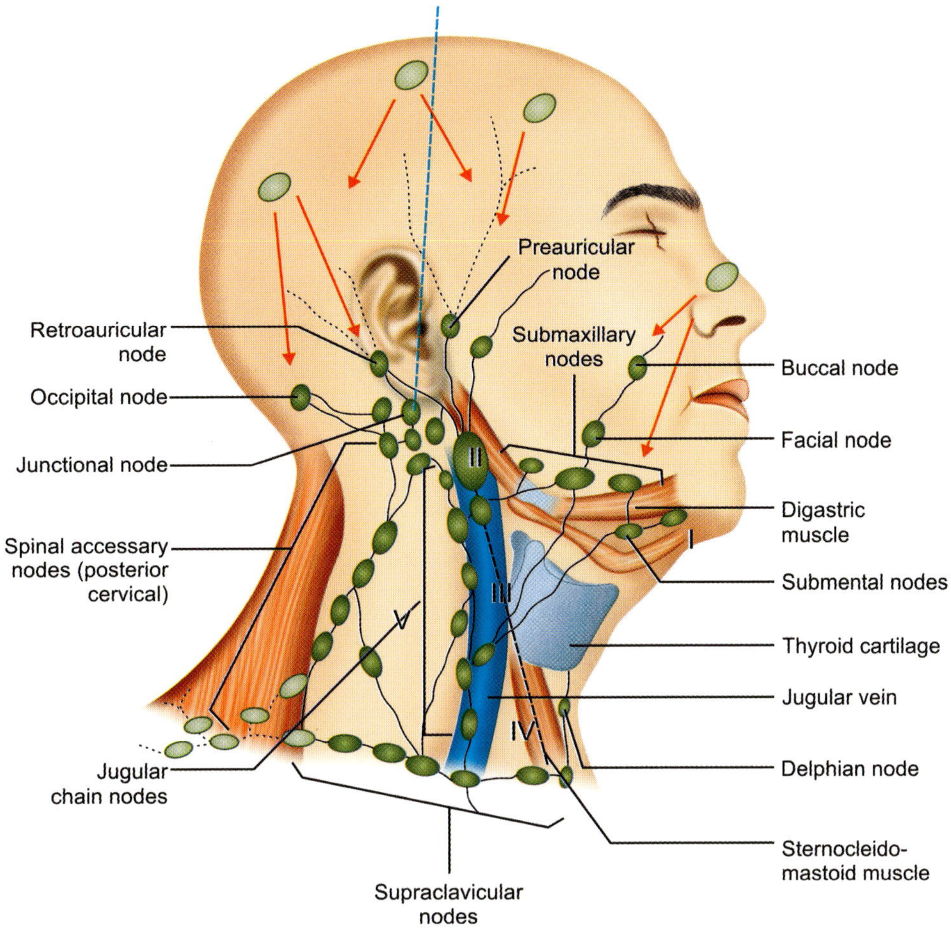

Fig. 26.6: Lymphatic drainage patterns of cutaneous melanomas located on the anterior as compared to the posterior scalp. Cutaneous melanomas of the scalp anterior to the coronal plane bisecting the external auditory canals (dotted line) typically drain to the parotid and jugulodigastric lymph nodes. From there, regional spread can be variable but typically involves the anterolateral cervical lymph nodes (levels I–IV). Cutaneous melanomas of the posterior scalp and occiput (posterior to the coronal plane describe above) can drain to the suboccipital and postauricular lymph node basins before continuing on to the posterolateral cervical lymph nodes (levels II–V). Understanding these well-described lymphatic drainage patterns helps one plan the appropriate completion neck dissection in the care of sentinel lymph node-positive cutaneous melanoma of the head and neck.

which is often composed of multiple surgeries resulting in prolonged recovery time to achieve an oncologically sound, functional, and cosmetically acceptable result. Reconstructive efforts most often take the form of a skin graft, local flap, regional flap, or other advanced closure technique. The success of these reconstructions is highly dependent on the vascularity of the surrounding tissue. As a result, these wounds are at high risk for vascular compromise and potential infection. Some amount of superficial nerve injury is to be expected when performing a cutaneous melanoma resection, most often resulting in sensory deficit. Larger nerves, like the facial and spinal accessory nerves, however, are not usually encountered unless a SLNB or lymphadenectomy is performed.

Parotidectomies are frequently performed in cases of cutaneous melanoma of the head and neck. Any time this procedure is performed, a risk of facial paresis or paralysis exists due to the intraparotid course of the facial nerve, though the risk of permanent injury is very low.[29] Anterolateral, lateral, and posterolateral neck dissections are also regularly performed based on clinical presentation or SLNB results. When performing neck dissections, careful attention should be paid to the preservation of all major nerves including the spinal accessory, vagus, recurrent laryngeal, hypoglossal, phrenic, and brachial plexus. De-spite the many nerves encountered during functional neck dissections, cranial nerve complication rates have been reported as <2% when performed by experienced

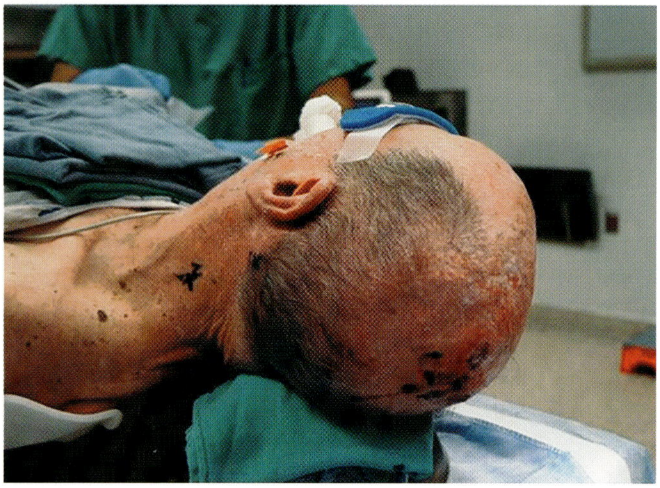

Fig. 26.7: Preparation for sentinel lymph node biopsy. The patient is positioned in neck extension with a gel roll under the left shoulder to allow adequate exposure of left suboccipital and posterior neck lymph node basins. Sites of sentinel lymph nodes previously found by lymphoscintigraphy with single-photon emission computerized tomography–computerized tomography and marked by the nuclear medicine physician with "x's" are included in the surgical field.

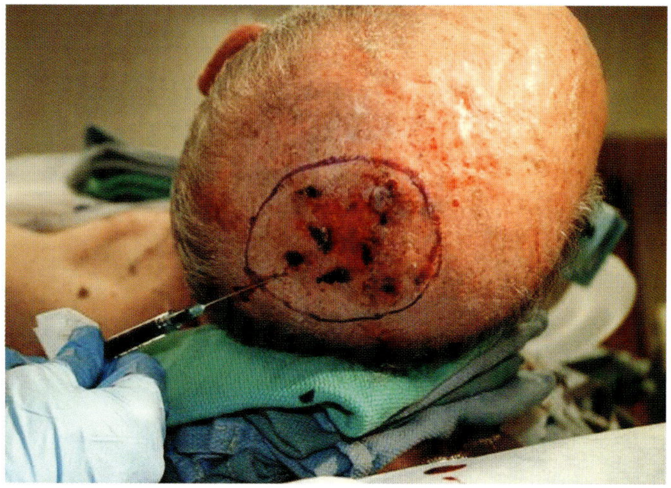

Fig. 26.8: Intradermal injection of Lymphazurin 1% (isosulfan blue dye). Isosulfan blue dye is shown being injected intradermally in the posterior (6 o'clock) quadrant. This was repeated in the anterior and both lateral quadrants of the tumor. Dye was allowed to penetrate the deeper layers of skin and lymphatic channels for approximately 5–10 minutes with gentle massage over the injection sites prior to initiating the primary resection. If desired, methylene blue can be substituted for isosulfan blue.

head and neck surgeons.[38] Rarer complications that are also associated with neck dissections include chyle leak from thoracic duct damage, pneumothorax, and jugular vein and carotid artery injuries. Although potential complications are numerous, lymphadenectomy remains a strongly recommended procedure in the presence of macroscopic and microscopic lymph node metastases.[6]

POSTOPERATIVE AND FOLLOW-UP CARE

Following surgical management of a cutaneous melanoma of the head and neck, the length of a patient's stay in the hospital is heavily dependent on the type and breadth of the surgery. Patients with low-stage melanoma (stage I or IIA) will often undergo their WLE in an outpatient setting under local anesthesia. However, patients who undergo SLNB or neck dissections tend to stay in the hospital overnight or 1–2 days depending on the recovery of the patient, as these are more extensive procedures performed under general anesthesia.

Although the immediate postoperative care is relatively straightforward and largely case dependent, the long-term follow-up for cutaneous melanoma is a topic of some debate. Although the risk of developing recurrence or a second primary melanoma is significantly increased after the first diagnosis, as of January 1, 2014 a well-accepted consensus did not exist as to how melanoma should be followed after primary resection.[39] Rather, the major cancer societies have their own recommendations regarding follow-up visits and imaging. Despite many minor differences, a few general concepts are illustrated in many of the societies' recommendations. First and foremost, the primary goal of follow-up is to identify local, regional, and distant recurrence as early as possible. The most agreed-upon facet of long-term follow-up is the need for regular examinations, both by a physician and by the patient themselves; a majority of melanoma recurrence is not found by the physician but rather by the patient between follow-up appointments.[22,39] The recommended frequency of follow-up skin and lymph node examinations varies from every 3–12 months, with more regular visits being recommended for those at high risk for recurrence (stage IIB or greater).[39] The utility of regular follow-up imaging (e.g. chest X-ray, CT, PET, MRI) in diagnosing disease recurrence has been found to be relatively limited due to the high false-positive rate.[22] Many societies suggest surveillance imaging for those with more advanced disease or those who become symptomatic postresection.[39] Regardless of what follow-up plan is chosen, it is imperative that patients are well educated about the risks, signs,

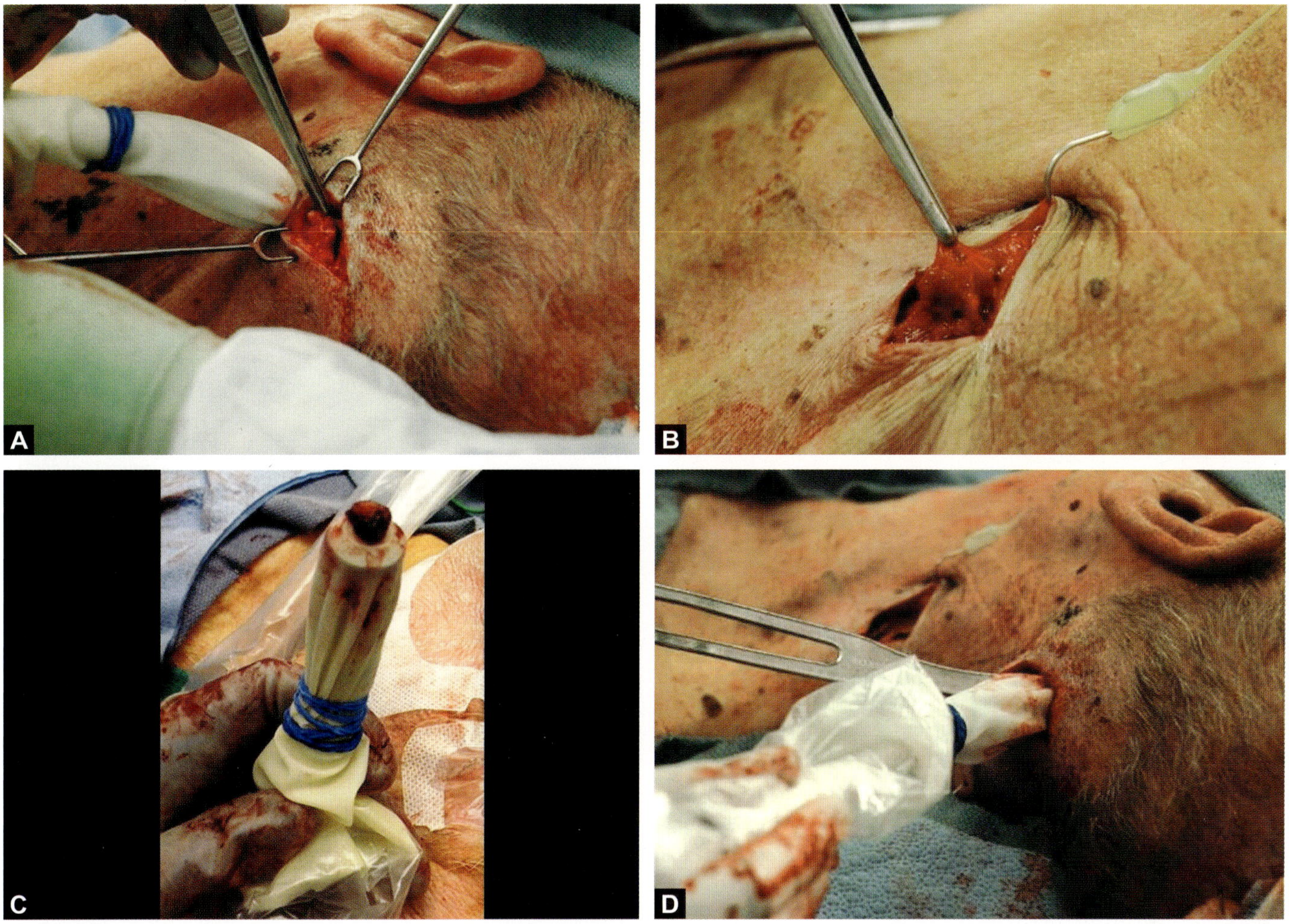

Figs. 26.9A to D: Evaluation and excision of sentinel lymph nodes. (A) Suboccipital and (B) level Va sentinel lymph nodes previously identified via lymphoscintigraphy with single-photon emission computerized tomography–computerized tomography are shown dissected out during the sentinel lymph node biopsy. (A) The gamma probe is shown being used intermittently during the dissection to localize the sentinel lymph nodes (SLNs) in vivo by continually reorienting the focus of the dissection toward the area of greatest radioactivity (the "hottest" area) as determined by the gamma probe. (B) A "hot and blue" level Va SLN is shown here after having been dissected with care to maintain the capsular integrity as well as the lymphovascular pedicle. The lymphovascular pedicle is later sealed with electrocautery and divided with scissors completing the sentinel lymph node biopsy. (C) The "hot and blue" SLN is shown here being measured ex vivo with the gamma probe (oriented away from the patient) to obtain a 10-second cumulative count of radioactivity. Ten percent of this 10-second count is used as the threshold for evaluating the remaining lymph node basins for the continued presence of SLNs. (D) The gamma probe is shown here within the wound bed following removal of the "hottest" SLN to obtain a 10-second cumulative background count. When the count is ≥ 10% of the cumulative 10-second ex vivo count of the "hottest" node, continued exploration for remaining sentinel lymph nodes is performed until the background count is <10% of the cumulative 10-second ex vivo count of the "hottest" SLN. When the background count is <10% of that of the "hottest" node, it can be safely assumed that all sentinel lymph nodes have been removed from this nodal basin.

and symptoms of melanoma recurrence so that prompt action can be taken when necessary.

CONCLUSION

Melanoma is a relatively common cutaneous malignancy with potentially serious ramifications, as it accounts for more than half of all skin cancer-related mortality.[1] The frequent occurrence of melanoma in the sun-exposed head and neck skin makes it an issue of significant import to the head and neck surgeon. Surgical resection, using WLE, is the mainstay of treatment of cutaneous melanoma of the head and neck. SLNB is recommended to determine which high-risk melanoma patients harbor occult regional lymph node metastases, thus making them candidates for completion lymphadenectomy. SLNB

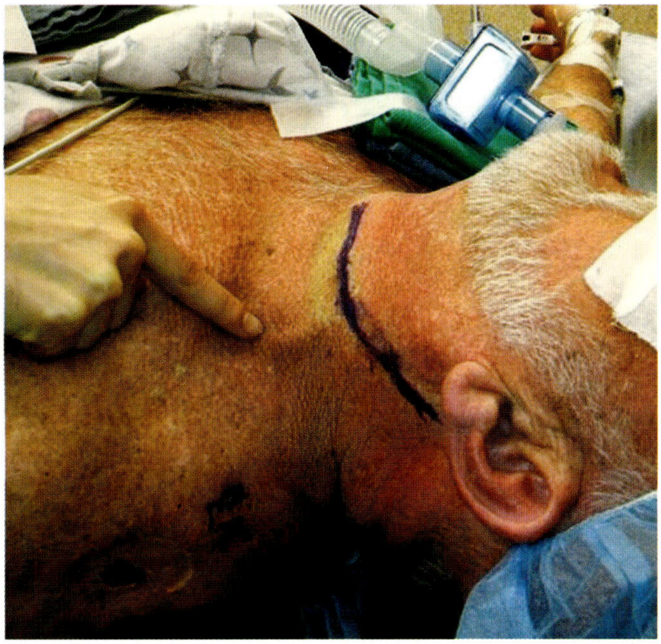

Fig. 26.10: Preparation for completion left neck dissection. Shown here is a patient with a history of a T4bN3M0 left posterior shoulder melanoma that underwent wide local excision and sentinel lymph node biopsy (SLNB) at another institution but was then referred for completion lymphadenectomy given that melanoma was found in the left level IV sentinel lymph node. The assistant is pointing out the scar from the prior SLNB. Note the proposed incision for the planned left level II–V neck dissection. The "x" demarcates where a subcutaneous nodule was excisionally biopsied by the outside surgeon and came back positive for an in-transit metastasis of melanoma, which will be excised with wide margins at the time of the neck dissection.

with subsequent completion lymphadenectomy for sentinel node positivity significantly increases the 10-year disease-free survival in patients with melanomas thicker than 1.2 mm.[6] Management of cutaneous melanoma of the head and neck is often complex and requires multiple procedures, commonly with delayed definitive reconstruction to achieve an oncologically sound, functional, and cosmetically acceptable result. Comprehensive multidisciplinary care involving head and neck oncologic surgery, plastic and reconstructive surgery, medical oncology, radiation oncology, and dermatology should be employed as indicated in the management of high-risk cutaneous melanoma of the head and neck. Patient education about and investment in the recommended treatment and post-treatment surveillance is critical to the long-term success of a carefully crafted and comprehensive treatment plan for this challenging disease.

REFERENCES

1. Siegel R, Naishadham D, Jemal A. Cancer statistics, 2013. CA: A Cancer Journal for Clinicians. 2013;63:11-30.
2. Clark WH, Elder D, Guerry D, et al. A study of tumor progression: the precursor lesions of superficial spreading and nodular melanoma. Hum Pathol. 1984;15:1147-65.
3. Skender-Kalnenas TM, English DR, Heenan PJ. Benign melanocytic lesions: risk markers or precursors of cutaneous melanoma? J Am Acad Dermatol. 1995;33:1000-7.
4. Miller AJ, Mihm M. Mechanisms of disease: melanoma. New Engl J Med. 2006;355:51-65.
5. Morton DL, Wen DR, Wong JH, et al. Technical details of intraoperative lymphatic mapping for early stage melanoma. Arch Surg. 1992;127:392-9.
5a. Alitalo K, Tammela T, Pertova T. Lymphangiogenesis in development and human disease. Nature. 2005;438(7070): 946-53.
6. Morton DL, Thompson JF, Cochran AJ, et al. Final trial report of sentinel-node biopsy versus nodal observation in melanoma. New Engl J Med. 2014;370(7):599-609.
7. Schmid-Wendtner MH, Brunner B, Konz B, et al. Fractionated radiotherapy of lentigo maligna and lentigo maligna melanoma in 64 patients. J Am Acad Dermatol. 2000;43: 477-82.
8. Kaufman HL, Kirkwood J, Hodi FS, et al. The Society for Immunotherapy of Cancer consensus statement on tumour immunotherapy for the treatment of cutaneous melanoma. Nature Rev Clin Oncol. 2013;10:588-98.
9. Grob JJ, Dreno B, de la Salmonière P, et al. Randomised trial of interferon alpha-2a as adjuvant therapy in resected primary melanoma thicker than 1.5 mm without clinically detectable nodal metastases. French Cooperative Group on Melanoma. Lancet. 1998;351:1905-10.
10. Hansson J, Aamdal S, Bastholt L, et al. Two different durations of adjuvant therapy with intermediate-dose interferon alfa-2b in patients with high-risk melanoma (Nordic IFN trial): a randomised phase 3 trial. Lancet Oncol. 2011;12: 144-52.
11. Kirkwood JM, Manola J, Ibrahim J, et al. A pooled analysis of eastern cooperative oncology group and intergroup trials of adjuvant high-dose interferon for melanoma. Clin Cancer Res. 2004;10:1670-7.
12. Davar D, Tarhini AA, Kirkwood JM. Adjuvant immunotherapy of melanoma and development of new approaches using the neoadjuvant approach. Clin Dermatol. 2013;31: 237-50.
13. Chen JY, Hruby G, Scolyer RA, et al. Desmoplastic neurotropic melanoma: a clinicopathologic analysis of 128 cases. Cancer. 2008;113(10):2770-8.
14. Burmeister BH, Henderson MA, Ainslie J, et al. Adjuvant radiotherapy versus observation alone for patients at risk of lymph-node field relapse after therapeutic lymphadenectomy for melanoma: a randomised trial. Lancet Oncol. 2012;13(6):589-97.

15. Chapman PB, Hauschild A, Robert C, et al. Improved survival with vemurafenib in melanoma with BRAF V600E mutation. N Engl J Med. 2011;364:2507-16.
16. Balch CM, Gershenwald J, Soong Sj, et al. Final version of 2009 AJCC Melanoma Staging and Classification. J Clin Oncol. 2009;27:6199-206.
17. Tarhini AA, Edington H, Butterfield LH, et al. Neoadjuvant ipilumimab in patients with stage IIIB/C melanoma: immunogenicity and biomarker analysis. J Clin Oncol. 2012;30[Abstract 8536].
18. Abbasi NR, Shaw H, Rigel D, et al. Early diagnosis of cutaneous melanoma: revisiting the ABCD criteria. JAMA. 2004; 292:2771-6.
19. Lengele B, Hamoir M, Scalliet P, et al. Anatomic basis for the radiological delineation of lymph node areas. Major collecting trunks, head and neck. Radiother Oncol. 2007;85: 146-55.
20. White DC, Schuler FR, Pruitt SK, et al. Timing of sentinel lymph node mapping after lymphoscintigraphy. Surgery. 1999;126(2):156-61.
21. Kalady MF, White DC, Fields RC, et al. Validation of delayed sentinel lymph node mapping for melanoma. Cancer J. 2001;7(6):503-8.
22. Bichakjian CK, Halpern A, Johnson T, et al. Guidelines of care for the management of primary cutaneous melanoma. J Am Acad Dermatol. 2011;65:1032-47.
23. Gershenwald JE, Ross MI. Sentinel-lymph-node biopsy for cutaneous melanoma. New Engl J Medicine. 2011;364(18): 1738-45.
24. Melanoma. (Version 3.2014). National Comprehensive Cancer Network Guidelines in Oncology. Retrieved March 19, 2014, from http://www.nccn.org/professionals/physician_gls/pdf/melanoma.pdf
25. Kupferman ME, Kubik MW, Bradford CR, et al. The role of sentinel lymph node biopsy for thin cutaneous melanomas of the head and neck. Am J Otolaryngol. 2014;35(2):226-32.
26. Pasquali S, Spillane AJ, de Wilt JH, et al. Surgeons' opinions on lymphadenectomy in melanoma patients with positive sentinel nodes: a worldwide web-based survey. Ann Surg Oncol. 2012;19:4322-9.
27. Gyorki DE, Boyle JO, Ganly I, et al. Incidence and location of positive nonsentinel lymph nodes in head and neck melanoma. EJSO. 2014;40:305-10.
28. Haigh PI, DiFronzo LA, McCready DR. Optimal excision margins for primary cutaneous melanoma: a systematic review and meta-analysis. Can J Surg. 2003;46(6):419-26.
29. Gaillard C, Périé S, Susini B, et al. Facial nerve dysfunction after parotidectomy: the role of local factors. Laryngoscope. 2005;115(2):287-91.
30. McKean ME, Lee K, McGregor IA. The distribution of lymph nodes in and around the parotid gland: an anatomical study. Br J Plast Surg. 1985;38(1):1-5.
31. O'Brien CJ, Gianoutsos MP, Margan MJ. Neck dissection for cutaneous malignant melanoma. World J Surg. 1992;16:222-6.
32. O'Brien CJ, Petersen-Schaefer K, Ruark, et al. Radical, modified and selective neck dissection for cutaneous malignant melanoma. Head Neck. 1995;17:232-41.
33. O'Brien CJ, Petersen-Schaefer K, Stevens GN, et al. Adjuvant radiotherapy following neck dissection and parotidectomy for metastatic malignant melanoma. Head Neck. 1997;19:589-94.
34. Balch CM, Soong SJ, Bartolucci AA, et al. Efficacy of an elective regional lymph node dissection of 1 to 4 mm thick melanomas for patients 60 years of age and younger. Ann Surg.1996;224:255-66.
35. Morton DL, Cochran AJ, Thompson JF, et al. Sentinel-node biopsy for early stage melanoma: accuracy and morbidity in MSLT-1, an international multicenter trial. Ann Surg. 2005;242:302-11.
36. Morton DL, Thompson JF, Cochran AJ, et al. Sentinel-node biopsy or nodal observation in melanoma. N Engl J Med. 2006;355:1307-17.
37. Scolyer RA, Murali R, McCarthy SW, et al. Pathologic examination of sentinellymph nodes from melanoma patients. Semin Diagn Pathol. 2008;25(2):100-11.
38. Prim MP, DeDiego JI, Verdaguer JM, et al. Neurological complications following functional neck dissection. Head Neck Oncol. 2006;263(5):473-6.
39. Trotter SC, Sroa N, Winkelmann R, et al. Global review of melanoma follow-up guidelines. J Clin Aesth Dermatol. 2013;6:18-26.

Index

Note: Page numbers followed by *f* and *t* indicate figures and tables, respectively.

E

F

G

H

I

J

K

L

M

N

T

U

V

W

Z